Survey Methods in
Community Medicine

For Eleanor

Survey Methods in Community Medicine

Epidemiological Research
Programme Evaluation
Clinical Trials

J. H. Abramson

Emeritus Professor of Social Medicine
The Hebrew University-Hadassah School of Public Health and
Community Medicine
Jerusalem

Z. H. Abramson MD MPH

Director
Beit Hakerem Community Clinic (Kupat Holim Clalit)
Jerusalem

FIFTH EDITION

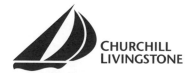

CHURCHILL
LIVINGSTONE

EDINBURGH LONDON NEW YORK PHILADELPHIA
SYDNEY TORONTO 1999

CHURCHILL LIVINGSTONE
An Imprint of Harcourt Brace and Company Limited

Churchill Livingstone, 1–3 Baxter's Place, Leith Walk,
Edinburgh EH1 3AF

First edition 1974   Fourth edition 1990
Second edition 1979   Fifth edition 1999
Third edition 1984

ISBN 0443 061637

British Library of Cataloguing in Publication Data
A catalogue record for this book is available from the British
Library.

Library of Congress Cataloging in Publication Data
A catalog record for this book is available from the Library of
Congress.

Medical knowledge is constantly changing. As information
becomes available, changes in treatment, procedures, equipment and the use of drugs become necessary. The authors
and publisher have, as far as it is possible, taken care to
ensure that the information given in the text is accurate and
up-to-date. However, readers are strongly advised to confirm
that the information, especially with regard to drug usage,
complies with current legislation and standard of practice.

For Churchill Livingstone:
Commissioning editor: Michael Parkinson
Project editor: Barbara Simmons
Production controller: Frances Affleck
Design direction: Erik Bigland

The
publisher's
policy is to use
**paper manufactured
from sustainable forests**

Printed in China
NPCC/01

Preface

The purpose of this book is to provide a simple and systematic guide to the planning and performance of investigations concerned with health and disease and with health care, whether they are studies designed to widen the horizons of scientific knowledge or whether they have more directly practical aims, such as the provision of information needed as a basis for immediate decisions and action. It is not a compendium of detailed techniques of investigation or of statistical methods, but an ABC to the design, conduct and analysis of studies.

Two new chapters have been added in this edition, one dealing with rapid epidemiological methods and one with the selection of cases and controls for case-control studies; a checklist for use in appraising a community's health needs has been added as an appendix. The whole book – text, notes and references – has again been thoroughly revised and updated, and it has grown by 80 pages. A number of references to Internet sites have been incorporated. Until these sites become inaccessible, they will be helpful as accessory sources.

We hope the book will be useful in the planning of investigations of groups and populations, such as health surveys, cohort studies, comparisons of cases and controls, prophylactic and therapeutic trials, studies of the use of medical services, and other epidemiological and evaluative research. It may also be helpful to readers who wish only to enhance their capacity for the judicious appraisal of medical literature.

Most of the chapters have relevance to studies of all the above kinds, both experimental and observational. Some deal with special types of study, e.g. case-control studies, clinical trials and programme trials. The chapter on community-oriented primary care was written to meet the needs of practitioners of primary health care (doctors, nurses, health educators, managers and others) who try to 'treat the community as a patient' by appraising the health needs of a population and establishing programmes to deal with these in a systematic way, as well as caring for the needs of its individual members or their families.

To maintain continuity, we have retained 'Survey Methods' in the title, although 'Research Methods' would better reflect the book's coverage of experimental as well as observational studies of various kinds. The original decision to use 'Survey Methods' was motivated by a wish not to repel readers who, despite an interest in conducting investigations aimed at pragmatic purposes, might conceive of 'research' as an ivory-tower activity, far removed from their own mundane activities.

'Making Sense of Data', a self-instruction manual by J. H. Abramson on the interpretation of data (Oxford University Press, 1994) may be regarded as a companion volume.

Jerusalem   J.H.A.
1999   Z.H.A.

Contents

1 First steps

The purpose of most investigations in community medicine, and in the health field generally, is the collection of information that will provide a basis for action, whether immediately or in the long run. The investigator perceives a problem that requires solution, decides that a particular study will contribute to this end, and embarks upon the study. Sound planning—and maybe a smile or two from Lady Luck—will ensure that the findings will be useful, and possibly even of wide scientific interest. Only if the problem has neither theoretical nor practical significance and the findings serve no end but self-gratification may sound planning be unnecessary.

Before planning can start, a problem must be identified. It has been said that 'if necessity is the mother of invention, the awareness of problems is the mother of research'.[1] The investigator's interest in the problem may arise from a concern with practical matters or from intellectual curiosity, from an intuitive 'hunch' or from careful reasoning, from personal experience or from that of others. Inspiration often comes from reading, not only about the topic in which the investigator is interested, but also about cognate topics. An idea for a study on alcoholism may arise from the results of studies on smoking (conceptually related to alcoholism, in that it is also an addiction) or delinquency (both it and alcoholism being, at least in certain cultures, forms of socially deviant behaviour).

While the main purpose is to collect information which will contribute to the solution of a problem, investigations may also have an educational function, and may be carried out for this purpose. A survey can stimulate public interest in a particular topic (the interviewer is asked: 'Why are you asking me these questions?'), and can be a means of stimulating public action. A community self-survey, carried out by participant members of the community, may be set up as a means to community action; such surveys may collect useful information, although it is seldom very accurate or sophisticated.

This chapter deals with the purpose of the investigation, use of the literature, ethical aspects, and the formulation of the study topic.

First steps

- Clarifying the purpose
- Use of the literature
- Ethical considerations
- Formulating the topic

CLARIFYING THE PURPOSE

The first step then, before the study is planned, is to clarify its purpose—the 'why' of the study. (We are not speaking here of the researcher's psychological motivations—a quest for prestige, promotion, the gratifications of problem-solving, etc.—which may or may not be at a conscious level.) Is it 'pure' or 'basic' research with no immediate practical applications in health care, or is it 'applied' research? Is the purpose to obtain information that will be a basis for a decision on the utilization of resources, or is it to identify persons who are at special risk of contracting a specific disease in order that preventive action may be taken; or to add to existing knowledge by throwing light on (say) a specific aspect of aetiology; or to stimulate the public's interest in a topic of relevance to its health? If an evaluative study of health care is contemplated, is the motive a concern with the welfare of the people who are served by a specific practice, health centre or hospital, or is the main purpose to see whether a specific treatment or kind of health programme is good enough to be applied in other places also?

The reason for embarking on the study should be clear to the investigator. In most cases it will in fact be so from the outset; but sometimes the formulation of the problem to be solved will be less easy. In either instance, if an application is made for facilities or funds for the study it will be necessary to describe this purpose in some detail, so as to justify the performance of the study. The researcher will need to review previous work on the subject, describe the present state of knowledge, and explain the significance of the proposed investigation. This is the 'case for action'.

Preconceived ideas introduce a possibility of biased findings, and an honest self-examination is always desirable, to clarify the purposes. If the reason for studying a health service is that the investigator thinks it is atrocious and wants to collect data that will condemn it, extra-special care should be taken to ensure objectivity in the collection and interpretation of information. In such a case the researcher would be well advised to 'bend over backwards' and consciously set out to seek information to the credit of the service. Regrettably, not all evaluative studies are honest.[2]

REVIEWING THE LITERATURE

The published experiences and thoughts of others may not only indicate the presence and nature of the research problem, but may be of great help in all aspects of planning and in the interpretation of the study findings. At the outset of the study the investigator should be or should become acquainted with the important relevant literature, and should continue with directed reading throughout. References should be filed in an organized way,[3] manually or in a computerized database. It is of limited use to wait until a report has to be written, and then read and cite (or only cite) a long list of publications to impress the reader with one's erudition—a procedure that may defeat its own ends, since it is often quite apparent that the papers and books listed in the extensive bibliography have had no impact on the investigation.

Papers should be read with a healthy scepticism; in Francis Bacon's words, 'Read not to contradict and confute, not to believe and take for granted ... but to weigh and consider'.[4] Several guides to critical reading are available.[5]

If the title and abstract suggest that the paper may be of interest, you should appraise the methods used in the study (which requires the kind of familiarity with research methods and their pitfalls that this book attempts to impart), assess the accuracy of the findings, judge whether the inferences are valid, and decide whether the study has relevance to your own needs and interests. Do not expect any study to be completely convincing, or reject a study because it is not completely convincing; avoid 'I am an epidemiologist' bias (repudiation of any study containing any flaw in its design, analysis or interpretation) and other forms of what has been called 'reader bias'.[6]

Electronic databases (on computer discs, CD-ROMs and the Internet) have both eased the task of finding references and made it harder. The explosive growth in published material in recent years means that a simple manual search is inevitably both laborious and incomplete; on the other hand, a computer search may find so many references (and so many of them irrelevant) that sifting them can be a demanding chore, to the extent that one may be tempted to rely on the abstracts provided by most databases instead of tracking papers down and reading them.

Conducting a computer search in such a way that you get what you want—and don't get what you don't want—is not always easy. Until you have the requisite skill it may be worth enlisting the help of a librarian. The best database is Medline, which covers millions of medical articles. It is searched by looking for specified words (in the title, abstract, author's names, or institution) or Medical Subject Headings (the *MeSH* terms by which the entries are classified); various procedures for widening or narrowing the selection are available.[7] If a key paper is known, a search can be conducted for related articles in MedLine, or the Science Citation Index can be used to identify recent papers that cite it; with luck, some of these will have extensive relevant bibliographies. Very recent papers can be found by using Current Contents, which provides the contents pages of hundreds of journals.

Medline and some other useful databases are available on the Internet.[8]

ETHICAL CONSIDERATIONS

Before embarking on a study the investigator should satisfy himself that it is ethical to do it, and that it can be done in an ethical way. Ethical questions arise in both experimental and non-experimental studies.

There is an obvious ethical problem if an experiment to test the benefits or hazards of a treatment is contemplated. However beneficial the trial may turn out to be for humanity at large, some subjects may be harmed either by the experimental treatment or by its being withheld. There is also an ethical problem in *not* performing a clinical trial, since this may lead to the introduction or continued use of an ineffective or hazardous treatment. 'Where the value of a treatment, new or old, is doubtful, there may be a higher moral obligation to test it critically than to continue to prescribe it year-in-year-out with the support merely of custom or wishful thinking.'[9] But, it has been pointed out, 'this ethical imperative can only be maintained if, and to the extent that, it is possible to conduct controlled trials in an ethically justifiable way'.[10] The heinous medical experiments conducted on helpless victims in the first part of the 20th century should never be forgotten.[11]

For an experimental study to be ethical, the subjects should be aware that they are to participate in an experiment, should know how their treatment will be decided and what the possible consequences are, should be told that they may withdraw from the trial at any time, and should freely give their *informed consent*. In clinical settings these requirements are not always easily accepted, and are sometimes circumvented by medical investigators who feel that they have a right to decide their patient's treatment. Studies have shown that patients (especially poorly educated ones) who sign consent forms are often ignorant of the most basic facts. Special problems concerning consent arise in trials where a total community is exposed to an experimental procedure or programme (see p. 376), and when experiments (such as trials of new vaccines) are performed in developing countries.[12]

Ethical objections to clinical trials are reduced if there is genuine uncertainty about the value of the treatment tested or the relative value of the treatments compared—for some investigators it is sufficient that there is genuine uncertainty in the health profession as a whole, whatever their own views—and if controls are given the best established treatment. 'The essential feature of a controlled trial is that it must be ethically possible to give each patient *any* of the treatments involved'.[13]

Decisions on the ethicality of trials are not simple.[14] Bradford Hill has said that there is only one Golden Rule, namely 'that one can make no generalization ... the problem must be faced afresh with every proposed trial'.

The goals of the research should always be secondary to the well-being of the participants. The Helsinki declaration states, 'Concern for the interests of the subject must always prevail over the interests of science and society ... every patient—including those of a control group, if any—should be assured of the best proven diagnostic and therapeutic method'. But researchers sometimes argue that obtaining an answer to the research question is the primary ethical obligation, so that they then 'find themselves slipping across a line that prohibits treating human subjects as means to an end. When that line is crossed, there is very little left to protect patients from a callous disregard of their welfare for the sake of research goals'.[15] This has raised debates about possible 'scientific imperialism', characterized by the performance of trials, sometimes with lowered ethical standards, in countries that are unlikely to benefit from the findings—'Are poor people in developing countries being exploited in research for the benefit of patients in the developed world where subject recruitment to a randomised trial would be difficult?'[16]

In 1997 a furore was aroused at the disclosure that in developing countries controls were receiving placebos in trials, sponsored by the United States, of regimens to prevent the transmission of HIV (human immunodeficiency virus) from mothers to their unborn children, although there was an effective treatment that had been recommended for all HIV-infected pregnant women in the United States and some other countries. A debate ensued, the main issue being whether the Helsinki declaration's requirement that controls should be given the best current treatment was outweighed by the claims that a comparison with placebo was the best way of finding out whether the relatively cheap experimental regimens would be helpful in countries that cannot afford optimal care, and that the investigators were simply observing what would happen to the infants of the controls, who would anyway not have received treatment if there had been no study.[17]

In nonexperimental studies[18] ethical problems are usually less acute, unless the study involves hazardous test procedures or intrusions on privacy. But here too there is a need for informed consent[19] if participants are required to answer questions, undergo tests that carry a risk (however small), or permit access to confidential records. The investigators should give an honest explanation of the purpose of the survey when enlisting subjects, and respondents should be told what their participation entails and be assured that they are free to refuse to answer questions or continue their participation. Pains should be taken to keep information confidential. Any promises made to participants, say about anonymity or the provision of test results, should of course be kept.

Of particular importance is the question of what action should be taken if a survey reveals that participants would benefit from medical care or other intervention. This is a real dilemma in studies involving HIV antibody testing—should subjects with positive results be notified? Each of the possible strategies (mandatory or optional notification, anonymous or blind testing, etc.) may have adverse effects on willingness to participate or other factors affecting the soundness of the study.[20]

The notorious Tuskegee study in Alabama is a horrible illustration of an unethical survey.[21] It began in 1932, with the aim of throwing light on the effects of untreated syphilis. Some 400 untreated Black syphilitics (mostly poor and uneducated) were identified and then followed up; their course was compared with that of apparently syphilis-free age-matched controls. Treatment of syphilis was withheld. By 1938–1939 it was found that a number of the men had received sporadic treatment with arsenic or mercury, and a very few had had more intensive treatment. In the interests of science 'fourteen young untreated syphilitics were added to the study to compensate for this'. Treatment was withheld even when penicillin was found to be effective and became easily available in the late 40s and early 50s. Participants received free benefits, such as free treatment (except for syphilis), free hot lunches, and free burial (after a free autopsy). By 1954 it was apparent that the life expectancy of the untreated men aged 25–50 was reduced by 17%. By 1963, 14 more men per 100 had died in the syphilitic than in the control group. In 1972 there was a public outcry, and compensation payments were later made.

In many countries informed consent is mandatory for studies of human subjects unless there are valid contraindications, such as qualms about alarming fatally ill patients with doubts about the efficacy of treatment. Many institutions have ethical committees that review and sanction proposed studies. Some investigators feel that this control is too permissive, but there are some who think it is too restrictive ('stops worthwhile research');[22] a fanciful account of the rise and fall of epidemiology between 1950 and 2000 AD—printed in 1981[23]—attributes the fall to ethical committees and regulations designed to protect the confidentiality of records.

At a different ethical level, consideration should be given to the justification for any proposed study in the light of the availability of resources and the other ways in which these might be used. Does the possible benefit warrant the required expenditure of time, manpower and money? Is it ethical to perform the study at the expense of other activities, especially those that might directly promote the community's health?

An honest endeavour to clarify the purpose of the study may lead to second thoughts—is the study really worth doing? A great deal of useless research is conducted. This wastes time and resources, and exposes the scientific method to ridicule.[24]

How well the study is planned and performed is also important: 'Scientifically unsound studies are unethical. It may be accepted as a maxim that a poorly or improperly designed study involving human subjects—one that could not possibly yield scientific facts (that is, reproducible observations) relevant to the question under study—is by definition unethical. Moreover, when a study is in itself scientifically invalid, all other ethical considerations become irrelevant. There is no point in obtaining "informed consent" to perform a useless study'.[25]

FORMULATING THE TOPIC

When the purpose and moral justification of the study are clear, the investigator can formulate the topic he proposes to study, in general terms. In many cases this is easily done and almost tauto-logical. For example, if the reason for setting up the study is that infant mortality is unduly high in a given population and there is insufficient information on its causes for the planning of an action programme, the topic of the study can be broadly stated as 'the causes of infant mortality in a defined population in a given time period'. If the reason for the investigation is that health education on smoking has been having little effect, and that it is considered that certain new methods may be more effective, the investigation will be a comparative study of defined educational techniques for the reduction of smoking.

In other instances the formulation of the topic may be less easy, since the researcher may have difficulty in deciding precisely what study is needed to solve the research problem, taking account of practical limitations. As an illustration, a problem arose in a tuber-culosis programme; the extent of public participation in X-ray screening activities fell short of what was desired, and there were indications that the tuberculosis rate was higher among people who did not come for screening. It was decided to seek information that would help to improve the situation, but considerable thought was required before a study topic could be formulated. The alternative topics were the reasons for non-participation and those for partici-pation. For a variety of reasons it was decided that the latter approach would be more useful.[26]

As another example, a researcher interested in the possibility that eating fish reduces the risk of coronary heart disease has several alternative approaches. He may for instance decide to study the previous dietary habits of people with and without coronary heart disease; or he may follow up groups of people whose diets differ, to determine the occurrence of the disease during a defined period; or he may examine statistics on the disease rates and average fish consumption of different countries. His decision will be based both on the ease with which the required information can be obtained and on the probability of obtaining convincing evidence, one way or the other.

At this early stage, the formulation of the topic of study may be regarded as a provisional one. When planning and the pretesting of methods get under way, it frequently happens that unpredicted difficulties come to light, requiring a change in the topic or even leading to a decision that there is no practical way of solving the research problem.

NOTES AND REFERENCES

1. Geitgey D A, Metz E A 1969 Nursing Research 18: 339.
2. A dishonest evaluation of health care may be *eyewash* (an appraisal limited to aspects that look good), *whitewash* (covering up failure by avoiding objectivity, e.g. by soliciting testimonials), *submarine* (aimed at torpedoing a programme, regardless of its worth), a *postponement ploy* (noting the need to seek facts, in the hope that the crisis will be over by the time the facts are available), etc. Providers of care who evaluate services that they themselves provide should take pains to confute the criticism that this is like 'letting the fox guard the chicken house'. (Spiegel A D, Hyman H H 1978 Basic health planning methods. Aspen Systems, Germantown, Md. pp 324, 355).
3. Numerous computer programs for storing references are available. Over 20 freeware or shareware programs, some of which can accept information from Medline, can be easily downloaded from the Internet (try visiting www. shareware.com and searching for 'bibliographic', 'papers' or 'literature').
   Otherwise, a card index is a great help (one reference per card). Full bibliographic details should be included (names of all authors, first and last page numbers, etc.) to avoid another hunt when a bibliography is prepared for the report. If photocopies, reprints, printouts or tear-out copies of articles or abstracts are collected they should be filed and indexed in an orderly way. The planning of a filing system is described in detail by Haynes R B, McKibbon K A, Fitzgerald D, Guyatt G H, Walker C J, Sackett D L 1986 (How to keep up with the medical literature. Annals of Internal Medicine 105: 149, 309, 574, 636, 810, 978).
4. Bacon F 1620 Novum organum. English translation: Open Court Publishing 1994.
5. Guides to the critical reading of papers about health care include: (a) Greenhalgh T 1997 (How to read a paper: the basics of evidence based medicine. BMJ Publishing Group, London)—ten excerpts appeared in successive issues of the British Medical Journal [vol 315] from July 19 1997; (b) Sackett D L, Richardson W S, Rosenberg W, Haynes R B 1997 (Evidence-based medicine: how to practice and teach EBM. Churchill

Livingstone, New York, pp 81–117); (c) A series of 'Users' Guides to the Medical Literature', commencing in the Journal of the American Medical Association of Nov. 3, 1993; (d) on the Internet: Oxman A D, Sackett D L, Guyatt G H, the Evidence Based Medicine Working Group 1997 (Users' guides to the medical literature): hiru.hirunet.mcmaster.ca/ebm/;(e) Sackett D L, Haynes R B, Tugwell P 1991 (Clinical epidemiology: A basic science for clinical medicine, 2nd edn. Lippincott-Raven).

Checklists are provided by: Polgar S, Thomas S A 1988 (Introduction to research in the health sciences. Churchill Livingstone, Melbourne, p. 279); Crombie I K 1996 (The pocket guide to critical appraisal: a handbook for health care professionals. BMJ Publishing Group, London); for case-control studies, by Lichtenstein M J, Mulrow CD, Elwood P C 1987 (Guidelines for reading case-control studies. Journal of Chronic Diseases 40: 893); for clinical trials, by Chalmers T C, Smith H, Blackburn B, Silverman B, Schroeder B, Reitman D, Ambroz A 1981 (A method for assessing the quality of a randomized control trial. Controlled Clinical Trials 2: 31); and, for programme trials, by Smith P J, Moffatt M E K, Gelskey S C, Hudson S, Kaita K 1997 (Are community health interventions evaluated appropriately? A review of six journals. Journal of Clinical Epidemiology 50: 137).

Also, see Riegelman R K, Hirsch R P 1996 (Studying a study and testing a test: How to read the health science literature, 3rd edn. Little, Brown Boston); and Abramson J H 1994 (Making sense of data: a self-instruction manual on the interpretation of epidemiologic data, 2nd edn. Oxford University Press, New York).

6. Forms of 'reader bias' include rivalry bias (pooh-poohing a study published by a rival), personal habit bias (over-rating or under-rating a study to justify the reader's habits, e.g. a jogger favouring a study showing the health benefits of running), prestigious journal bias (over-rating study results because the journal has an illustrious name), and pro-technology and anti-technology bias (over-rating or under-rating a study owing to the reader's enchantment or disenchantment with medical technology). (Owen R 1982 Reader bias. Journal of the American Medical Association 247: 2533).

For entertaining and instructive examples of 'repudiation of any study containing any flaw in its design, analysis or interpretation', visit the Junk Science page on the Internet ('All the junk that's fit to debunk'; www.junkscience.com), where studies are pilloried (sometimes justifiably) because of flaws, but their positive aspects are ignored. A study that showed that depressed people were 80% more likely to suffer heart attacks, for example, was condemned because: (a) the association was weak ('i.e, less than 100%'); (b) the researchers failed to look into whether treating the depression removed the additional risk; and (c) they had no biological explanation for the association. The verdict: 'Three strikes and it's junk science!'.

7. For aids to the use of Medline, see Greenhalgh T 1997 (The Medline database. British Medical Journal 315: 180) [this is an excerpt from the book cited in note 6] and Sackett et al 1997 ([see note 5] pp 56–63), who promise that 'If you enjoy puzzles, MEDLINE is great fun'.

The MeSH (Medical Subject Headings) terms and their use are explained by Lowe H J, Barnett G O 1994 (Understanding and using the medical subject headings [MeSH] vocabulary to perform literature searches. Journal of the American Medical Association 271: 1103). On the Internet, PubMed (see note 8) provides a MeSH browser permitting the identification of appropriate MeSH terms for a specific search.

8. At the time of writing, free access to Medline is available through PubMed (www.ncbi.nlm.nih.gov/PubMed/), Internet Grateful Med (igm.nlm.nih.gov/),

which accesses PubMed and other resources, and numerous other services, links to which can be found in tan.net/medline.html

Other bibliographic databases and sources of information are best sought by using a multisearch engine—such as Dogpile (www.dogpile.com) or Metafind (www.metafind.com)—that makes simultaneous use of a number of search engines.

One useful source is the Combined Health Information Database maintained by US governmental agencies, which supplies information (including references to monographs, chapters, articles, bibliographies, programme descriptions, and reports) on selected diseases and such topics as cancer prevention, school health, health promotion and education, maternal and child health, oral health and weight control (URL: chid.nih.gov/).

9. Green F H K, cited by Hill (1997) (see note 13).
10. Roy D J 1986 Controlled clinical trials: an ethical imperative. Journal of Chronic Diseases 39: 159.
11. Seidelman W E 1988 (Mengele Medicus: medicine's Nazi heritage. Milbank Quarterly 66: 221) cites the horrors committed by Mengele and other Nazi physicians as warnings against 'ethical compromise where human life and dignity become secondary to personal, professional, scientific, and political goals'. Also, see Seidelman W E 1996 (Nuremberg lamentation: for the forgotten victims of medical science. British Medical Journal 313: 1463) and Annas G J, Grodin M A (eds) 1995 (The Nazi doctors and the Nuremberg Code: human rights in human experimentation. Oxford University Press, New York).

    Experiments on prisoners in the United States are described by Hornblum A M 1997 (They were cheap and available: prisoners as research subjects in twentieth century America. British Medical Journal 315: 1437).
12. Proposed International Guidelines for Biomedical Research Involving Human Subjects have been published by the World Health Organization and the Council for International Organizations of Medical Sciences (Geneva: CIOMS, 1982).

    These guidelines state that in community-based research—e.g. health services research and trials undertaken on a community basis—'individual consent on a person-to-person basis may not be feasible, and the ultimate decision to undertake the research will rest with the responsible public health authority. Nevertheless, all possible means should be used to inform the community concerned of the aims of the research, the advantages expected from it, and any possible hazards or inconveniences. If feasible, dissenting individuals should have the option of withholding their participation. Whatever the circumstances, the ethical considerations and safeguards applied to research on individuals must be translated, in every possible respect, into the community context'.

    Regarding *research in developing countries*, the international guidelines state: 'Rural communities in developing countries may not be conversant with the concepts and techniques of experimental medicine ... Where individual members of a community do not have the necessary awareness of the implications of participation in an experiment to give adequately informed consent directly to the investigators, it is desirable that the decision whether or not to participate should be elicited through the intermediary of a trusted community leader. The intermediary should make it clear that participation is entirely voluntary, and that any participant is free to abstain or withdraw at any time from the experiment'. It may also be practicable to obtain the subjects' informed consent as a second stage, after consent has been received from a community leader, as demonstrated in a vaccine trial in Senegal (Preziosi M-P, Yam A, Ndiaye M, Simaga A, Simondon F, Wassilak S G F

1997 Practical experiences in obtaining informed consent for a vaccine trial in rural Africa. New England Journal of Medicine 336: 370).

Ethical considerations in field trials in developing countries are reviewed by Smith P G, Morrow R H (eds) 1991 (Methods for field trials of interventions against tropical diseases: a 'toolbox'. Oxford University Press, Oxford, pp 71–94).

13. Hill A B 1977 A short textbook of medical statistics. Hodder and Stoughton, London, p. 223.

14. The basic principle is neatly summarized in the following exchange: 'Mr Ederer: "If you could give only one bit of advice to a clinician planning a clinical trial, what would you tell him?" Dr Davis: "A one-word answer might be 'don't'. If you are determined to do it, my advice would be from the beginning put yourself in the patient's position and develop the protocol so you would be happy to be one of the subjects. If you cannot do that, you'd better not start." ' (Davis M D 1975 American Journal of Ophthalmology 79: 779).

See the Helsinki declaration (Declaration of Helsinki IV, 41st World Medical Assembly, Hong Kong, September 1989. In: Annas and Grodin 1995 [see note 11] pp 339–342). Internet sources include www.csu.edu.au/learning/ncgr/gpi/odyssey/privacy/HelDec.html An older version and the British Medical Research Council's statement on investigations of human subjects are in Hill A B 1977 (A short textbook on medical statistics. Hodder and Stoughton, London, pp 248–253).

Useful Internet sources on ethical aspects include Ethics in Biomedicine (www.mic.ki.se/Diseases/k1.316.html) and Online Bioethics Resources (biomednet.com/hmsbeagle/20/webres/institu.htmww.jir.com).

15. Angell M 1997 Editorial: The ethics of clinical research in the Third World. New England Journal of Medicine 337: 847.

16. Wilmshurst P 1997 Editorial: Scientific imperialism. British Medical Journal 314: 840. Other extracts: 'Should research be conducted in a country where the people are unlikely to benefit from the findings because most of the population is too poor to buy effective treatment? ... Drug companies have performed research on children and adults in countries such as Thailand and the Philippines that do not conform to the Declaration of Helsinki and could not be conducted in the developed world. Reasons quoted for conducting research in Africa rather than developed countries are lower costs, lower risk of litigation, less stringent ethical review, the availability of populations prepared to give unquestioning consent, anticipated underreporting of side effects because of lower consumer awareness ... In some experiments in developing countries it is difficult for patients to refuse to participate ... participation in a trial may be the only chance of receiving any treatment'.

17. For both sides of the debate on whether these AIDS trials in developing countries are ethical, see: Angell 1997 (see note 15); Lurie P, Wolfe S M 1997 (Unethical trials of interventions to reduce perinatal transmission of the human immunodeficiency virus in developing countries. New England Journal of Medicine 337: 853); and Halsey N A, Sommer A, Henderson D A, Black R E 1997 (Editorial: Ethics and international research. British Medical Journal 315: 965).

'Stopping trials in Africa that are trying to improve the health of poor people so that those in affluent countries can have peace of mind seems a tortured form of ethical logic' (Gambia Government/Medical Research Council Joint Ethical Committee 1998 Ethical issues facing medical research in developing countries. Lancet 351: 286).

18. For ethical aspects of epidemiological research, see: Coughlin S S, Beauchamp T L (eds) 1996 (Ethics and epidemiology. Oxford University Press, New York); and Susser M, Stein Z, Kline J 1978 (Ethics in epidemiology. Annals

of the American Academy of Political and Social Science 437: 128 [reprinted in Susser M 1987 Epidemiology, health and society: Selected papers. Oxford University Press, New York, pp 13–22]).

19. A specimen 'informed consent' form for use in an interview survey is provided by Stolley P D, Schlesselman J J 1982 (Planning and conducting a study. In: Schlesselman J J, ed. 1982 Case-control studies: design, conduct, analysis. Oxford University Press, New York, pp 69–104).

20. The 'To tell or not to tell' dilemma in studies involving HIV testing, and possible solutions, are discussed by Avins A, Lo B 1989 (To tell or not to tell: the ethical dilemmas of HIV test notification in epidemiologic research. American Journal of Public Health 79: 1544); Kegeles S, Coates T J, Lo B, Catania J 1989 (Mandatory reporting of HIV testing would deter men from being tested. Journal of the American Medical Association 261: 1989); and Avins A, Woods W, Lo B, Hulley S 1993 (A novel use of the link-file system for longitudinal studies of HIV infection: practical solution to an ethical dilemma. AIDS 7: 109).

21. Thomas S B, Quinn S C 1991 The Tuskegee syphilis study, 1932 to 1972: implications for HIV education and AIDS risk education programs in the Black community. American Journal of Public Health 81: 1498.

22. Waters W E 1985 Ethics and epidemiological research. International Journal of Epidemiology 14: 48.

23. Rothman K J 1981 The rise and fall of epidemiology, 1950–2000 A.D. New England Journal of Medicine 304: 600.

24. 'Time, talent, and money are sometimes squandered on the measurement of the trivial, the irrelevant, and the obvious ... A friend of mine who has a gift for felicitous expression has distinguished between "ideas" research on the one hand and "occupational therapy for the university staff" on the other, and once referred to a research project as "squeezing the last drop of blood out of a foregone conclusion" ' (Lord Platt 1967 Medical science: master or servant. British Medical Journal 2: 439).

See an amusing compilation by Hartston W 1988 (The drunken goldfish: a celebration of irrelevant research. Unwin Hyman) of actual research results (Do rats prefer tennis balls to other rats? Can pigeons tell Bach from Hindemith? Does holy water affect the growth of radishes?) that serves 'to drop a gentle hint that there might be too much research going on, and much of that is taken far too seriously'. Useless research is satirized in the Journal of Irreproducible Results (for details and a sample of contents, visit www.jir.com on the Internet).

25. Rutstein D D 1972 In: Freund F A (ed) 1972 Experimentation with human subjects. George Allen & Unwin, London.

26. Rosenstock I M, Hochbaum G M 1961 Some principles of research design in public health. American Journal of Public Health 51: 266.

2 Types of investigation

Before discussing the detailed planning of a study we will consider the types of investigation and their nomenclature. The primary distinction is between surveys (or observational studies) and experiments (trials). The various types of epidemiological and evaluative studies will be reviewed in this chapter.

SURVEYS AND EXPERIMENTS

Since a survey is most easily defined negatively, as a nonexperimental investigation, we will start by defining an experiment.

An *experiment* is an investigation in which the researcher, wishing to study the effects of exposure to or deprivation of a defined factor, himself decides which subjects (persons, animals, towns, etc.) will be exposed to, or deprived of, the factor. Experiments are studies of deliberate intervention by the investigators. If the investigator compares subjects exposed to the factor with subjects not exposed to it, this is a *controlled experiment*; the more care that is taken to ensure that the two groups are as similar as possible in other respects, the better controlled is the experiment. In a controlled experiment on the effect of vitamin supplements, for example, it is the investigator who decides who will and who will not receive such supplements; in a survey, by contrast, people who happen to be taking vitamin supplements are compared with people who do not take them.

A study is a true experiment only if decisions about exposure to the factor under consideration (e.g. to whom will vitamin supplements be offered?) are made by the experimenter. A researcher who wants to conduct an experiment does not always have full control over the situation, and may be unable to make such decisions. It may be possible, however, to construct a study that resembles an experiment although in this respect it falls short of being a true one. For example, it may be feasible to make observations before and after some intervention not under the investigator's control (medical treatment, exposure to a health education programme, etc.) and to make parallel observations in an unexposed group. The study may then be called a *quasi-experiment*[1] (although some experts prefer to regard such studies as nonexperimental). This term is also sometimes used if the allocation to experimental and control groups (even if under the experimenter's control) is not random (see *Randomization*, p. 359).

Although they are sometimes given the unflattering appellation of 'pseudo-experiments', quasi-experiments are often well worth doing when a true experiment is not feasible (see pp 376 and 378); but their findings must be interpreted with caution—it is difficult to be sure that the outcome is in fact attributable to the intervention.

The term *natural experiment* is often applied to circumstances where, as a result of 'naturally' occurring changes or differences, it is easy to observe the effects of a specific factor. A famine may permit a study of the effects of starvation. Snow's classic comparison of cholera rates in homes with different water sources, some more contaminated than others, in London in the middle of the 19th century may be termed a 'natural experiment'.[2] 'Natural experiments' are surveys or, at most (if they examine the effects of man-made changes), quasi-experiments. They have also been termed 'experiments of opportunity'.

Manipulations of animals or human beings are not synonymous with experiments. An investigator who studies bacteriuria in pregnancy by needling the bladders of pregnant women through their abdominal walls in order to collect urine for examination is conducting a survey, not an experiment. An experiment is always a study of change.

A *survey* (or *observational study*)[3] is an investigation in which information is systematically collected, but the experimental method is not used—that is, there is no active intervention by the investigators. In this book 'survey' is used in a broad sense to mean a nonexperimental study of any kind, and does not have the narrow connotations sometimes associated with the term, such as a public opinion survey, a questionnaire survey, a descriptive study of population characteristics, a field survey, or a household survey. Surveys are not necessarily brief operations; they may involve long-term surveillance (see p. 29) or repeated interviews or examinations.

DESCRIPTIVE AND ANALYTIC STUDIES

Studies may be descriptive or analytic. A *descriptive* study sets out to describe a situation, e.g. the distribution of a disease in a population in relation to age, sex, region, etc. An *analytic* (or *explanatory*) study tries to find explanations and examine causal processes (Why does the disease occur in these people? Why do certain people fail to make use of health services? Can the decreased incidence of the disease be attributed to the introduction of preventive measures? Does treatment reduce the risk of complications?). This is done by formulating and testing hypotheses, which may have various sources,[4] including the findings of previous descriptive studies. An analytic survey may be used to explain a local situation in a specific population in which the investigator is interested, or to obtain results of a more general applicability, e.g. new knowledge about the aetiology of a disease.

All descriptive studies are surveys, but surveys can also be analytic; experiments are obviously analytic. The distinction between a descriptive and an analytic survey is not always clear, and many surveys combine both purposes.

CROSS-SECTIONAL AND LONGITUDINAL STUDIES

Studies, whether descriptive, analytic or both, can be usefully categorized as cross-sectional or longitudinal, depending on the time period covered by the observations. A *cross-sectional* ('instantaneous', 'simultaneous', 'prevalence') study provides information about the situation that exists at a single time, whereas a *longitudinal* ('time-span') study provides data about events or changes during a period of time.

A survey in which children are measured in order to determine the distribution of their weights and heights, or to compare heights at different ages, is cross-sectional; the children are examined once, at about the same time (not necessarily on the same day). A survey in which the same children are examined repeatedly in order to appraise their growth is longitudinal. If the influence on child growth of parents' smoking habits is investigated in any of these surveys, the study is an analytic one. Most experiments are longitudinal studies that follow up different groups to measure events or changes; some only compare the status of the groups after the experimental exposure ('postmeasure only' trials), without measuring their initial status.

A longitudinal survey in which a group (or 'cohort') of individuals (however selected) is followed up for some time may be called a *cohort* ('follow-up', 'panel') study; but the term 'cohort study' is generally used more restrictively, to refer to an analytic longitudinal study (see p. 22). 'Cohort study' should not be confused with 'cohort analysis'.[5] A study of the occurrence of new cases of a disease is an *incidence* study, and a follow-up study of persons born in a defined period is a *birth-cohort* study.

Note that the distinction between cross-sectional and longitudinal studies depends only on whether the information collected refers to a particular time. The *timing* of the study—*when* it is conducted, i.e. at the same time as the events studied (a *concurrent* study) or afterwards (a *historical* study)—is not relevant. Nor does it matter whether the study uses previously recorded data, or data collected after the start of the study; these two kinds of data are best termed *retrolective* and *prolective* respectively (from the Latin root of the word 'collect')[6] rather than 'retrospective' and 'prospective', to avoid confusion with other meanings of the latter terms. Note also that the term 'cross-sectional' is sometimes used in other senses, e.g. for studies of total populations or representative samples ('cross-sections') of them.

In some studies, data that refer to the present time are treated as if they referred to the past. Reported disease in the subject's relatives, for example, may be taken as evidence of his or her prior exposure to genetic or other familial factors; or in a study of the association between lead poisoning and behavioural problems in school, the lead content of milk teeth may be used as an indicator of lead poisoning in early childhood.[7] It has been suggested that such studies should be called *pseudolongitudinal*.

EPIDEMIOLOGICAL STUDIES

Epidemiology is the study of the occurrence, distribution and determinants of states of health and disease in human groups and populations, and the application of this study to the control of health problems.[8]

Epidemiological studies have three main uses. First, they serve a diagnostic purpose. Just as a diagnosis of the patient's state of health is a prerequisite for good clinical care, so a *community diagnosis*[9] or *group diagnosis*, leading to a *needs assessment*, provides a basis for the care of a community (or other defined group of people). Epidemiological studies—descriptive and analytic—provide the required information about health status and the determinants of health in a specific community or group. Secondly, epidemiological studies (mainly analytic surveys) can throw light on aetiology, prognostic factors, the natural history of disease, and growth and development. Such knowledge is of general interest and has a wide applicability, in addition to the help it provides in the care of specific patients and in specific local situations. Thirdly, epidemiological studies (surveys and experiments) contribute to the evaluation of health care both in specific local situations (How well is this accident prevention programme working?) and in general (Does this vaccine prevent disease?) Surveys of population health, it has been said, 'can be both the alpha and omega of health care by being the vehicle for both the discovery of need and the evaluation of the outcome of care and treatment'.[10]

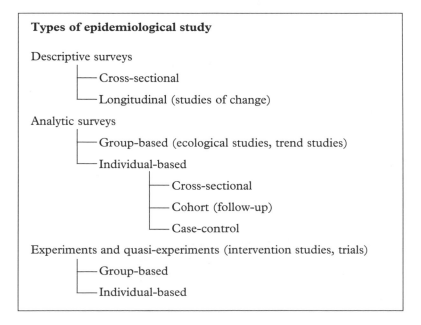

Types of epidemiological study

Descriptive surveys
- Cross-sectional
- Longitudinal (studies of change)

Analytic surveys
- Group-based (ecological studies, trend studies)
- Individual-based
  - Cross-sectional
  - Cohort (follow-up)
  - Case-control

Experiments and quasi-experiments (intervention studies, trials)
- Group-based
- Individual-based

The role of epidemiological studies in community-oriented primary care, which integrates the care of individuals with the care of the community as a whole, will be described in Chapter 34.

Descriptive epidemiological surveys may be cross-sectional (how many blind people are there in the population?) or longitudinal. Longitudinal surveys investigate *change*, e.g. studies of child growth and development, or a changing suicide rate, or the 'natural history' of disease (what is the course of events after infection with AIDS virus?), or the occurrence of new cases of disease or deaths in the population. They include *clinical follow-up studies* that monitor the progress of groups of patients. Descriptive epidemiological surveys do not aim to find explanations, but their findings are often presented by age, sex, region, and other demographic variables.

Analytic epidemiological surveys may be group-based or individual-based.

Group-based analytic surveys

A *group-based* analytic survey[11] is a comparison of groups or populations. It is a study of a group of groups, not a group of individuals. As an example, a group of countries could be compared with respect to their death rates from cirrhosis of the liver, on the one hand, and the average consumption of alcohol and various nutrients on the other.[12] Such studies are sometimes termed *ecological* or *correlation* studies.

We could also conduct a *trend* or *time-series* study, by comparing the findings of descriptive studies performed in the same group at different times, e.g. by analyzing the changing mortality rate from a disease in relation to changes in average fat intake and per capita tobacco consumption.[13] Such studies often produce results of considerable interest, like the doubling of the rate of fractures of the proximal femur in Oxford between 1956 and 1983.[14] Comparisons of trends in different populations may be instructive: a study of liver cirrhosis mortality in 25 European countries between 1970 and 1989 showed different trends in different regions but, in all regions, rates declined a few years after a decrease in per capita alcohol consumption; there was also evidence of a birth-cohort effect,[5] portending a future decrease in mortality in western and southern Europe, and an increase in eastern and northern Europe.[15]

Group-based studies are sometimes denigrated, on two main grounds. First, because they sometimes yield misleading results as a result of the inaccuracy, inappropriateness or unavailability of data, often obtained from national statistical offices or other official sources. But even then, they may serve to draw attention to differences or trends meriting further investigation. The strong positive correlation between infant mortality and the number of doctors per 10 000 population demonstrated in a comparison of 18 developed countries in Europe and North America[16] does not necessarily mean that infants should be kept away from doctors, but it raises important questions, even if the correlation is a reflection of other (unknown) factors for which data were not available. Doll & Peto have pointed out that although the striking correlations between colon cancer and meat consumption and between breast cancer and fat consumption, observed in international comparisons, may not mean that eating meat or fat is a major aetiological factor, they certainly show that the large international differences in the rates of these neoplasms are not chiefly genetic in origin, and suggest that these cancers are largely avoidable.[17]

Secondly, it may be misleading to apply the findings of a group-based study at an individual level; this has been termed the *ecologic fallacy*, a type of *cross-level bias*. If we find that populations with a high consumption of beer tend to have a high death rate from cancer of the rectum,[18] this does not necessarily mean that *individuals* who drink more beer are prone to develop this tumour; this should be tested in an individual-based survey, or maybe in a rather pleasant experiment.

The term 'ecologic fallacy' has unfortunately tended to throw ecologic studies into disrepute. But the findings of group-based studies can be important in their own right, and there is no reason to expect that their findings will necessarily be valid at an individual level[18] (or, conversely, that findings at an individual level will necessarily be valid at a group level, which has been called the '*atomistic fallacy*'.)[19] A comparison of villages in Mexico showed a strong association between dengue infection (the presence of antibodies) and exposure to *Aedes aegyptii* mosquitoes, which was a useful finding although no such association existed at an individual level.[20] Similarly, the observation that after floods in Bangladesh there was an increase in the proportions of children who manifested aggressive behaviour and enuresis is of interest, although the behaviour of individual children did not vary according to the danger of drowning they experienced.[21]

Group-based studies are sometimes the only appropriate study design, for example in comparisons of groups exposed to different environmental influences[22] or differing with respect to processes of intra-group transmission or interaction, and sometimes they facilitate the study of relationships with environmental exposures that are difficult to measure at an individual level. Group-based studies have assumed greater importance with the resurgence of interest in the influence of societal and other group processes on health, and in the determinants of the health status of human populations.[23]

Individual-based analytic surveys

Individual-based analytic surveys are of course (like all epidemiological studies) studies of groups, but they utilize information about each individual in the group. In their simplest form, such surveys are performed to test a hypothesis that a specific causal factor is a determinant of a specific disease (or other outcome), by measuring each individual's exposure to the postulated causal factor and the presence of the disease in each individual.

Most individual-based analytic surveys can be categorized as cross-sectional, cohort or case-control[23] studies, or as combinations of these types. (This classification diverges from the one used in previous editions of this book.)[24]

An analytic *cross-sectional study* examines the associations that exist in a group or population (or a sample of a group or population) at a given time. The study may be based on retrolective (previously-recorded) or prolective data.

A *cohort* study is an analytic *follow-up* or *prospective* study in which people who are (respectively) exposed and not exposed to the postulated causal factor(s), or who have different degrees of exposure, are compared with respect to the subsequent development of the disease (or other outcome under study); the people who are followed up are referred to as the cohort. If the disease is one that cannot be contracted twice, people who have it at the outset (before the follow-up) are generally excluded from the comparison.

Note two sources of possible terminological confusion: the term 'cohort study' is sometimes used for a descriptive (nonanalytic) follow-up study, and the term 'prospective' is often used to indicate the collection of data after the start of a study (prolective data; see p. 18), rather than a cohort-study design.

A cohort study resembles an experiment, except that exposure or nonexposure is not controlled by the investigator. Specific subjects may be chosen for follow-up because of their exposure or nonexposure to the causal factor, or a cohort may be selected in some other way (say, because of residence in a specific neighbourhood), characterized with respect to exposure status, and followed up. As an example, baseline information about drinking habits and other characteristics was obtained for a population sample of Finnish beer-drinkers; after a seven-year follow-up, a comparison of men who initially had different drinking habits showed that mortality was three times as high among men who had beer binges (six or more bottles per session) than among those who usually drank less than three bottles each time (allowing for differences in age, smoking, total alcohol consumption, and other factors that might affect mortality).[25]

Previously-collected (retrolective) and historical data are often used in cohort studies. An extreme example is a comparison of the mortality of obese and nonobese persons, the data being their weight when they originally took out life insurance policies and their survival from then until the time of the study. Such a study may be called a *historical prospective study* (among other terms).[26] As another example, a cohort study that started in 1976, in which 121 700 nurses were followed up by postal questionnaire every two years, was able to demonstrate that their weight at birth had a strong inverse relationship with the occurrence of coronary heart disease between 1976 and 1992, using birth weights reported in the 1992 questionnaire; the authors describe their design as 'retrospective self report of birth weight in an ongoing longitudinal cohort of nurses'.[27]

In a typical *case-control study* to examine the relationship between a suspected causal factor and a disease (or other outcome), people with the disease are compared with controls free of the disease, to determine whether they differ in their exposure to the causal factor. The controls should be representative of the population 'base' from which the cases came;[28] ideally, they are people who would have become cases in the study if they had developed the disease. This condition is most easily met in a case-control study performed within a defined population, where the cases can be compared with all, or a representative sample of, the non-cases. It can also be easily satisfied if the case-control study is performed in the framework of a cohort study, so that the experience of new cases identified in the study cohort can be compared with that of controls from the same cohort. This is a *nested case-control study*, where the controls are selected from cohort members who were free of the disease at the time the corresponding case developed it. If a case-control study is performed in a defined population or cohort, the controls can also represent the total population (*case-base* studies) or cohort (*case-cohort* studies), irrespective of the occurrence of the disease; the inclusion of cases-to-be in the control group is taken into account in the statistical analysis.

The selection of cases and controls for a case-control study will be considered in more detail in Chapter 9.

As a simple example of a case-control study, women students who acquired their first urinary tract infection were compared with sexually active women without a history of urinary tract infection, drawn from a random sample of all students at the same university. Questions about condom use in the previous fortnight indicated that use of an unlubricated condom strongly increased the risk of urinary tract infection (as compared with no birth control method); the increased risk was much smaller if the condom was lubricated or spermicide-coated.[29]

Two examples of nested case-control studies:

1. Men killed in road accidents during a 15-year cohort study of steelworkers were compared with control workers drawn from the same cohort. One of the findings was that exposure to high levels of noise at work was associated with an approximately doubled risk of being killed in a road accident.[30]
2. Participants in the cohort study of 121 700 nurses were asked in 1982 to submit toenail clippings—and 68 213 did so—in order to permit use of the concentrations of iron, arsenic, zinc and other trace elements in the clippings as measures of the intake of these elements. The toenail trace element levels of new cases of breast cancer identified between 1982 and 1986 were then compared with those of 459 individually matched controls. A simple cohort design would have required assays of clippings from 68 213 nurses, instead of about 900.[31]

Most case-control studies are 'time-span' (longitudinal) studies in which the measurements of cause and outcome refer, or are believed to refer (pseudolongitudinal studies—see p. 18) to different points in time. The data may be obtained retrolectively or prolectively.

In some case-control studies, however, no assumption can be made that the measurements can be attributed to different times, or (especially if the postulated causal factor and the postulated outcome may both have been present for some time before the study) there may be no certainty as to which came first (the 'cart-or-horse' problem); a study of the relationship between obesity and physical inactivity (measured at the same time) is an example. Also, in some instances it may not be conceptually clear that one of the variables can be considered a cause of the other.

A comparison of cases and controls that is based on associations existing at a single time should for practical purposes be classified as a case-control study rather than a cross-sectional one, since it is subject to the same considerations as other case-control studies with regard to (for example) the selection of subjects and how they may affect the analysis and interpretation of findings. For example, a study of a sample of 70-year-olds in which snorers are identified and compared with non-snorers in order to determine whether snoring is related to atherosclerotic manifestations[32] can be regarded as a case-control study in which the requirement that case and controls should be drawn from the same population base is well met.

It may be noted that not all case-control comparisons are case-control studies, i.e. studies in which cases of an outcome condition are compared with controls in order to investigate causal hypotheses. For example, a comparison of the birth weights of children born to samples of women who bleed during pregnancy (cases) and those who do not (controls) is a cohort study—the cases and controls are the subjects who are, respectively, exposed and not exposed to the postulated causal factor; this is a form of *clinical follow-up study*. Other case-control comparisons have nothing to do with the testing of an aetiological hypothesis (e.g. in evaluative studies of screening or diagnostic tests).

Combinations of the above three study types (hybrid designs) can be used.

Each of the above study designs has its advantages and disadvantages.[33] Case-control studies generally require less time than cohort studies and are relatively simple to perform, since (like cross-sectional studies) they avoid the difficult task of following up the subjects, and they usually require fewer subjects. They sometimes offer immediate solutions to a problem, e.g. in studies of disease outbreaks, where the cases studied are the very cases constituting the problem. But the fact that information about exposure to the 'cause' is generally obtained when the disease is already present may produce various kinds of bias. There may, for example, be *recall bias* (cases may be more likely to report exposure than controls, or vice versa) or *exposure suspicion bias* (the investigator's knowledge that the illness is present may stimulate an especially intensive search for evidence of exposure).[34] Appropriate controls are often difficult to find, and the use of inappropriate controls may distort the findings. Cohort studies are preferable in many ways. They generally leave less doubt about the time relationships between exposure and the disease, and can more easily provide information about the degree of risk associated with exposure, the natural history of the disease, and other effects of the exposure. But losses to follow-up are frequent, and may skew the results. Moreover, a cohort study may be impracticable if the disease is rare or if it develops very long after exposure to the cause. For example, the hypothesis that severe diarrhoea is conducive to the development of cataract many years later is easier to test in a case-control study.[35]

Experiments and quasi-experiments

Epidemiological experiments that are designed to test cause–effect hypotheses may be termed *intervention studies*.[36] They can be performed only if it is feasible and ethically justified to manipulate the postulated cause. ('The bearing of children, exposure to hazards, or personality type, are not normally subject to experiment'.)[37] Like surveys, intervention studies may be group-based or individual-based. When the effect of fluoride on dental caries was investigated by fluoridating the water supplies of some towns and comparing the subsequent occurrence of dental caries in these towns with that in control towns, this was a group-based experiment; data were not available on the fluoride consumption of each individual. On the other hand, when the hypothesis that the administration of oxygen to premature infants caused retrolental fibroplasia (a blinding disease) was tested by administering oxygen continuously to some babies and not to others,[38] this was an individual-based experiment.

Experiments and quasi-experiments conducted to appraise the value of treatments, preventive procedures and health care programmes are generally termed *trials*.

EVALUATIVE STUDIES

Evaluative studies[39] are those that appraise the *value* of health care —they set out to measure how 'good' care is. (The criteria used will be discussed in Chapter 5.)

Evaluative studies are of two main types. These may be termed *reviews* and *trials*, and are distinguished by their different purposes.

A *programme review* is motivated by concern with the welfare of the specific patients, community or population to whom care is given, and it evaluates the care given to them. It may evaluate a particular programme that operates in a defined setting, with well defined aims such as case-finding, immunization, the control of hypertension, fluoridation of water supplies, etc. (A programme may be defined as 'any enterprise organized to eliminate or reduce one or more problems').[40] It may also evaluate a specific health service (a national or regional service, a health centre, a group practice, a hospital, etc.), a part or aspect of a service, or even the work of an individual practitioner, and may be called a 'service review'. Medical audit (see p. 243) is a form of programme review.

Types of evaluative study

1. Programme reviews
2. Trials
    a. Of care given to groups and populations:
        Programme trials
    b. Of care given to individuals:
        Clinical trials (of curative or preventive care)
        Trials of screening and diagnostic tests

An essential feature of a programme review is that the findings should be helpful to whoever makes decisions about the specific programme or service. It follows that the evaluation can be conducted within the framework of the assumptions accepted by the decision maker or makers, e.g. the assumption that the performance of certain procedures will have beneficial effects. These assumptions, on which the programme is based, are not necessarily questioned or tested. The evaluation results can be useful without necessarily being found convincing by those who doubt the validity of the assumptions on which the programme is founded. Programme and service reviews are akin to a physician's periodic reviews of the treatment given to a specific patient, which enable him to decide whether to continue, modify or stop therapy. These assessments are an indispensable part of the clinical process, although the clinician can seldom obtain convincing evidence of the extent to which changes in the patient's condition can be attributed to the treatment. Programme reviews are generally descriptive surveys, sometimes with an analytic component.

A *programme trial*, by contrast, sets out to obtain generalizable knowledge, that can be applied in other settings, about the value of a *type* of health care provided for a group or population. To meet its purpose a trial must yield conclusions that are well enough substantiated to be generally convincing. It is not enough merely to demonstrate a beneficial effect, but there must be evidence that the effect can be attributed to the care given. To this end, pains must be taken to eliminate or allow for the possible influence of other factors.

It is important to distinguish between programme reviews and programme trials, since the questions they ask and the methods they use are different. In a review, basic assumptions are not in question, and definitive tests of cause–effect hypotheses are not required; it is wasteful and may be self-defeating to use excessively rigorous study techniques. A trial, on the other hand, may be inconclusive if methods are insufficiently rigorous. There are other differences as well, which also have implications for the planning of the study. To be useful, a review must usually be rapid and (if possible) ongoing. Changes in circumstances, personnel and policy results in frequent changes in the procedures used in a service, and there may be little practical benefit in evaluating a programme as it used to be some years previously. If appraisal is rapid, it can give early warning of inadequacies and provide an up-to-date factual basis for decisions. Speed is less important in a trial. Further, a review is carried out in a service-oriented setting—this is the review's *raison d'être*. Evaluation may not be seen as an important element, and little time and resources may be available for special information-collecting procedures. A trial, on the other hand, is more likely to be conducted as a specific investigative procedure. Not infrequently the programme is set up specially, as a test or demonstration. Programme trials may be experiments or quasi-experiments.

An evaluation of a programme may be of a hybrid type, e.g. when a programme trial is conducted in the context of a service review. This may happen if there is a call for the appraisal of an innovative feature of the service, or if certain of the assumptions on which the service is based are questioned, or if there is a wish to generalize from the experience of the service. In such instances there will be a need for the demanding methods of study that are appropriate to a trial, as well as for the less rigorous ones needed for a review of other aspects of the service. Difficulties often arise when a programme trial is conducted in the setting of an established service, since evaluation and service may make competing demands.

A *clinical trial* appraises the worth of a form of care—preventive, curative, educational, etc.—given to individuals, rather than to a group or population; it may be an experiment or a quasi-experiment. Trials may also be conducted to evaluate screening and diagnostic tests (see pp 197–199).

While programme and clinical trials require separate consideration (see Chs 32 and 33), there is a degree of overlap between them, as some programme trials are based on a comparison of individuals who are exposed and not exposed to the programme under study. Individual-based programme trials of this sort do not differ in their design from other clinical trials.

Some trials have double objectives: when testing a new form of treatment, the aim may be both to appraise its value for individuals and to evaluate the programme whereby it is provided to the public.

The use of case-control studies for the evaluation of preventive and therapeutic procedures is discussed on page 350.

The term '*inbuilt evaluation*' may be used if the evaluation is planned in advance and the requisite information is collected in a systematic way as an integral part of the provision of a service.

Medical audit is a technique used mainly in service reviews, whereby the quality of a service is evaluated by appraising the quality of the care given to individuals. It will be discussed in more detail in Chapter 21.

OTHER TERMS

Surveillance[41] denotes the maintenance of an ongoing watch over the status of a group or community. It yields information about new and changing needs, and provides a basis for appraising the effects of health care. A watch may be kept on health status—in terms of mortality, morbidity, nutritional status, child growth and development, or other indices—and on environmental hazards, health practices, and other factors that may affect health.

There is considerable confusion about the use of the terms 'surveillance' and 'monitoring', and they are often used interchangeably. *Monitoring* is probably best used to refer to the maintenance of an ongoing watch over the activities of a health service, e.g. the provision of answers to questions such as 'what are we doing at the present moment?'; 'what does it cost in resources to do what for whom?'[42]

Surveillance and monitoring may be based on ongoing data collection (often as a byproduct of the provision of a service) or a trend study, i.e. comparison of repeated cross-sectional surveys. The term 'inbuilt surveillance' may be applied if a health service has set up routine procedures for this purpose, such as the ascertainment and recording of births, deaths and movements, the notification of infectious diseases, and the use of records designed for the easy retrieval of diagnostic information, with periodic analysis of these data.

Demographic surveillance[43] refers to ongoing measurement of the size of the population, its age and sex composition, and other demographic characteristics. Apart from other purposes, this provides the *denominator data* without which rates and other meaningful measures of group health cannot be calculated.

The term *exploratory study* is often applied to a descriptive survey designed to increase the investigator's familiarity with the problem he wishes to study. The aim may be to formulate a problem for more precise investigation, to develop hypotheses, to clarify concepts, or to make the investigator more familiar with the phenomenon he wishes to investigate or with the setting in which he will study it. It is not always necessary to use quantitative methods in a survey of this sort; at this stage it may be sufficient, for example, to build up a simple list of the foodstuffs or dishes eaten in a community (with no numerical information) as a basis for the design of a questionnaire for use in the study proper. An exploratory study of this sort is sometimes called a *pilot study*; however, this term is better confined to another connotation, namely a dress rehearsal of an investigation performed in order to identify defects in the study design. A descriptive survey in which a very large number of characteristics are studied, i.e. in which the net is thrown wide, performed in the hope that the results will provide hypotheses for subsequent testing, is sometimes unflatteringly referred to as a *fishing expedition*.

A *methodological study* is one performed with the purpose of collecting information on the feasibility or accuracy of a research method (see Chs 16 and 17). In community medicine the aim of such a study is usually the evaluation of an investigative procedure for use in community diagnosis.

A *morbidity survey* is a study, usually descriptive, of the occurrence and distribution of a disease, or diseases, in a population. It may be a *prevalence study*, concerned with all cases of the disease present in the population at a given point in time or during the period of the survey, or an *incidence study*, concerned only with new cases (patients, or episodes of illness) occurring or diagnosed during a given period. A *two-stage morbidity study* is one in which screening tests (see p. 197) are used to identify persons who may have the disease, and the presence of the disease is then determined by more exact tests.

The term *household survey* usually refers to a descriptive survey of illnesses and disability, performed by interviewing persons in their own homes, often by questioning a single informant about other members of his household.

KAP studies are studies of knowledge, attitudes and practices.

Outbreak investigations,[44] or epidemiological field investigations, are surveys that aim to determine the causes of an outbreak in order to control its spread. They may be descriptive, analytic or both.

Health practice research (health services research, operational research) is concerned with organizational problems—with the planning, management, logistics and delivery of health care services. It deals with manpower, organization, the utilization of facilities, the quality of health care, cost, the relationship between need and demand, and other topics. It makes use of systems analysis, computer simulation, and other sophisticated techniques of operations research.[45]

NOTES AND REFERENCES

1. *Quasi-experiments* are often used in evaluative studies. They compare groups, compare observations made at different times ('time-series design'), or both ('multiple-group time-series design').

Quasi-experimental designs are described by Trochim W M K 1997 (The knowledge base: an online research methods textbook. On the Internet: Trochim.human.cornell.edu/kb/kbhome.htm). Also, see Trochim W (ed) 1986 (Advances in quasi-experimental design and analysis. New Directions for Program Evaluation Series, Number 31. Jossey-Bass, San Francisco); Campbell D T, Stanley J C 1966 (Experimental and quasi-experimental designs for Research. Rand McNally, Chicago); Campbell D T 1969 (Factors relevant to the validity of experiments in social settings. In: Schulberg H C, Sheldon A, Baker F, eds. Program evaluation in the health fields. Behavioral Publications, New York); Cook T D, Campbell D T 1979 (Quasi-experimentation: design and analysis issues for field settings. Rand McNally, Chicago, Ill.); and Kleinbaum D G, Kupper L L, Morgenstern H 1982 (Epidemiologic research: principles and quantitative methods. Lifetime Learning Publications, Belmont, Cal., pp 44–47).

2. Snow J 1855 On the mode of communication of cholera. Churchill, London. Facsimile edition 1965: Hafner, New York.
3. The term 'observational study' does not imply that methods other than observation (questionnaires, documentary sources) are not used. Another term for non-experimental studies is 'naturalistic': Polgar S, Thomas S A 1988 (Introduction to research in the health sciences. Churchill Livingstone, Melbourne, p. 71).
4. How hypotheses about a possible cause are generated 'is little understood. They are products of their times, what is in the air, of what is known and being thought important, and of the prepared mind and individual imagination ... *Where* epidemiological hypotheses come from is also interesting: they emerge—from everywhere ... and from nowhere in particular' (Morris J N 1975 Uses of epidemiology, 3rd edn. Churchill Livingstone, Edinburgh, pp 233–249).
5. *Cohort analysis* refers to the investigation of data concerning people born in various specific time periods (e.g. 1940–1949) with a view to learning about the morbidity, mortality, etc. of each birth cohort or its various subgroups, and to comparing people born in different periods. This may reveal a cohort effect—i.e. there may be differences in morbidity, mortality, etc. when people of the same age in different birth cohorts are compared, as a result of differences in the experience of different cohorts. In a cross-sectional survey 50-year-olds may be shorter and have a lower mean IQ than 30-year-olds, not because they are older, but because they belong to different cohorts with different prior experiences.
6. Feinstein A R 1981 Clinical biostatistics: LVII. A glossary of neologisms in quantitative clinical science. Clinical Pharmacology and Therapeutics 30: 564.
7. Needleman H L, Gunnoe C, Leviton A, Reed R, Peresie H, Maher C, Barrett P 1979 Deficits in psychologic and classroom performance of children with elevated dentine lead levels. New England Journal of Medicine 300: 689.
8. Last J M, Abramson J H, Friedman G D, Porta M, Spasoff R A, Thuriaux M 1995 A dictionary of epidemiology, 3rd edn. Oxford University Press, New York. (A simpler definition: 'Epidemiology is what epidemiologists do'.)
9. For discussions and examples of community diagnosis in the context of community-oriented primary care, see Kark S L 1981 (The practice of community-oriented primary health care. Appleton-Century-Crofts, New York); Kark S L, Kark E, Abramson J H, Gofin J 1994 (Atencion primaria orientada a la comunidad. Doyma, Barcelona); and the references cited in note 1, page 400.

    Needs appraisal is reviewed by Mooney G, Leeder S R 1997 (Measuring health needs. In: Detels R, Holland W W, McEwen J, Omenn G S, eds. 1997 Oxford textbook of public health, 3rd edn, vol 3. The practice of public health. Oxford University Press, New York, pp 1553–1559); and Wright W (ed) 1998 (Health needs assessment in practice. BMJ Publishing Group, London; six excerpts appeared in successive issues of the British Medical Journal [vol 316] from April 25 1998). Needs appraisal in the context of community oriented primary care is discussed in Chapter 34.
10. Acheson R M, Hall D J 1976 In: Acheson R M, Hall D, Aird L (eds) Seminars in community medicine, vol 2: health information, planning, and monitoring. Oxford University Press, London, pp 145–164.
11. *Group-based (ecologic) studies* are discussed in depth by (among others) Susser M 1994a (The logic in ecological: II. The logic of analysis. American Journal of Public Health 84: 825) and 1994b (The logic in ecological: II. The logic of design. American Journal of Public Health 84: 830); and Morgenstern H 1998 (Ecologic studies. In: Rothman K J, Greenland S 1998 Modern epidemiology, 2nd edn. Lippincott-Raven, Philadelphia, pp 459–480).

Biases in ecologic studies are discussed by Diez-Roux 1998 (Bringing context back into epidemiology: variables and fallacies in multilevel analysis. American Journal of Public Health 88: 216); and Greenland S, Robins J 1994 (Invited commentary: Ecologic studies—biases, misconceptions, and counterexamples. American Journal of Epidemiology 139: 747) and in the commentaries that follow the latter paper. Cross-level bias may have various causes; for example, if risk to an individual is caused only by very high exposures to a causal factor (a *threshold effect*) the average exposure of a group of people may not reflect the average risk of its members.

12. Qiao Z-K, Halliday M L, Coates R A, Rankij J G 1988 (Relationship between liver cirrhosis death rate and nutritional factors in 38 countries. International Journal of Epidemiology 17: 414). The authors found that a higher average intake of protein, vitamins A and B2 and calcium (none of which was related to average alcohol consumption) was associated with a lower mortality from liver cirrhosis. They concluded that these relationships were not necessarily causal, but indicated a need for further studies.

13. After analyzing trends in New Zealand, for example, Jackson & Beaglehole (1987) concluded that changes in fat and tobacco consumption provided a biologically plausible explanation for at least part of the decline in coronary mortality between 1968 and 1980 (Jackson R, Beaglehole R 1987 Trends in dietary fat and cigarette smoking and the decline in coronary heart disease in New Zealand. International Journal of Epidemiology 16: 377).

14. Boyce W J, Vessey M P 1985 Rising incidence of fracture of the proximal femur. Lancet i: 150.
    A newer study showed an increase in hospital admissions for fractured femur between 1968 and 1986 both in Oxford and in England as a whole; the findings suggested a cohort effect (Evans J G, Seagroatt V, Goldacre M J 1997 Secular trends in proximal femoral fracture, Oxford record linkage study area and England 1968–86. Journal of Epidemiology and Community Health 51: 424).

15. Corrao G, Ferrari P, Zambon A, Torchio P, Arico S, Decarli A 1997 Trends of liver cirrhosis mortality in Europe, 1970–1989: age-period-cohort analysis and changing alcohol consumption. International Journal of Epidemiology 26: 100.

16. The correlation between infant mortality and the number of doctors may be a distortion produced by the effect of other (confounding) factors. The authors were not able to find an explanation: 'we must admit defeat and leave it to others to extricate doctors from their unhappy position' (Cochrane A L, St Leger A S, Moore F 1978 Health service 'input' and mortality 'output' in developed countries. Journal of Epidemiology and Community Health 32: 200; reprinted in 1997 in Journal of Epidemiology and Community Health 51: 344).
    McPherson K 1997 (Health services and mortality in developed countries: a comment. Journal of Epidemiology and Community Health 51: 349) points out the value of the study in 'raising questions whose importance might not otherwise have been appreciated'.

17. Doll R, Peto R 1981 The causes of cancer. Oxford University Press, Oxford, pp 1204–1205.

18. Breslow N E, Enstrom J E 1974 Geographic correlations between cancer mortality rates and alcohol-tobacco consumption in the United States. Journal of the National Cancer Institute 53: 531. Individual-based studies yield conflicting findings on this issue.

19. Schwartz S 1994 The fallacy of the ecological fallacy: the potential misuse of a concept and the consequences. American Journal of Public Health 84: 819. The converse fallacy is termed 'atomistic' by Diez-Roux A V 1998 (see note 11). It has also been called the 'individualistic' fallacy.

20. Koopman J S, Longini I M Jr 1994 The ecological effects of individual exposures and nonlinear disease dynamics in populations. American Journal of Public Health 84: 836.
21. Durkin M S, Kahn N, Davidson L L, Zaman S S, Stein Z A 1993 The effects of a natural disaster on child behavior: evidence for posttraumatic stress. American Journal of Public Health 83: 1549.
22. For example, Katsouyami K, Spix C, Schwartz J et al 1997 (Short term effects of ambient sulphur dioxide and particulate matter on mortality in 12 European cities: results from time series data from the APHEA project. British Medical Journal 314: 1658).
23. The importance of social and ecological processes is stressed by (among others) Susser M, Susser E 1996 (Choosing a future for epidemiology: II. From black box to Chinese boxes and eco-epidemiology. American Journal of Public Health 86: 674); Krieger N 1994 (Epidemiology and the web of causation: has anyone seen the spider? Social Science and Medicine 39: 887); and Diez-Roux A V 1998 (see note 11).
24. This edition adopts a simple and widely-used *classification of individual-based analytic studies*. In previous editions these studies were categorized as prospective (cohort), retrospective or cross-sectional on the basis of their *directionality* (starting with the postulated cause and going to the outcome, vice versa, or neither).

   To 'unconfound' confusion in the classification and nomenclature of these study designs, Kramer and Boivin suggested a three-way classification by (1) the *directionality* in which exposure and outcome are investigated (cohort, case-control, or cross-sectional), (2) *sample selection* criteria (by exposure, outcome, or other criteria), and (3) *timing* of the study proper with respect to the calendar times of exposure and outcome. In some studies, distinctions based on directionality are artificial or blurred: in studies of population samples, for example, the results can often be analyzed using either a forward- or backward-looking approach (Kramer M S, Boivin J-F 1987 Toward an 'unconfounded' classification of epidemiologic research design. Journal of Chronic Diseases 40: 683).

   Bailar et al define longitudinal studies as prospective or retrospective, depending on whether the selection of study subjects is based on the occurrence of putative causes or outcomes. They subclassify prospective and retrospective investigations: studies of deliberate intervention by the investigators, observational studies (including studies of deliberate interventions not under the control of the investigators), and pseudolongitudinal (pseudoretrospective and pseudoprospective) ones (Bailar J C III, Lewis T A, Lavori P W, Polansky M et al 1984 New England Journal of Medicine 311: 1482).

   Opponents of classifications based on directionality aver that these are 'founded on nonsense' (Miettinen O S 1988 Steps to deconfound the fundamentals of epidemiologic study design. Journal of Clinical Epidemiology 41: 709), since the reasoning is from cause to effect even when one compares cases and controls (see note 28).

   Debates on alternative classifications appeared in the Journal of Clinical Epidemiology 1988: 41, 705 and 1989: 42, 819. For defences of the utility of directionality as an axis of classification, see the following papers in that journal: Kramer M S, Boivin J-F 1988 The importance of directionality in epidemiologic research design 41: 717; Kramer M S, Boivin J-F 1989 Directionality, timing and sample selection in epidemiologic research design 42: 827; Abramson J H 1989 Classification of epidemiologic research 42: 819; and Feinstein A R 1989 Directionality and scientific inference 42: 829.

   Other terms used for case-control studies include retrospective, case-comparison, and case-referent studies (Last et al 1995; see note 8).

25. Kauhanen K, Kaplan G A, Goldberg D E, Salonen J T 1997 Beer binging and mortality: results from the Kuopio ischaemic heart disease risk factor study, a prospective population based study. British Medical Journal 315: 846. Beer binging was strongly associated with fatal myocardial infarction, as well as with fatal injuries and other external causes. The effects of differences in age, smoking, total alcohol consumption, and other factors that might affect mortality were taken into account.

26. A historical prospective study may be called a *nonconcurrent prospective study*, a *retrospective cohort study*, a *prospective study in retrospect*, or a *retrospective design with forward directionality* (all this in the interest of greater clarity!).

27. Rich-Edwards J W, Stampfer M J, Manson J E et al 1997 Birth weight and risk of cardiovascular disease in a cohort of women followed up since 1976. British Medical Journal 315: 837. For references to numerous other studies demonstrating that foetal malnutrition may affect health in adult life, see Scrimshaw N S 1997 (Editorial: The relation between fetal malnutrition and chronic disease in later life. British Medical Journal 315: 825).

28. An essential principle of case-control studies is that cases and controls should be drawn from the same population 'base': 'If a case-control study enrols cases and controls from the same underlying population at risk of the outcome and can measure exposure status validly in them, the results obtained will be identical to those from a properly performed cohort study' (Weiss N S 1997 Case-control studies. In: Detels R, Holland W W, McEwen J, Omenn G S, eds. 1997 Oxford textbook of public health, 3rd edn, vol 2. The methods of public health. Oxford University Press, New York). 'The case-control design can be considered a more efficient form of the follow-up study, in which the cases are those that would be included in a follow-up study and the controls provide a fast and inexpensive means of inferring the person-time experience according to exposure in the population that gave rise to the cases' (Rothman K J 1986 Modern epidemiology. Little, Brown, Boston, p. 64). (The 'person-time' concept is explained in note 3, p. 122.)

     Case-cohort and nested case-control methods are compared by Langholz B, Thomas D C 1990 (Nested case-control and case-cohort methods of sampling from a cohort: a critical comparison. American Journal of Epidemiology 131: 169).

29. Foxman B, Marsh J, Gillespie B, Rubin N, Koopman J S, Spear S 1997 Condom use and first-time urinary tract infection. Epidemiology 8: 637.

30. Barreto S M, Swerdlow A J, Smith P G, Higgins C D 1997 Risk of death from motor-vehicle injury in Brazilian steelworkers: a nested case-control study. International Journal of Epidemiology 26: 814.

31. Garland M, Morris J S, Colditz G A et al 1996 Toenail trace element levels and breast cancer: a prospective study. American Journal of Epidemiology 144: 653. Note the description of this case-control study as 'prospective'. The results provided no evidence of an important effect of arsenic, copper, chromium, iron or zinc on breast cancer risk.

32. Snoring was not found to be associated with atherosclerotic manifestations (Jennum P, Schultz-Larsen K, Christensen N J 1996 Snoring and atherosclerotic manifestations in a 70-year-old population. European Journal of Epidemiology 12: 285). Other good news for snorers is that snoring in pregnancy does not endanger the fetus, according to a cohort study (Loube D, Poceta J S, Morales M C, Peacock M D, Mitler M M 1996 Self-reported snoring in pregnancy: association with fetal outcome. Chest 109: 885).

33. Cohort, case-control and cross-sectional studies are discussed in all textbooks of epidemiology. Their uses and limitations are described in Detels R et al 1997 (see note 9), in the following chapters: Feinleib M, Breslow N E, Detels R: Cohort studies, pp 557–570; Weiss N S: Case-control studies, pp 547–555; Abramson J H: Cross-sectional studies, pp 517–535. The pros

and cons of numerous study designs, including hybrid ones, are discussed by Kleinbaum et al 1982 (see note 1 and Ch. 5).

For classic examples of cohort and case-control studies, see Buck C, Llopis A, Najera E, Terris M (eds) 1988 (The challenge of epidemiology. Pan American Health Organization, Washington D C, pp 584–725 and 458–583 respectively).

Case-control studies are discussed in detail in a symposium edited by Armenian H K 1994 (Applications of the case-control method. Epidemiologic Reviews 16: 1), which includes papers on applications in genetic epidemiology, demography, occupational health and other fields. See also: Schlesselman J J 1982 (Case-control studies: design, conduct, analysis. Oxford University Press, New York); Ibrahim M A (ed). 1979 (The case-control study: consensus and controversy. Journal of Chronic Diseases 32: 1); and Breslow N 1982 (Design and analysis of case-control studies. Annual Review of Public Health 3: 29).

34. Sackett D L 1979 Bias in analytic research. Journal of Chronic Diseases 32: 51.

35. An association between severe diarrhoea and cataract has been shown by case-control studies in India and England (Minassian D C, Mehra V, Jones B R 1984 Dehydrational crises from severe diarrhoea or heatstroke and risk of cataract. Lancet i: 751); and Harding J J, Harding J S, Egerton M 1989 (Risk factors for cataract in Oxfordshire: diabetes, peripheral neuropathy, myopia, glaucoma and diarrhoea. Acta Ophthalmologica 67: 510).

36. For classic examples of epidemiological experiments, see Buck C et al 1988 (see note 33) pp 726–806.

37. Susser M, Stein Z, Kline J 1978 Ethics in epidemiology. Annals of the American Academy of Political and Social Science 437: 128.

38. Kinsey V E, Hemphill F M 1955 Etiology of retrolental fibroplasia: preliminary report of a cooperative study of retrolental fibroplasia. American Journal of Ophthalmology 40: 166.

39. Texts on *evaluative studies* include: Fink A 1993 (Evaluating fundamentals: guiding health programs, research, and policy. Sage Publications, Beverly Hills); and St Leger A S, Schnieden H, Walsworth-Bell J P (eds) 1991 (Evaluating health services' effectiveness: a guide for health professionals, service managers, and policy makers. Open University).

40. Kane R L, Henson R, Deniston O L (1974) In: Kane R L (see note 8).

41. *Surveillance.* See: Berkelman R L, Stroup D F, Buehler J W 1997 (Public health surveillance. In: Detels R et al 1997 [see note 9] pp 735–750); Buehler J W 1998 (Surveillance. In: Rothman K J, Greenland S 1998 [see note 11] pp 435–457).

42. The meanings of the terms 'surveillance' and 'monitoring' are discussed by Acheson R M, Hall D J 1976 ([see note 10] p. 126). 'Monitoring' often denotes not only watching, but using the observations as a basis for continual modification of goals, plans or activities; Knox E G (ed) 1979 Epidemiology in health care planning. Oxford University Press, Oxford, pp 18–19, 127–129.

43. Accurate information on the size and composition of a population is seldom easy to obtain. See page 392.

44. *Outbreak investigations.* See: Gregg M B 1997 (The principles of an epidemic field investigation. In: Detels R et al 1997 [see note 9] pp 527–546); Dwyer D M, Strickler H, Goodman R A, Armenian H K 1994 (Use of case-control studies in outbreak investigations. Epidemiologic Reviews 16: 109).

For descriptions of classic studies of epidemics, see Buck C et al 1988 ([see note 33] pp 415–557).

45. *Health services research* methods are described by (among others) Crombie I K, Davies H T O 1996 (Research in health care: design, conduct and

interpretation of health services research. John Wiley, Chichester); and Shi L 1996 (Health services research methods [Delmar series in health services administration]. Delmar Publications).

For operations research, see: Cretin S 1997 (Operational and system studies. In: Detels R et al 1997 [see note 9] pp 873–888); Beech R 1995 (Using operational research modelling to improve the provision of health services: the case of DNA technology. International Journal of Epidemiology 24: S90); Kwak N K, Schmitz H H, Schniederjans M J 1984 (Operations research: applications in health care planning. University Press of America, Lanham, Md.).

For a treasure-house of papers on health services research (concepts, methods and implications for health policy), see White K L, Frenk J, Ordonez C, Paganini J M, Starfield B (eds) 1992 (Health services research: an anthology. Pan American Health Organization, Washington D C). A number of classic studies are collected in Buck C et al 1988 ([see note 33] pp 809–964).

3 Stages of an investigation

1. Preliminary steps; see Chapter 1
   a. Clarifying the purpose
   b. Reviewing the literature
   c. Ethical considerations
   d. Formulating the topic
2. Planning; see Chapters 2–23
3. Preparing for data collection; see Chapter 24
4. Collecting the data; see Chapter 25
5. Processing the data; see Chapter 26
6. Interpreting the results; see Chapters 27–29
7. Reporting the findings; see Chapter 30

The stages of an investigation may be listed in a logical sequence, in which each phase is dependent on the preceding one. After the investigator has clarified the purpose of the study and formulated its topic in general terms, a detailed plan can be prepared. Preparations for data collection can then be made, by testing the methods and making practical arrangements. The data are then collected and processed. The researcher can then sit down to make sense of the findings and decide on their theoretical and practical implications; and, finally, the world can be told.

In practice, this scheme is seldom followed rigidly, even by the most obsessional of researchers. There are two main reasons for this. First, it may be convenient for certain stages to overlap. For example, some of the preparations for the collection of data may be made before the study plan is complete, or it may be possible to collect and even analyze some types of information before other aspects have been fully planned. Secondly, and more important, the various phases may be influenced not only by the preceding phases, but also by subsequent ones. As one example, unforeseen snags may appear when the methods are tested, or even after data collection has commenced, sending the investigator 'back to the drawing board'. As another example, in the above scheme the interpretation of findings follows their processing, which seems logical; but a basic element of the scientific method is that inferences are drawn from facts, and these inferences are then tested by obtaining further facts; this means that usually, except in the simplest of investigations, the researcher interprets the data that have been processed, decides what further analyses are needed, interprets the new facts, and so on; processing and interpretation have a two-way influence on each other, and usually proceed hand in hand.

Although 'reviewing the literature' is shown as a preliminary step in the above scheme, directed reading usually continues throughout the study. The published experiences and thoughts of others may not only indicate the presence and nature of the research problem, but may be of great help in all aspects of planning and in the interpretation of the findings.

Needless to say, the value of any investigation depends on sound planning, which may necessitate a considerable amount of effort. The closer the attention to detail, the better the prospects of a fruitful study. The planning phase may take more of the investigator's time, or even of the total duration of the investigation, than any other phase of the study.

A dilemma frequently faced by investigators seeking research funds is that the success of the application may depend on the quality of the study plan, so that a considerable investment of time is required for planning, without any assurance that the study will actually be performed.

The first step in planning is to formulate the objectives of the investigation. The investigator already knows *why* the study is being undertaken, and has formulated the topic in general terms (see Ch. 1). The detailed study objectives must now be formulated —what knowledge is the study designed to yield? (Note that the term 'objective' is sometimes used to indicate what we have called the 'purpose' of the study on page 2; we are specifically excluding this connotation.) This decision determines the further planning of the investigation, and the methods of the study can be judged by their appropriateness to these study objectives.

> **The planning phase**
>
> 1. Formulation of study objectives; see Chapters 4 and 5
> 2. Planning of methods
>   a. The study population (whom?); see Chapters 6–9
>   Selection and definition
>   Sampling
>   Size
>   b. Variables (what to measure?); see Chapters 10–14
>   Selection
>   Definition
>   Scales of measurement
>   c. Methods of collecting data; see Chapters 15–21
>   d. Methods of recording and processing; see Chapters 22 and 23

The second step is to plan the methods. Consideration must be given to:

1. *The study population* (see Chs 6–9): Whom is it proposed to study? Will a sample or samples be used? How will sampling be done? What will be the sample size?
2. *The variables to be studied* (Chs 10–14): What characteristics will be measured? How will the variables be defined? What scales of measurement will be used?
3. *Methods of data collection* (Chs 15–21): Will data be collected by direct observation, from documentary sources, or by interviews or self-administered questionnaires? What are the detailed procedures and questions to be used?
4. *Methods of recording and processing* (Chs 22–23): How will the data be recorded? What data-processing techniques will be used? What is the analysis plan?

The various elements of planning are interdependent, and should be regarded as different aspects on which attention must be focused, rather than as discrete entities. A decision on the characteristics to be measured, for example, may depend not only on the study objectives, but on the nature of the study population and on the practicability of various methods of data collection; or a detailed consideration of the methods required to satisfy the study objectives may lead to a reformulation of the objectives.

Some investigators see their main planning task as the design of a 'form'—a schedule on which findings will be recorded, or a questionnaire—and make this their first (and sometimes only) planning activity. This approach cannot be recommended.

It is usually helpful to commit the study plan to writing, whether briefly or in detail, since human memory is fallible. The study objectives and an outline of the methods will in any case require to be described in the report of the study. If an application is made for research funds the objectives and methods may have to be stated in a detailed study protocol.

It may not be frivolous to suggest that, as the plan of the study begins to take form and a clearer picture emerges of the effort and cost involved, the investigator should ask himself whether the investigation is still seen as worthwhile—is its performance warranted by the importance of the problem which was its starting-point? It is better to scrap a study at the outset than to decide afterwards that it was not worth doing.

MUST A STUDY BE PERFECT?

In the pages which follow, a great deal of attention will be paid to various aspects of sound planning—the careful choice of definitions, the use of standardized and accurate methods of collecting information, etc. The better the techniques of investigation, the greater are the prospects of producing useful findings, and the more certain the researcher can be that his findings will be reproducible. However, there are very few perfect studies. Almost invariably, practical difficulties, oversights and accidents produce methodological imperfections. What is important is that the investigator should be aware of these imperfections, examine their impact, and take them into account in interpreting his findings; if this is done, the study will still be a sound and possibly a useful one. While striving for perfection, the investigator should from the outset realize that his reach will almost certainly be shorter than his grasp, and be prepared to make compromises with reality. In fact, an undue insistence on impeccable techniques at all costs may well ruin a study. There is much truth in the statement that 'in science as in love a concentration on technique is quite likely to lead to impotence'.[1]

REFERENCE

1. Berger P L 1969 Invitation to sociology: a humanistic perspective. Penguin Books, Harmondsworth, p. 24.

4 Formulating the objectives

Having decided *what* to study and *why* (i.e. the study's topic and purpose), the investigator can now formulate the study objectives—what knowledge should the study yield—*what questions* should it answer? Serendipity apart—and accidental discoveries are more common than some researchers may care to admit[1]—one is likely to learn only what one sets out to learn.

The explicit formulation of study objectives is an essential step in the planning of a study. It may be an exaggeration to say that 'a question well-stated is a question half-answered',[2] but a question that is poorly stated or unstated is unlikely to be answered at all. The specification of objectives determines the whole subsequent planning of the study. 'If you don't know where you're going, it is difficult to select a suitable means for getting there.'[3] In fact, 'if you're not sure where you're going, you're liable to end up someplace else'.[3]

OBJECTIVES OF DESCRIPTIVE SURVEYS

The objectives of a descriptive survey of a specific group or population—a survey carried out with a diagnostic purpose—are usually easy to formulate. The investigator needs only to state the characteristics he wants to measure. These may be diseases, deaths, or other 'disagreeable Ds' (disabilities, discomforts, dissatisfactions, deviations from statistical or social norms); they may be positive aspects of health (e.g. physical fitness, life expectancy, quality of life); or they may be somatic or psychological character-

43

istics (body weight, biological markers,[4] behaviour patterns, left-handedness[5] etc.) that are not necessarily negative or positive, but are seen as elements of health status or expressions of health. There are numerous health indicators and health indices, serving different ends and appropriate in different circumstances.[6] The investigator may also want to study other characteristics of the group (demographic, biological, behavioural, social or cultural), or environmental features. He may also be interested in the health services provided for the population, or in their use.

Such objectives are easily stated, e.g. 'to determine the infant mortality rate in population Y during period Z', 'to measure the incidence rate of rabies', 'the prevalence rate of scabies', 'the case fatality rate of tabes', 'the distribution of head circumference in babies', etc.

Objectives may be stated in general terms, e.g. 'to measure the prevalence of disability (in population Y at time Z)', or may be phrased more specifically, e.g. in terms of mobility, capacity to work, ability to perform activities of daily living, or other selected functions. The more specifically the objectives are stated, the more helpful they will be in the further planning of the study. A formulation that is too general, e.g. 'to study the health status of ...' will not be helpful at all. If general objectives are stated, more specific ones should be listed as well. Careful thinking about specific objectives may help to ensure that the study meets its purposes.

Even in a simple descriptive survey there is usually interest in obtaining separate information for different groups—for specific age groups, for the two sexes, for ethnic groups or parts of a city, etc. The objective might be stated as 'to measure X in population Y by age, sex (etc.)'. In a survey of the 'community diagnosis' type, findings may provide pointers to the different health needs of different parts of the population. If alcoholics are concentrated in one neighbourhood, that neighbourhood may need a special programme.

Not uncommonly, a descriptive survey centres not on the characteristic (say, disease D) in which interest actually lies, but on something that is known to be associated with this characteristic. The main circumstances in which the study may focus on an associated characteristic or characteristics (C) are as follows:

1. If it is easy to obtain information about C and difficult to obtain information about D, C may be used as a *proxy measure* of D. As an example, an investigator may be interested in the occurrence

of prostatic hypertrophy in a community; if examinations to establish the diagnosis are not feasible, the proxy may be the prevalence of a specific symptom pattern, believed to be associated with the disease. It may be possible to estimate the prevalence rate of D from the prevalence rate of C.[7] If C is a poor proxy measure many individuals will be misclassified, and problems of interpretation may arise (see p. 188).

2. The presence of C may be of use as a *screening test*—that is, to discriminate between people who are likely and those who are unlikely to have D. Once people who have C (say a high casual blood pressure measurement) have been identified, they can be invited to be examined more fully in order to determine whether D (hypertensive disease) is present. To warrant such use of the association, C must be easier to study than D; C and D must be present at the same time; and certain other conditions (see p. 199) must be met. The study objective might be stated as 'to measure the prevalence rate of C' or 'to identify people with positive screening tests for D'.

3. If C precedes D in time, it may be of use as a *risk marker*—that is, to distinguish between people who are likely and those who are unlikely to develop D in the future. The presence of C identifies vulnerable individuals or groups (*at risk* or *high risk* groups) who are especially likely to develop the disorder, and who hence have a special need for preventive care. C *points to* the increased risk, it does not necessarily *cause* it. It may be a cause, or it may be a precursor or early manifestation of the disorder, or it may itself be an effect or correlate of the factor that increases the risk. Bald men have an increased risk of dying of coronary heart disease,[8] and elderly men with impaired memories have an increased risk of dying in the next five years.[9] These are certainly not causal relationships—any special preventive care given to these high-risk men would not include prescribing a toupee or a course of memory training. In one study, elderly subjects who did not respond to a postal questionnaire had a more than two-fold risk of dying in the next year—not, presumably, cause and effect.[10] On the other hand, a high diastolic blood pressure, another risk marker for mortality in elderly men,[9] is presumably also a risk *maker*, i.e. one reason for the high risk. Whether a risk marker affects risk is often unclear.[11] A descriptive study might aim to 'determine the prevalence of a (specified) risk marker' or 'to identify people who are at special risk of a (specified) disorder'.

Health risk appraisal[12] is a particular instance of the use of risk markers.

4. C may also be of interest because it is a *cause* of D—that is, its presence or degree influences the risk of developing D. If C is amenable to change, and if a change in C will reduce the risk of D, there may be a case for intervention directed at C. In such instances C is possibly best termed a *modifiable risk factor* (the adjective 'modifiable' refers both to the factor and to the risk). The unqualified term '*risk factor*' is generally used, but unfortunately this has more than one meaning; it is also often used to denote *any* cause of a disorder (modifiable or not), and sometimes to denote a risk marker. A causal factor may or may not be of use as a risk marker; it may or may not be possible to modify it, and modifying it may or may not modify the risk—often, in the words of the American humorist Will Rogers, 'We know lots of things we used to dident know but we don't know any way to prevent em happening'.[13] The general objective of a descriptive study of modifiable risk factors might be formulated as 'to determine the prevalence of' or 'to identify people who have' specified factors.

OBJECTIVES OF ANALYTIC STUDIES

Experiments and analytic surveys seek information about associations between variables—that is, about whether and how different characteristics 'hang together'. The aim may be to explain the health status of a specific group or population, to seek new knowledge about factors affecting health and disease, or to test the value of tools used in health care, e.g. screening or diagnostic tests or risk markers, etc.

Analytic surveys commonly have a descriptive as well as an analytic element. A survey of elderly people with foot problems, for example, aimed to discover the extent to which they used chiropody services—useful descriptive information in its own right —and also whether their use was related to age, sex, living alone, the number and type of foot problems, etc.[14]

Possible formulations of the study objective, when an association is to be investigated, include 'To examine the association between infant mortality rates and region', 'To determine whether there is a difference between the rates in regions A and B', and 'To test the hypothesis that the rates in regions A and B differ'. *Hypotheses* are suppositions that are tested by collecting facts that lead to their acceptance or rejection. They are not assumptions that are to be taken for granted, neither are they beliefs that the investigator sets out to prove. They are 'refutable predictions' (T H Huxley wrote of 'the great tragedy of Science—the slaying of a beautiful hypothesis by an ugly fact').

A hypothesis may be stated as a positive declaration (sometimes called the *research hypothesis, study hypothesis*, or *substantive hypothesis*), e.g. 'The infant mortality rates in regions A and B are different' or 'The rate is higher in region A than in region B', or as a negative declaration (*null hypothesis*), e.g. 'There is no difference between the rates' or 'The rate is not higher in region A than in region B'. Statistical testing of an association requires the formulation of a null hypothesis, which is tested against a specific alternative,[15] this alternative ('that there is a difference between the two regions', or 'that the rate is higher in region A') is the 'research hypothesis'. If statistical testing is intended it is advisable to make the hypotheses as specific as possible at this stage, and not to leave them implicit (as in 'to study the association between mortality and region').

In a case-control study designed to examine a possible causal relationship between smoking and a disease, typical specific hypotheses might be that the proportion of smokers is higher among cases than among controls, that the proportion of heavy smokers is higher among cases than among controls, that the average age at starting smoking is earlier among cases than among controls, etc. In a cohort study set up for the same purpose the hypotheses would relate to the relative incidence of the disease among persons with different smoking habits. The value of epidemiological hypotheses is enhanced if they deal not only with the combined occurrence of the postulated cause and effect (i.e. when one is present, does the other tend to be present?), but also with the quantitative *dose–response* relationship between cause and effect (e.g. when there is more intensive exposure to the cause, is the disease more frequent or more severe?) or with the *time–response* relationship (the relationship to the time interval since exposure).

As will be seen later (in Ch. 28), if we want to know *why* there is an association between two variables, we will usually need analyses that take account of the way the association is influenced by other characteristics. The selection of these other variables will be discussed on pages 116–119. If the investigator wishes he may make mention of them when formulating the study objectives, e.g.

by saying that the association will be tested 'holding sex and eth-nic group constant' or 'controlling for' these variables, or that the hypothesis will be tested separately in each sex and ethnic group, or by listing the 'modifying' and 'confounding' variables that he will take into account (these terms will become clearer later).

Remember there is still lots of time for these decisions; the planning of the study is still in its early stages, and study objectives can be rethought and reformulated as often as we wish.

SPELLING OUT THE OBJECTIVES

It is usually helpful to formulate the study objectives explicitly in writing, as a guide to the planning of appropriate study methods. They may or may not be published in the ultimate study report.

For convenience the objectives are often first stated in fairly general terms, followed by a more detailed statement of the relevant specific objectives. In a study whose general objective is to determine the incidence of cancer by occupation in New Zealand in 1972–1984,[16] a specific objective might be 'to determine the incidence rates of cancer (separate and combined sites) in occupational categories and selected specific occupations, controlling for age and socioeconomic status'. In a study with a general objective of examining the association between the mental health status of mothers and the nutritional status of their children,[17] specific objectives might be 'to compare the mental health status of mothers of malnourished children and mothers of well-nourished children, controlling for mother's age, education and number of children, income, and the child's birthweight' and 'to test the hypothesis that educational status affects the association between mother's mental health and child's nutritional status'.

Requirements of study objectives

1. They must meet the purposes of the study
2. They should be formulated clearly
3. They should be expressed in measurable terms

The stated objectives should satisfy three requirements. First, they must meet the requirements of the study. This is usually easily achieved in a descriptive survey, but in planning an analytic survey or experiment there may be considerable difficulty in the formulation of a hypothesis; this is where the creative researcher comes into his own. Secondly, the objectives should be phrased clearly—unambiguously and very specifically—leaving no doubt as to precisely what has to be measured. Thirdly, they should be phrased in measurable terms. That is, the objectives should be realistic (answerable questions, testable hypotheses) and formulated in operational terms, which can be applied in practice. 'Any fool can ask a question; the trick is to ask one that can be answered.'[18]

A few imaginary and actual examples follow.

1. 'To improve the community's health' and 'To plan a programme for improving the community's health' are not appropriate study objectives for a community health survey. They explain *why* the study is being conducted (the *purpose* of the study), but do not stipulate what knowledge the study is designed to yield. 'To determine the community's health needs' might be an appropriate general objective, but a much more detailed formulation is required. Does the researcher propose, for example, to determine the community's perceived needs, or to examine the availability or use of health services, or to determine the incidence of specified disorders or the prevalence of specified disorders or risk factors?

2. A survey of diabetes was conducted in an English community.[19] Its first objective was '1. To establish exactly the number of diabetics'. This is a clear statement; but the formulation is incomplete, since the investigators also measured the prevalence *rate* of diabetes and established the age and sex distribution of cases. The second objective was '2. To discover the undiagnosed cases of diabetes'. This is not a complete statement, as the investigators also wanted to answer questions about the hitherto unknown cases. It should go on: 'and to compare their age and sex distribution with that of known cases'. The next objective was '3. To investigate the possible hereditary factors'. This is far too non-specific to be helpful as a blueprint in planning the study. Did the investigators intend to examine familial clustering among the people they examined? Did they want to see if prevalence was higher among the offspring of consanguineous marriages? Did they want to look for an association with the occurrence of diabetes-related genes? Or (as was actually the case) did they want to compare the frequency of positive family histories of diabetes among known diabetics, newly discovered diabetics, and non-diabetics, controlling for age and sex? One

last example from this study: '6. To repeat the whole survey at a future date'. This is hardly a study objective.

3. A report on a national study of cerebral palsy in adolescence and adulthood[20] states: 'The primary objectives of the study were: 1. To learn about the extent and nature [of the problem] and the specific needs of cerebral palsied youngsters and adults through a sociomedical study. 2. To collect epidemiological data on the cerebral palsied'. These formulations may be useful as starting points in planning a study, or as summary statements in a report, but would not be very useful as blueprints. Much further detail is needed for this purpose. (The study itself is a good one, and it is clear that the investigators actually did have specific and well thought out objectives.) Another stated objective, 'To evoke the interest of local communities and public agencies in the problems and needs of the cerebral palsied', is a laudable *purpose* for a study, but not what we have called a study objective. It might be stated as an objective of an action programme.

4. The objective of a study was stated to be 'to study the effects of vaccination against measles'. This formulation is completely nonspecific, and could have given the investigator little help in the planning of his study. Was he interested in the development of serological changes, or in differences in antibody titre between groups of vaccinated and non-vaccinated children, or in differences in the subsequent incidence of measles? The study turned out to be a descriptive survey of the incidence of fever, pain at the injection site, and other manifestations immediately after vaccination.

5. A hypothesis including the word 'cause', such as one that the habitual drinking of coffee is a cause of cancer of the bladder, must be made more specific before it can be tested. Is it proposed to determine whether the incidence rate of the disease in different countries or at different times is correlated with the average consumption of coffee per head (group-based analytic surveys), or to determine whether patients drink more coffee than controls (a cross-sectional or retrospective survey), or to determine whether the incidence of new cases is higher among persons who drink much coffee than among those who take less coffee, and lowest among those who drink no coffee at all (a prospective survey or a rather unlikely experiment)? 'Controlling for age, sex, smoking habits (etc.)' would probably be specified in the hypothesis.

6. The hypothesis that the occurrence of a disease 'is associated with diet' is not sufficiently specific. The investigator may aim to compare the dietary histories of cases and controls, or compare incidence rates in vegetarians and others, or seek correlations between national disease rates and food consumption data. Neither is it stated in operational terms. In what aspect of diet is the investigator interested: in the average daily intake of calories, proteins, fats and other specific nutrients, or in the average amounts consumed of milk, meat, and other specific foodstuffs, or in the number of days a week that meat, fish, etc. are usually eaten, or in the average number of meals taken per day? It may be felt that such decisions can be postponed until later in the planning phase. There is no great harm in this, but it is arguable that since these decisions may be very close to the nub of the research problem, they should be made at an early stage of planning. They are of a different order of importance from decisions on various methods of measurement, such as the choice of a technique for measuring the daily caloric intake (questioning, self-maintained dietary records, weighing of dishes and leftovers, etc.). Similar considerations arise when other vague terms are used, such as 'nutritional status', 'disability', 'emotional health', or 'stress'.

NOTES AND REFERENCES

1. 'One sometimes finds what one is not looking for', said Sir Alexander Fleming, the serendipitous discoverer of penicillin (see Henderson J W 1997 The yellow brick road to penicillin: a story of serendipity. Mayo Clinic Proceedings 72: 683). Other discoveries based on unplanned 'chance' observations (immunization with attenuated pathogens, anaphylaxis, the connection between the pancreas and diabetes, etc.) are listed by Comroe J H Jr 1997 (Roast pig and scientific discovery: parts I and II. American Review of Respiratory Disease 115: 853 and 1035) and Beveridge W I B 1957 (The art of scientific investigation, 3rd edn. Vintage Books, New York). The latter book, which stresses that 'the most important instrument in research must always be the mind of man', concentrates on the 'mental skills' of scientific investigation, such as the ability to recognize the importance of a chance or unexpected observation, to interpret the clue and develop a hypothesis, and to follow up the initial finding in a systematic way.
2. Isaac S, Michael W B 1977 Handbook in research and evaluation for education and the behavioural sciences. EdITS, San Diego, p. 2.
3. Mager R F 1975 Preparing instructional objectives. Fearon, Belmont, California.
4. *Biological markers*, or *biomarkers*, are biochemical, molecular, genetic, immunological or other indicators (often quantitative) of past exposure, biological changes, disease processes, or predisposition to disease. Examples: lead content of blood, creatinine clearance, human leucocyte antigens, alpha-fetoprotein, antibody titres. Their uses in epidemiological research are discussed by Schulte P A 1987 (Methodologic issues in the use of biologic

markers in epidemiologic research. American Journal of Epidemiology 126: 1006).

See: Suk W A, Collman G, Damstra T 1996 (Human biomonitoring: research goals and needs. Environmental Health Perspectives 104 [suppl 3]: 479); Vine M F 1996 (Biologic markers of exposure: current status and future research needs. Toxicology and Industrial Health 12: 189); Hemminki K, Kumar R, Bykov V J, Louhelainen J, Vodicka P 1996 (Future research directions in the use of biomarkers. Environmental Health Perspectives 104 [suppl 3]: 459).

5. Left-handedness is mentioned in the text as a reminder of the wide gamut of questions that surveys may ask. Not that left-handedness is necessarily trivial—it may increase the risk of hand injuries, fractures, injuries in general, and kyphosis (Taras J S, Behrman M J, Degnan G G 1995 Left-hand dominance and hand trauma. Journal of Hand Surgery 20: 1043; Stellman S D, Wynder E L, DeRose D J, Muscat J E 1997 The epidemiology of left-handedness in a hospital population. Annals of Epidemiology 7: 167; Wright P, Williams J, Currie C, Beattie T 1996 Left-handedness increases injury risk in adolescent girls. Perceptual and Motor Skills 82: 855; Nissinen M, Heliovaara M, Seitsamo J, Poussa M 1995 Left handedness and risk of thoracic hyperkyphosis in prepubertal schoolchildren. International Journal of Epidemiology 24: 1178).

6. *Health indicators* for use in health surveys, population monitoring, health policy evaluations and other contexts are reviewed by Ware J E Jr 1995 (The status of health assessment 1994. Annual Review of Public Health 16: 327). For applications in clinical practice, see a symposium (Advances in health status assessment: proceedings of a conference) in Medical Care 1992 (May: suppl): MS1.

Indicators that are useful for comparing populations or individuals are not always suitable for detecting changes; see *'responsiveness'*, page 196.

'Health index' may be a synonym for 'health indicator', or may refer to a numerical index based on two or more indicators, such as the *Health Problem Index* ('Q value') devised by the Division of Indian Health in the United States. This is based mainly on the mortality rate, the average age at death, and the numbers of outpatient visits and hospital days per head; see Haynes M A 1972 (In: Reinke W A, ed. Health planning: qualitative aspects and quantitative techniques. Johns Hopkins University, Baltimore, Md., p. 158).

7. For methods of estimating the confidence limits of the prevalence of a disease in a population from the prevalence of a proxy attribute in the population or a sample, see Peritz E 1971 Estimating the ratio of two marginal probabilities in a contingency table. Biometrics 27: 223 (correction note: 27: 1104) and Rogan W J, Gladen B 1978 Estimating prevalence from the results of a screening test. American Journal of Epidemiology 107: 71.

8. Ford E S, Freedman D S, Byers T 1996 Baldness and ischemic heart disease in a national sample of men. American Journal of Epidemiology 143: 651.

9. Abramson J H, Gofin R, Peritz E 1982 Risk markers for mortality among elderly men: a community study in Jerusalem. Journal of Chronic Diseases 35: 565.

A cohort study in Holland showed a similar association (Gussekloo J, Westendorp R G J, Remarque E J, Lagaay A M, Heeren T J, Knook D L 1997 Impact of mild cognitive impairment on survival in very elderly people: cohort study. British Medical Journal 315: 1053).

10. Hebert R, Bravo G, Korner-Bitensky N, Voyer L 1996 Refusal and information bias associated with postal questionnaires and face-to-face interviews in very elderly subjects. Journal of Clinical Epidemiology 49: 373.

11. Cohort studies of elderly men have found that little walking, despite ability to walk, was predictive of more future physical disability and earlier death. Do

these findings express a protective effect, as the researchers suggest, or is 'little walking' only a risk marker? (Clark D O 1996 The effect of walking on lower body disability among older Blacks and Whites. American Journal of Public Health 86: 57; Hakim A A, Petrovitch H, Burchfiel C M et al 1998 Effects of walking on mortality among nonsmoking retired men. New England Journal of Medicine 338: 94).

12. *Health risk appraisal* is the use of a battery of information on health-related behaviour, exposure to environmental hazards and personal characteristics in order to estimate an individual's chances of acquiring specific diseases, of dying, etc. It has been mainly used to enable individuals to identify hazards and to motivate them to lessen them. The technique offers promise as a tool for use in community medicine, both for identifying high-risk individuals and as a way of gauging a group or population's risk of preventable diseases and other outcomes. Many programmes over-reach existing scientific knowledge in order to accomplish the former aim. An important criticism is that the message generated for the client is based on the sometimes questionable assumption that changes made by the individual will necessarily change the risk—i.e. that risk markers are modifiable risk factors. Health risk appraisal may be offered as an incentive to make participation in a health survey attractive. *Health hazard appraisal* usually refers to environmental exposures.

13. Cohen J M, Cohen M J 1976 The Penguin dictionary of modern quotations. Penguin Books, Harmondsworth, p. 194.

14. Harvey I, Frankel S, Marks R, Shalom D, Morgan M 1997 Foot morbidity and exposure to chiropody: population based study. British Medical Journal 315: 1054.

15. See note 9, page 322.

16. Firth H M, Cooke K R, Herbison G P 1996 Male cancer incidence by occupation: New Zealand, 1972–1984. International Journal of Epidemiology 25: 14.

17. De Miranda C T, Turecki G, Mari J D J et al 1996 Mental health of the mothers of malnourished children. International Journal of Epidemiology 25: 128.

18. Lemkau P V, Pasamanick B 1957 Problems in evaluation of mental health programs. American Journal of Orthopsychiatry 27: 55.

19. Walker J B, Kerridge D 1961 Diabetes in an English community: a study of its incidence and natural history. Leicester University Press, Leicester.

20. Margulec I (ed) 1966 Cerebral palsy in adolescence and adulthood: a rehabilitation study. Jerusalem Academic Press, Tel Aviv, p. 8.

5 The objectives of evaluative studies

When we evaluate a treatment or other health care procedure we are making a value judgement. To reduce the subjective element in this judgement we should base the appraisal on facts, using explicit criteria. An evaluative study sets out to collect these facts, and the facts to be collected should be specified in the study objectives.

Evaluative studies may be descriptive, analytic, or both, and their objectives should be formulated accordingly, along the lines suggested in Chapter 4. This chapter will review the basic questions commonly asked in evaluative studies of all kinds, and will then discuss their application to programme reviews. Consideration will be given in later chapters to their application to other evaluative studies—clinical and programme trials (Chs 32 and 33) and evaluations of screening and diagnostic tests (p. 197) and risk markers (p. 199).

The need for objective data should be reflected in the wording of the specific study objectives. The challenge faced by the evaluator is to translate a 'How satisfactory is ...?' question into a set of study objectives that are free of terms requiring value judgements. In an evaluation of routine medical examinations of schoolchildren, for example, the specific objectives might be to determine the prevalence of previously undiagnosed chronic disorders or the number of children treated, or successfully treated, as a consequence of the routine examinations. Words like 'good', 'bad', 'should' and 'ought' have no place here.

The basic questions that are commonly asked in evaluative studies are listed below. These questions specify the dimensions of care that are commonly appraised, whether as separate issues or as components of global appraisals. They provide a framework for the formulation of specific study objectives. In these questions 'care' refers to whatever procedure is being evaluated—care directed at individuals or populations, screening and other diagnostic activities, or environmental health programmes.

We will discuss each of the basic questions separately, and consider its role as a basis for the formulation of clear-cut study objectives.

The basic questions of evaluative studies

1. Requisiteness
   To what extent is care needed?
2. Quality
   a. How satisfactory is the *outcome*?
      Attainment of desirable effects (*effectiveness*)?
      Absence of undesirable effects (*harmlessness*)?
   b. How satisfactory is the *process*?
      Performance of activities by the providers of care?
      Compliance and the *utilization of services* by the recipients of care?
   c. How satisfactory are the *facilities* and *settings*?
3. Efficiency
   How efficiently are resources used?
4. Satisfaction
   How satisfied are the people concerned?
5. Differential value
   How do the above features differ in different categories or groups or in different circumstances?

REQUISITENESS

The first question is the *requisiteness* ('appropriateness', 'relevance') of care. To what extent is care *needed*?[1] It can hardly be of value if there is no need for it. This question may be asked in reviews of well established programmes and services, which may have outlived their need. It is not asked in trials—the need for care is a precondition for a trial rather than a question the trial sets out to answer.

The appraisal by health professionals of the need for care generally requires, inter alia, facts about the nature, extent and severity of the problem or problems that the programme aims to solve, and of other problems that compete for the available resources, as well as facts about the availability of resources. Account may also be taken of *perceived need* (as stated by patients or public) and *expressed demand* (e.g. requests for care, as reflected by the use of services, waiting-lists for treatment, etc.). When formulating study objectives, thought should be given to the specific facts required for these purposes.[1]

QUALITY

The quality of health care may be judged from information about effects (*outcome evaluation*), about the performance of activities (*process evaluation*), or about facilities and settings (*structure evaluation*). In each instance, the question asked is 'How satisfactory?'), and the evaluative study aims to yield the objective facts required to answer this question.

Numerous schemes of evaluation have been proposed, and it may not greatly matter which is used. Beware of schemes that focus only on an appraisal of the structural and organizational context within which health care is provided, while neglecting the actual care given and its effects. Appraisals of such attributes as the availability, accessibility, comprehensiveness and co-ordination of services, continuity of care, and accountability—if based on hard facts rather than impressions—may indicate whether the setting is conducive to a satisfactory quality of care. But (unless inadequacies are striking) firm conclusions about the quality of care generally require evaluation of the process and outcome of care as well.

Outcome

Both desirable and undesirable effects should always be measured, since a full appraisal of *outcome* depends on the balance between these, a judgement that may not be easy since it requires decisions on the relative weight to be given to qualitatively different outcomes (effects on mortality, morbidity, working capacity, the quality of life, etc.). The popular term *risk–benefit ratio*[2] should be avoided, unless desirable and undesirable effects can be measured on the same scale, as in a comparison of the numbers of deaths that might be caused and prevented by a new treatment (a ratio is one number divided by another).

Effectiveness refers to the degree of achievement of desirable effects. These may be expressed at the individual level (recovery from disease, restoration of function, etc.) or at the group or community level (changes in mortality and morbidity rates, changes in a community's knowledge or practices, environmental changes, etc.).

Effectiveness is sometimes distinguished from *efficacy*. While definitions vary, 'efficacy' may be used to refer to the benefits observed when a procedure is applied as it 'should' be, and with full compliance by all concerned, i.e. 'under ideal conditions'. The term is usually reserved for benefits at the individual level, as measured by a clinical trial. 'Effectiveness' then refers to the benefits observed at the population level, or among people to whom the procedure or service is offered. 'Efficacy' answers the question, '*can* the procedure or service work?' whereas 'effectiveness' answers the question, '*does* it work?'[3] A programme for the control of hypertension in a community would use drugs known to be efficacious; the community programme might or might not be effective. In Gambia, trials of insecticide-treated bednets (to reduce malaria) showed that under ideal conditions these could prevent 63% of child mortality, but in a practical community programme context the reduction was only 25%.[3]

Clear-cut explicit criteria of effectiveness (or efficacy) are readily available if the activities under evaluation have well defined predetermined goals, i.e. situations or conditions whose attainment was set up as an aim. (We will refer to these as 'goals' rather than 'objectives', so as not to confuse them with study objectives; some authors distinguish between the 'goals' and 'objectives' of health care programmes.[4]) The extent of accomplishment of these aims is a realistic measure of effectiveness. With this method of evaluation in mind, effectiveness is sometimes defined as the extent to which pre-established goals are attained as a result of the activity.

This 'goal attainment' approach (which will be further discussed on p. 374) can be used only if predetermined goals are known or can be inferred, and if it is possible to measure their attainment. For the latter purpose, they must be expressed in clear and specific terms. It is not easy to appraise the effectiveness of an antenatal programme if its goal is expressed in such general terms as 'to promote the health of the mother and baby'. If the goals are 'to reduce the stillbirth rate', 'to reduce the number of babies born with Down's syndrome', etc., evaluation is easier. It is especially easy if precise quantitative targets are stated, e.g. 'to reduce the stillbirth rate to 15 per 1000 births'.

If the goal attainment model cannot be used, the investigator will need to formulate his own criteria, or to use standards[5] or criteria formulated by experts. The need for such (additional) criteria should be considered even when the goal attainment model is used, so as to avoid the danger of 'tunnel vision'—an investigator who concentrates only on the present goals may not see beneficial outcomes that were not specified as goals, and may be blind to adverse effects.

When possible, *end results*—i.e. effects on health status—should be used as criteria of effectiveness, even if the production of these effects is not a direct aim of the procedure or programme under evaluation. A highly 'successful' case-finding programme may merit a negative evaluation if the detection of new cases resulted in no improvement in health status. The ultimate criterion of effectiveness is the extent to which the underlying problem is alleviated or prevented. This is sometimes referred to as the *adequacy* of the intervention. A programme that deals with only a small part of a large problem may be regarded as inadequate, however effectively it does what it *does* do.

Adverse effects[6] may be missed unless they are sought. These include not only side-effects of medication ('The children crippled by thalidomide are on their slow procession through the special schools for the handicapped, following those made deaf by streptomycin who succeeded the infants blinded by oxygen'[7]), but overdependence, anxiety, and other less obvious effects. An editorial entitled 'The menace of mass screening' in a public health journal points to the morbidity caused among children with innocent heart murmurs who falsely perceive themselves as having heart disease, and the disability caused to children as a result of being identified as carriers of the sickle-cell trait.[8] Being labelled as hypertensive may produce symptoms of depression,[9] and being told that one is 'at-risk' (especially with the current expansion of genetic testing) may have far-reaching consequences.[10]

Process

An appraisal of the *performance of activities* requires information on the services provided—what kinds, and how much? If there is a programme plan that lays down what activities *should* be performed, these requirements provide ready-made yardsticks. If the stated intention was to make contact with every known blind person at least once a year, or to examine the developmental status of all year-old children, or to X-ray the chests of all patients with pneumonia after their treatment, to what extent were these things done? In some programmes, *coverage*[11] may be a useful criterion—what proportion of the people who can or should receive a service (the target population) actually receive it? A third approach, especially in studies of the quality of medical care, is to make a detailed formulation of the activities that it is believed *should* be carried out, usually in relation to a specific diagnosis or other medical problem, and to compare actual performance with this set of standards (see 'Medical audit' in Ch. 21).

A further basis for evaluation is provided by information on the activities of patients or public—the *utilization of services* (what services, and how much?), the degree of *compliance* with advice or instructions (taking of medicines, keeping of appointments, dietary changes, etc.) and the degree of *community participation* in the programme. Clear-cut criteria are not usually available. The appraisal of activities (by providers and recipients of care) may be extended to studies of knowledge and attitudes that may influence overt behaviour, and of relationships and communication between providers and recipients.

Structure

Finally, information on *facilities and settings* also provides a basis for the appraisal of quality. Are equipment, accommodation, suitably qualified personnel, laboratory facilities etc. available? Recommended norms[5] are sometimes used as criteria, e.g. for numbers of hospital beds. How accessible are services to those who need them? (What are the organizational and fiscal arrangements? Transport facilities? Are there language barriers? etc.) Is the service accountable, and to whom? Are there organizational arrangements to permit continuity of care, teamwork and co-ordinated functioning, co-ordination and co-operation with other agencies (including arrangements for patient referrals and information transfer), and community participation?

EFFICIENCY

Efficiency[12] (or *economic efficiency*) is a measure of the cost in resources that is incurred in achieving results. It is determined by the balance between what is put in (in time, manpower, equipment, etc. or their monetary equivalent) and what is got out. Collecting the required facts on inputs and outputs is a major task of a study of efficiency. The recent burgeoning of *managed care*,[13] a term used for 'a variety of methods of financing and organizing the delivery of comprehensive health care in which an attempt is made to control costs by controlling the provision of services', has led to an intensified interest in economic evaluation.

Efficiency may be expressed as the average cost per unit of care (cost per test, per day in hospital, per patient treated, etc.) for comparison with other programmes or recommended standards. More usefully, the input can be balanced against measures of effectiveness (*cost-effectiveness analysis*), permitting comparisons of the costs of alternative ways of achieving similar effects on health—e.g. costs per year of life gained, or per quality-adjusted life-year (QALY)[12] or healthy years equivalents (HYE)[12]—or comparisons of the benefits that may be obtained at the same cost by different means. As an example, a comparison of three ways of reducing heart disease by controlling cholesterol levels in children—*A* population-wide intervention centred on health education, *B* universal screening, and *C* selective screening for children with a family history of coronary heart disease—indicated that *A* would cost 2.6 times as much per year as *B*, and 17.5 times as much as *C*. But *A* would save 6.8 times as many years of life as *B*, and 32.6 times as many as *C*. *A* was thus the most cost-effective—its cost per year of life saved would be 32% of that of *B*, and 45% of that of *C*.[14] Smoking interventions vary widely in their cost per year of life saved: nicotine gum, $8481 to $13 331 (for men); nicotine patches, $1796 to $2949 (men); physician counselling, $1454 to $4244; nurse counselling, $241.[15] Detailed recommendations for the performance and reporting of cost-effectiveness analyses have been made by an expert panel.[16]

Cost–benefit analysis requires translation of the study's benefits (as well as its inputs) into monetary terms, so that inputs and outputs are measured on the same scale. Account should be taken of the cost of providing the service and the cost of *not* providing it, taking account of all known outcomes, both desirable and undesirable. The collection of adequate data and the conversion of benefits to monetary units present considerable theoretical and practical difficulty.[17] Over half the so-called cost–benefit studies reported in the health-care literature do not meet the definition of a cost–benefit study as one that compares the costs and benefits (in monetary terms) of two or more programmes; most of the studies are cost comparisons, with no accounting of benefits.[18]

SATISFACTION

If patients or public are satisfied with their health care, this does not necessarily mean that their care is of high quality. Satisfaction does, however, enhance the prospects of compliance and the continued utilization of services, and it is also an important additional end-result in its own right. The measurement of satisfaction[19] requires a survey of attitudes or of overt acts from which attitudes can be inferred, such as changes of physician, or the lodging of complaints.

Attention may also be paid to the satisfaction of health professionals. Although the gratification of health workers can hardly be regarded as a central purpose of health care, 'it is reasonable to assume that the best technical care cannot be maintained if the persons who provide it are unhappy with the work they do and the conditions under which it is done'.[20]

DIFFERENTIAL VALUE

The value of a procedure or programme may differ in different patients, population groups, or circumstances. This possible nonuniformity appears as a separate item in our list (Question 5) because of its importance and the frequency with which it is forgotten. This question could actually be asked as an extension of each of the other questions: To what extent is care needed by various groups of the population? How do effectiveness and safety vary in different categories of patients or population groups? Are services equally available to all parts of the population? Equality or (more importantly) equity may be among the touchstones in evaluating a programme.[21] Why was the rate of hysterectomies during a 20-year period consistently twice as high among young women in the southern United States as it was in the northeastern states?[22] Are the people who use a service the ones who need it? Women with a low risk of cancer of the cervix may participate in a screening programme, while high-risk groups may stay away; this tendency for people in most need of care to be those least likely to receive it has been called the 'inverse care law'.[23] Who is more compliant, who is less compliant? And so on. If such questions are to be asked, they must be formulated as study objectives.

OBJECTIVES OF PROGRAMME REVIEWS

A programme review (see p. 27) aims to provide a feedback that will be helpful to whoever makes decisions about the programme. To be useful, the findings must be provided rapidly, and in real time if possible. Since measurement of outcomes would often be relatively protracted or difficult, interest generally centres on the process rather than the outcome of care, and on requisiteness (especially in long-established programmes), the availability of equipment and other facilities, the public's satisfaction, and differences between population groups or categories in their need for care, use of services, and coverage. Programme reviews differ in this respect from programme trials, in which the central issue is usually the outcome (see Ch. 33).

The assumption (on which the programme is based) that the planned activities of the programme are beneficial is generally not in question; if it is, the more rigorous methods of a programme trial are required. The issue is whether these activities are conducted as planned, and their performance is used as a criterion of the quality of care. Data on activities can usually be obtained far more readily and rapidly than data on outcome, often as a byproduct of routine work, i.e. from inbuilt monitoring procedures. If there is no record of what activities were planned—as is often the case in a clinical service—arbitrary standards may be applied, e.g. by using medical audit techniques (see p. 243).

This emphasis on measures of 'process' and 'structure' does not mean that measures of outcome have no place in a programme review. On the contrary, information on outcomes may be valuable even without rigorous evidence that they are actually consequences of the programme. It is usually assumed that changes (or their absence) are, at least to some extent, reflections of the effectiveness of the programme. They are hence often used as a basis for decisions on the need for continuation or modification of the programme. At the very least, they may indicate whether there is a need for more detailed evaluative study.

Short-term outcomes are usually the easiest to measure. Measurement of long-term outcomes may require information about members of the target population with whom there is no routine contact, or with whom contact has ceased. It may also involve a long-term follow-up, with its attendant difficulty and delay. However, if surveillance procedures are available to provide data on relevant end-results, such as mortality rates, case fatality rates, or changes in the health status of patients or the population, this information is often especially helpful. If the programme has predetermined outcome goals, information on their accomplishment is of course particularly meaningful.

In a programme review the appraisal of efficiency, like that of quality, has special features. Although detailed studies of inputs may be undertaken, emphasis is often put on simple observations that can be used as a basis for decisions aimed at enhancing efficiency. Such observations relate especially to evidence of wasteful operation—the avoidable use of expensive or ineffective drugs, over-staffing, delays, the underexploitation of expensive equipment, superfluous activities, unnecessary hospitalization, unduly long institutional care, etc. Use is not necessarily made of explicit standards in appraising these observations. If cost-effectiveness studies are undertaken, cost is usually balanced against estimates or subjective appraisals of effectiveness, or against the performance of assumedly beneficial activities (used as a proxy measure of effectiveness).

The formulation of study objectives usually presents no difficulties in a simple programme review. If cause–effect hypotheses are to be tested (are the outcomes attributable to the programme?) the methods of a programme trial (Ch. 33) must be used.

NOTES AND REFERENCES

1. 'Program directors are concerned with appropriateness when they ask, "Are our program objectives worthwhile and do they have a higher priority than other possible objectives of this or other programs?"' (Deniston O L, Rosenstock I M, Getting V A 1968 Evaluation of program effectiveness. Public Health Reports 83: 323; reprinted in Schulberg H C, Sheldon A, Baker F, eds. 1969 Program Evaluation in the Health Fields. Behavioural Publications, New York, pp 219–239).

   For references to *needs appraisal* see note 9, p. 32. Needs appraisal in the context of community-oriented primary care is discussed in Chapter 34.
2. 'Risk-benefit ratio or risk-benefit nonsense' is the title of a report describing a Medline search that found many papers that used the term 'risk-benefit ratio' without explaining its meaning (Ernst E, Resch K L 1996 Journal of Clinical Epidemiology 49: 1203).
3. Lengeler C, Snow R W 1996 From efficacy to effectiveness: insecticide-treated bednets in Africa. Bulletin of the World Health Association 74: 325.
4. Dictionary definitions: *objective*, 'the precisely stated end to which efforts are directed'; *goal*, 'a desired state to be achieved within a specified time'; *target*,

'an aspired outcome that is specifically stated, e.g. what a health promotion program will achieve by a specified date' (Last J M, Abramson J H, Friedman G D, Porta M, Spasoff R A, Thuriaux M 1995 A dictionary of epidemiology, 3rd edn. Oxford University Press, New York). But the terms may be used very differently, e.g. 'goals are ... expressed as quantifiable, timeless aspirations', whereas 'objectives should express particular levels of expected achievement ... by a specific year' (Bureau of Health Planning and Resources Development 1970 Guidelines concerning the development of health systems plans and annual implementation plans. US Department of Health, Education & Welfare)

5. *Norms* and *standards* prescribed by an authority as 'what is desirable' may be used as criteria for evaluating facilities, performance, outcome, and cost. A distinction is sometimes made between norms and standards; definitions of 'norms', 'standards' and 'criteria' are discussed by Donabedian A 1981 (Criteria, norms and standards of quality: what do they mean? American Journal of Public Health 71: 409). Standards may be normative or empirical (see p. 243). They may specify a 'minimum' (minimum acceptable), an 'ideal' level, the 'desired achievable' level, or a 'maximum'.

6. Methods of studying adverse reactions to therapy are briefly reviewed by Sartwell P E 1974 (Iatrogenic disease: an epidemiologic perspective. International Journal of Health Services 4: 89). The 'current iatrogenic pandemic' is described and copiously documented by Illich I 1977 (Limits to medicine: medical nemesis: the expropriation of health. Penguin Books, Harmondsworth).

7. Morris J N 1975 Uses of epidemiology, 3rd edn. Churchill Livingstone, Edinburgh, p. 92.

8. Bergman A B 1977 American Journal of Public Health 67: 601.

9. A community survey in California identified people who were normotensive and not receiving medical care for hypertension, but had previously been told they were hypertensive. These 'mislabelled' people had more symptoms of depression and reported being in poorer health than other normotensives. Possible confounding by age, sex, education, marital status and ethnicity was controlled by matching, and the presence of other disorders was controlled in the analysis. The mislabelled hypertensives had as many symptoms of depression as correctly labelled hypertensives. (Bloom J R, Monterossa S 1981. Hypertension labeling and sense of well-being. American Journal of Public Health 71: 1228.)

   A study of a US national sample yielded similar findings: normotensives whose doctors had told them they had high blood pressure had lower 'general wellbeing' scores than other normotensives, as did 'correctly labelled' hypertensives, whether under treatment or not (Monk M 1980 Psychologic status and hypertension. American Journal of Epidemiology 112: 200.)

10. Kenen R H 1996 The at-risk health status and technology: a diagnostic invitation and the 'gift' of knowing. Social Science and Medicine 42: 1545. Reprinted in Sidell M, Jones L, Katz J, Peberdy A 1997 (Debates and dilemmas in promoting health: a reader. MacMillan Press, Houndmills, pp 306–313).

11. The evaluation of health service *coverage* is discussed by Tanahashi T 1978 (Health service coverage and its evaluation. Bulletin of the World Health Organization 56: 295). The importance of 'measuring what we do not do— the gap between what is done and what could and should be done', and the potential for such studies in general practices with stable populations is stressed by Hart J T 1982 (Measurement and omission. British Medical Journal 284: 1686).

12. For reviews of the *economic evaluation* of health care, see Donaldson C, Shackley P 1997 (Economic evaluation. In: Detels R, Holland W W,

McEwen J, Omenn G S, eds. 1997 Oxford Textbook of public health, 3rd edn, vol 2. The methods of public health. Oxford University Press, New York, pp 849–871); Bowling A, Jones I R 1997 (Costing health services: health economics. In: Bowling A 1997 Research methods in health: investigating health and health services. Open University Press, Buckingham, pp 78–98); and Jefferson T, Demicheli V, Mugford M 1996 (Elementary economic evaluation in health care. BMJ Publishing Group, London. Part of this book is available on the Internet in the Epidemiology Supercourse at www.pitt.edu/~super1/main/index.htm).

Donaldson and Shackley (pp 860–867) explain the use of *quality-adjusted life-years* (QALYs) and *healthy year equivalents* (HYEs), which convert years of unhealthy life to healthy years (only arithmetically, alas). To calculate these measures, weights are allotted to different degrees of disability and distress; account may be taken of the individual's or the community's preferences when determining weights. Problems in the use of QALYs are discussed in the first report by Russell et al 1996 (see note 16).

13. The definition of *managed care* is cited from Inglehart J K 1994 (Physicians and the growth of managed care: health policy report. New England Journal of Medicine 331: 1167). Managed care is explained in three articles in the British Medical Journal, which point out that 'it seeks to cut the costs of health care while maintaining its quality, but the evidence that it is able to achieve these aims is mixed … all its permutations have in common an attempt to influence and modify the behaviour and practice of doctors and other health professionals towards cost effective care' (Fairfield G, Hunter D J, Mechanic D, Rosleff F 1997a Managed care: origins, principles, and evolution. British Medical Journal 314: 1823; Fairfield G, Hunter D J, Mechanic D, Rosleff F 1997b Managed care: implications of managed care for health systems, clinicians, and patients. British Medical Journal 314: 1895; Hunter D J, Fairfield G 1997 Managed care: disease management. British Medical Journal 315: 50).

Despite the potential benefits of these approaches, many clinicians and other health professionals are concerned by possible negative consequences of an overemphasis on economic factors (see: Silver G 1997 Editorial: The road from managed care. American Journal of Public Health 87: 8). According to a probably fictional report, Hippocrates turned down an appointment in a health maintenance organization on ethical grounds—'a medical system that has minimal concern for ethics … and is run by financial people instead of doctors, nurses, or anyone else who cares for the patients' (Pruchnicki A 1997 First, do no harm [pending prior approval]. New England Journal of Medicine 337: 1627).

14. The cited study of options for controlling children's cholesterol levels made extensive use of *sensitivity analysis*, by seeing how results would be affected by different estimates of the risk associated with cholesterol level, the stability of cholesterol level, the degree of compliance, the change of cholesterol with diet, and the costs of screening and dietary intervention; these variations did not affect the ranking of the three programmes; Berwick D M, Cretin S, Keeler E 1985 Cholesterol, children, and heart disease: an analysis of alternatives. Pediatrics 68: 721.

15. Cheung A M, Tsevat J 1997 Commentary: economic evaluations of smoking interventions. Preventive Medicine 26: 271.

16. The consensus statement of the Panel on Cost-Effectiveness in Health and Medicine is described in three reports: Russell L B, Gold M R, Siegel J E, Daniels N, Weinstein M C 1996 (The role of cost-effectiveness analysis in health and medicine. Journal of the American Medical Association 276: 1172); Weinstein M C, Siegel J E, Gold M R, Kamlet M S, Russell L B 1996 (Recommendations of the Panel on Cost-effectiveness in Health and

Medicine. Journal of the American Medical Association 276: 1253); Siegel J E, Weinstein M C, Russell L B, Gold M R 1996 (Recommendations for reporting cost-effectiveness analyses. Journal of the American Medical Association 276: 1339). *Quality-adjusted life-years* (QALYs) are explained in the first report.

Also, see Gold M R (ed) 1996 (Cost-effectiveness in health and medicine. Oxford University Press, New York).

17. The less tangible costs of illness (i.e. other than impaired productivity) are seldom taken into account in cost–benefit studies, and estimates of the effects of preventive programmes are often speculative because of the paucity of epidemiological evidence (Drummond 1985 Survey of cost-effectiveness and cost-benefit studies in industrialized countries. World Health Statistics Quarterly 38: 383).

An analysis of recent economic evaluation studies revealed that in only 14% was uncertainty taken into account satisfactorily; in another 25% the handling of uncertainty was 'adequate' (Briggs A, Sculpher M 1995 Sensitivity analysis in economic evaluation: a review of published studies. Health Economics 4: 355).

A sceptical reader may find that the methods of estimation used in some cost–benefit studies are reminiscent of the method of weighing a pig attributed to John Burns: Find a plank that is absolutely straight, balance it at dead centre so that it is absolutely level, place the pig on one end, and pile stones on the other end until the plank is exactly level again. Then carefully guess the weight of the stones. This is the weight of the pig.

18. Zarnke K B, Levine M A H, O'Brien B J 1997 Cost-benefit analyses in the health-care literature: don't judge a study by its label. Journal of Clinical Epidemiology 50: 813.

19. *Patient satisfaction.* Issues and concepts are reviewed in detail by Sitzia J, Wood N 1997, who point out that very few patients express dissatisfaction, and that maybe a report of satisfaction 'should not be interpreted as indicating that care was "good" but simply that nothing "extremely bad" occurred' (Patient satisfaction: a review of issues and concepts. Social Science and Medicine 45: 1829).

Nine methods of measuring patient satisfaction are contrasted by Ford R C, Bach S A, Fottler M D 1997 Methods of measuring patient satisfaction in health care organizations. Health Care Management Review 22: 74.

20. Donabedian A 1966 Evaluating the quality of medical care. Milbank Memorial Fund Quarterly 44 (3, part 2): 166.

21. Cochrane A L 1972 Effectiveness and efficiency. Nuffield Provincial Hospitals Trust, London. The distinction between equality and *equity* ('Equity is about fairness and justice') is discussed by Calman K C, Downie R S 1997 (Ethical principles and ethical issues in public health. In: Detels R, Holland W W, McEwen J, Omenn G S, eds. 1997 Oxford Textbook of public health, 3rd edn, vol 1. The scope of public health. Oxford University Press, New York, pp 391–402). Also, see Mooney G 1987 (What does equity in health mean? World Health Statistics Quarterly 40: 296).

22. Pokras R, Hufnagel V G 1987 Hysterectomies in the United States, 1965–84. Vital and Health Statistics series 13 no 92.

23. Hart J T 1971 The inverse care law. Lancet i: 495.

6 The study population

The *study population* is the group that is studied, either *in toto* or by selecting a sample consisting of individual members of the group for investigation. The units in the group may be persons, families, medical records, certificates, nursery schools, specimens of milk, or dustbins. In the following discussion emphasis will be placed on human study populations. If a sample is chosen, the study population from which it is selected may also be called the *sampled population* or the *parent population*.

There may be more than one study population, e.g. in a group-based epidemiological study that compares countries or an evaluative study that compares health-care organizations. A cohort study may be performed in a single population, or more than one. In a case-control study, cases and controls should ideally be drawn from the same study population (the selection of subjects for a case-control study will be discussed in Ch. 9).

At an early stage in the planning of any study, a number of issues concerning the study population (or populations) may require consideration.

Study population and selection of subjects

1. What study population? What are its characteristics?
2. Does the study population represent a broader reference population?
3. Will sampling be used? (See Ch. 8)
4. Will controls be used? (See Ch. 7)

SELECTING THE STUDY POPULATION

Often the investigator will have implicitly chosen his study population when he defined the topic of his investigation, through his interest in a specific community, a specific health programme, or the testing of a treatment for a specific category of patient. In other instances he may require purposefully to select a study population. Appropriateness and practicability should be taken into account.

The appropriateness of the study population refers mainly to its suitability for the attainment of the objectives of the study. If the hypothesis is that cancer is related to the consumption of carrots, is the population one where it can be expected that there will be sufficient variation in carrot intake to permit the hypothesis to be tested? On the other hand, there may be too much variation in a population, and the objectives may be such that they can be best met by restricting the study to a selected category, such as one sex or a single age group or families of a standard size and composition, in order to avoid the effects of characteristics that may confuse the issue. Maybe the study would best be performed in a very special kind of population—among vegetarians or monks—or in an occupational group subjected to seasonal emotional stress; the choice of a suitable study population is one of the factors making for originality in research. Paradoxically, some aetiological processes may best be investigated in a population where the disease under study is rare; it would be difficult to study the possibility that asymptomatic urinary tract infection may be an occasional cause of anaemia in a population with a high prevalence of anaemia due to hookworm disease or dietary iron deficiency.

A specific study population may also be chosen because it is believed to be typical of a broader reference population to which the investigator wishes to generalize the findings.

Practical questions may arise. Is the proposed study population one about which it will be possible to obtain the required information? Is it an 'accessible' population to which the investigator already has an *entrée*? Is it likely to co-operate in the study so that a low nonparticipation rate can be expected, or will it be a resistant one, possibly as a result of having been over-researched in the past? If patients with a specific disease are to be studied, will it be possible to identify enough cases to yield useful conclusions? If a long-term follow-up study is planned, is the population so mobile that it may be difficult to maintain contact with the subjects? A preliminary exploratory survey may sometimes be required in order to answer such questions.

The study population or populations should be clearly and explicitly defined in terms of place, time and any other relevant criteria.[1]

In a longitudinal study the study population may be a *closed* or *fixed cohort*, which individuals cannot enter after the onset of follow-up. It can be regarded as closed even in cohort studies and trials where individuals enter, and their follow-up starts, at different calendar times, determined by the occurrence of some event (e.g. swimming in polluted water, or myocardial infarction). Alternatively, the study population may be a *dynamic* one (such as the population of a city) that individuals can enter or leave at any time. A dynamic population may or may not be *stable*, in the sense that its size and characteristics may or may not remain unchanged during the period of the study.

Denominator data—i.e. facts about the size and relevant characteristics (age, sex, etc.) of the study population—are essential for the computation of rates[2] and other meaningful measures of group health. As an illustration, a survey based on obituary columns in the British Medical Journal revealed that doctors of Indian origin tended to die young—at an average age of 61.8, compared with 75.2 for doctors born in the United Kingdom (a difference very unlikely to be due to chance; $P < 0.001$). This finding, it was suggested, might be due to a higher risk of coronary heart disease. But no denominator data were presented, without which the likeliest explanation is simply that doctors of Indian origin in Britain are relatively young. This was pointed out in letters to the editor.[3] When numbers of cases are presented instead of rates, they are sometimes referred to as *floating numerators*.

In studies where individuals remain in the study population for different periods it is important to obtain information on times of entry and exit, as a basis for the computation of a *person-time denominator* expressed in person-years[2] or other person-time units. This is the sum total of the periods during which individual members are in the study population.

Obtaining denominator data may present no special difficulty, e.g. in a morbidity survey where information is obtained about all subjects, irrespective of whether they have the disease under study. Sometimes, however, it may not be easy. The denominator data required for the above study of doctors' deaths, for example—the age distribution of living doctors of different origins—are not readily available. In some studies, numerator and denominator data come from different sources—e.g. in a study of correlates of infant mortality, from death and birth certificates respectively—and it becomes necessary to check whether the sources provide the required data and whether they use comparable definitions. These problems should be explored and tackled while the study is still on the drawing board.

Especially in studies requiring the co-operation of the subjects, *nonrespondents* or nonparticipants may bias the findings, since respondents and nonrespondents may differ with respect to whatever is being studied, and it may be difficult to apply the findings even to the study population, let alone a wider reference population. In a study of cardiovascular diseases in California nonrespondents were especially likely to be smokers, and were much less likely to have a family history of heart disease.[4] In Sweden, over half the nonparticipants in a health survey said their reason was that they were ill or in regular contact with a doctor; social insurance records revealed that nonparticipants in another Swedish study had over five times as many days of sickness, on average, as did participants;[5] in Switzerland, people who refused to participate in a health survey had particularly high health-care expenditures.[6] Exploration of the possibility of this kind of bias generally starts with a comparison of the demographic characteristics of the respondents with those of the nonrespondents (or those of the study population as a whole). From a practical point of view, the study plan should therefore include efforts to collect limited easy-to-get information concerning the nonrespondents, or a representative sample of them.

WHAT DOES THE STUDY POPULATION REPRESENT?

If a study population is believed to be typical of a broader population to which the findings may be generalized, the latter population may be termed the *reference population* or *external population*.[7] As an example, the study population may comprise the elderly people in a given neighbourhood, all or a sample of whom may be studied; the investigators may decide they can apply the findings to elderly people in the whole city or nation or world. There may be several possible reference populations: people with a given disease attending a given clinic during a given week may be studied with the intention of applying the findings to patients attending the clinic at other times, or to patients attending other clinics, or to all patients with the disease.

Consideration should be given to specific features of the study population that may affect the validity of generalizations of the findings to broader populations. For example:

1. *Volunteer populations*. Persons who volunteer to enter a study or submit to a procedure may differ in many respects from those who do not so volunteer—even in their chances of living or dying[8]—and therefore the findings in a volunteer population do not necessarily apply to the population at large. In some circumstances people who are anxious about their health may be those most likely to volunteer; in others, they may be the most reluctant. It is therefore wrong to evaluate an immunization procedure by immunizing volunteers and then comparing them with persons who have not been immunized. Studies of volunteers have their place: the finding, in a 17-year cohort study of 11 000 'vegetarians and other health conscious people' recruited through health food shops, vegetarian societies, and magazines, that daily consumption of fresh fruit was associated with a significantly reduced mortality may or may not be applicable to the general population (whose total mortality was double that of the cohort), but it is certainly of interest to vegetarians and other health conscious people.[9]

2. *Hospital or clinic populations*. Persons receiving medical care are obviously not representative of the general population or, necessarily, of all ill persons. People with rheumatoid arthritis who are treated in hospital may differ from those receiving ambulant care, and both groups may differ from patients with this disease who do not receive medical care for it. Expectant mothers who receive care from physicians may have different characteristics from those who do not—they may have higher incomes and include fewer teenagers,[10] or differ in other ways. Furthermore, the chance of entering a clinic population may vary for different diseases (or other characteristics) and for various combinations of characteristics, and this may produce spurious associations. For example, if people who have two specific diseases at the same time have an especially high chance of hospitalization, a study of hospital patients may reveal an association between the two diseases even if there is no such association in the population as a whole. If the two diseases carry different chances of

hospitalization, a third characteristic (another disease, or a suspected aetiological factor) might, for this reason, turn out to be more frequently associated with one of the two diseases than with the other. This problem of the interplay of admission rates, which is referred to as *Berkson's bias*[11] (admission rate bias) may arise in any population (not only hospital or clinic populations) in which individuals with different characteristics have different chances of inclusion. The use of hospital or clinic patients in case-control studies is discussed on page 110.

3. *Populations with good medical records.* It is often tempting to carry out studies in specific practices or clinics in which practitioners maintain good clinical records or are prepared to keep especially detailed records for the purposes of the study. This may be an essential condition for some studies, e.g. surveys of the work of general practitioners. But the doctors who are selected in this way may be singular in other respects also, and their practices may be atypical.

4. *People living at home.* A study population comprising people living at home necessarily excludes those who are in hospitals, old folks' homes, and other institutions; there may thus be a selective exclusion of persons with diseases and other conditions of interest to the investigator. Young adults who are unfit for army service may be over-represented in a country where such service is compulsory.

5. *Patients notified as having a disease.* Even if notification is compulsory, it is unlikely that all cases are notified, and the notified cases may not be representative. Socially unacceptable diseases, such as sexually transmitted ones, may be more fully notified by public agencies than by private physicians. A study in the United States showed under-reporting (particularly by private physicians) of hepatitis B patients who were homosexual.[12]

6. *Autopsy populations.* Persons submitted to autopsy are obviously not necessarily representative of all decedents. Also, Berkson's bias may occur. It played a role in a well known epidemiological blunder, the discovery in 1929 of an apparent 'antagonism' between tuberculosis and cancer, which led to the institution of a 'programme for treating cancer patients with tuberculin'.[13]

7. *Groups characterized by their behaviour or occupation* (smokers, joggers, migrants, bus drivers, etc.). It is often worth considering the selective factors that may have led to membership in these groups or exclusion from them, especially if health status may have played a role. This has been called *membership bias*.[14]

Persistent cigarette smokers may be healthier than ex-smokers, not because smoking is salubrious, but because people stop smoking because of illness. The mental health status of immigrants may be a reflection of the characteristics that led to migration, rather than of the stresses or rewards of migration. Since ill health interferes with work, workers are ipso facto healthier, on average, than nonworkers (this is termed the *healthy worker effect*).[15] Since having children may keep women away from work, working women may be relatively infertile (the *infertile worker effect*).[16] If there are many cases where ill health has led to, for example, the adoption of a sedentary occupation, or retirement from work, or weaning from the breast, relationships that are subsequently detected between health and sedentary work, retirement or breast feeding may be misinterpreted. Membership bias may crop up in unexpected places: a follow-up study in Finland showed that poor health at the age of 14 was predictive of a heavier coffee consumption at the age of 18, suggesting a 'sick drinker effect'.[17]

8. *Populations in which the same individuals appear more than once.* If the same individuals appear more than once in a study population, the findings in these individuals may have an undue effect on the results.[18] This may arise in a study of the correlates of gastroenteritis, based on an investigation of all cases of this disease treated in hospital, including repeated hospitalizations of the same patients. A list of women who received antenatal care may include repeated pregnancies of the same women. Similarly, patients who consult their doctor frequently will be over-represented in a study based on records of medical care; unless the study is focused on episodes of disease or medical visits it may be decided to limit each person to a single appearance, e.g. by using the first visit or a randomly selected one.

9. *Internet users.*[19] Employment of the Internet for conducting a study offers several potential advantages: inexpensive data collection, computerized data handling, easy follow-up, a worldwide base, and the use of explanatory pictures, e.g. showing portion sizes in a dietary survey or lesions in a study of a skin disease. But the study population is obviously a selected one; Internet users are computer-literate, and currently tend to be young, male and educationally and socio-economically advantaged. Nor will the study sample necessarily represent eligible Internet users in general, since inclusion depends on coming across an invitation to participate and volunteering to do so.

NOTES AND REFERENCES

1. A written record should be kept of the criteria for inclusion in the study population. These should be stated explicitly; e.g. if residents of a stated neighbourhood are to be studied, what is a 'resident'? (6 months' stay is often used as a criterion). If unforeseen problems of definition arise subsequently (e.g. students who live at home at weekends only) the new decisions should also be recorded, so that they can be applied uniformly.

2. See notes 2 and 3, pp 121–122.

3. Wright D J M, Roberts A P 1996 Which doctors die first? Analysis of BMJ obituary columns. British Medical Journal 313: 1581; Kaw K-T 1997 Which doctors die first? British Medical Journal 314: 1132; McManus C 1997 Which doctors die first? British Medical Journal 314: 1132.

4. Criqui M H, Barrett-Connor E, Austin M 1978 Differences between respondents and non-respondents in a population-based cardiovascular disease study. American Journal of Epidemiology 108: 367.

5. Janzon L, Hanson B S, Isacsson S-O, Lindell S-E, Steen B 1986 Factors influencing participation in health surveys: results from prospective population study 'Men born in 1914' in Malmo, Sweden. Journal of Epidemiology and Community Health 40: 174; Bergstrand R, Vedin A, Wilhelmsson C, Wilhelmsen L 1983 Bias due to non-participation and heterogeneous sub-groups in population surveys. Journal of Chronic Diseases 36: 725.

6. Etter J-F, Perneger T V 1997 Analysis of non-response bias in a mailed health survey. Journal of Clinical Epidemiology 50: 1123.

7. Other terms for the reference population are *target population* and *theoretical population*. The term 'target population' is best avoided in this context, since it is sometimes used for the sampled population and sometimes for the reference population. In the context of health care, it refers of course to the population at which a programme is directed. 'Target population' has also been used to refer to the population that the investigator wished to study or sample, before the loss of members through nonresponse or other reasons, leaving a study population not necessarily representative of the target population.

8. In Pennsylvania, respondents to an advertisement inviting people aged 65 or more to participate in an epidemiological study had a significantly lower mortality, over the next 6–8 years, than randomly selected subjects of the same age (Ganguli M, Lutle M E, Reynolds M D, Dodge H H 1998 Random versus volunteer selection for a community-based study. Journals of Gerontology, Series A, Biological Sciences and Medical Sciences 53: M39).

9. Key T J A, Thorogood M, Appleby P N, Burr M L 1996 Dietary habits and mortality in 11000 vegetarians and health conscious people: results of a 17 year follow up. British Medical Journal 313: 775.

10. Peoples-Sheps M D, Kalsbeek W D, Siegel E 1988 Why we know so little about prenatal care worldwide: an assessment of required methodology. Health Services Research 23: 361.

11. Real-life examples of *Berkson's bias*, from surveys in Ontario, include the detection of a strong association between diseases of the respiratory and locomotor systems in hospital data but not in the general population, and the finding that fatigue was positively associated with allergic and metabolic disease in the general population, but negatively in hospital data (Roberts R S, Spitzer W O, Delmore T, Sackett D L 1978 An empiric demonstration of Berkson's bias. Journal of Chronic Diseases 31: 119).

In a clinic, the rate of neurological disorders in boys was found to be double that in girls; this unusual finding was attributed to the fact that the ratio of boys to girls was 4:1 in this clinic (Brown G W 1976 Berkson fallacy revisited: spurious conclusions from patient surveys. American Journal of Diseases of Children 130: 56).

In a hospital, a problem arose in a study of a malignant disease because cancer was apparently regarded as a sufficient reason for hospitalization of patients, whereas noncancer patients with whom they might be compared tended to be admitted only if they had multiple diseases (Robertson S J, Grufferman S, Cohen H J 1988 Hospital versus random digit dialing controls in the elderly: observations from two case-control studies. Journal of the American Geriatric Society 36: 119).

Algebraic explanations of Berkson's fallacy are given by Fleiss J L 1981 (Statistical methods for rates and proportions, 2nd edn. John Wiley, New York, pp 8–13).

12. Alter M J, Mares A, Hadler S C et al 1987 The effect of underreporting on the apparent incidence and epidemiology of acute viral hepatitis. American Journal of Epidemiology 125: 133.

13. Lilienfeld A M, Lilienfeld D E 1980 Foundations of epidemiology, 2nd edn. Oxford University Press, New York, pp 203–204; Mainland D 1963 Elementary Medical Statistics, 2nd edn. W B Saunders, Philadelphia, pp 121–122.

14. For lists and descriptions of possible biases, see Sackett D L 1979 (Bias in analytic research. Journal of Chronic Diseases 32: 51), Schlesselman J J, Stolley P D 1982 (Sources of bias. In: Schlesselman J J ed. Case-control studies: design, conduct, analysis. Oxford University Press, New York, pp 124–143).

15. As an example of the *healthy worker effect*, a longitudinal study of a cohort of workers exposed to granite dust revealed that those who were still at work after five years had significantly less deterioration in their lung function than 'drop-outs' (Eisen E A, Wegman D H, Louis T A, Smith T J, Peters J M 1995 Healthy worker effect in a longitudinal study of one-second forced expiratory volume (FEV_1) and chronic exposure to granite dust. International Journal of Epidemiology 24: 1154).

16. Joffe M 1985 Biases in research in reproduction and women's work. International Journal of Epidemiology 14: 118.

17. Hemminki E, Rahkonen O, Rimpela M 1988 American Journal of Epidemiology 127: 1088.

18. Bias due to the over-representation of frequent attenders in a study that is based on records of medical visits can be controlled by a weighting procedure. This is described by Shepard D S, Neutra R 1977 (American Journal of Public Health 67: 743), who show how estimates of the numbers and characteristics of hypertensive patients attending a medical clinic can be derived from a study of visits.

19. A study of relationships between diet and breast cancer, the Epidemiologic Cyberspace Cohort Study, was possibly the first epidemiologic study to use the Internet. Its purpose was to examine the feasibility of using the Internet for a cohort study (Kushi L H, Finnegan J, Martinson B, Rightmyer J, Vachon C, Yochum L 1997 Epidemiology and the Internet. Epidemiology 8: 689). For detailed information on its aims and methods, visit www.epi.umn.edu/health_survey/

In the words of investigators who studied the correlates of atopic eczema by using an Internet questionnaire (completed by about 240 patients and healthy web surfers each month): 'Obviously, the web community is not a representative sample of the whole population, and results obtained with questionnaires on the web are biased towards self selection; thus they must be interpreted with care and verified in an unbiased population' (Eysenbach G, Diepgen T L 1998 Epidemiological data can be gathered with world wide web. British Medical Journal 316: 72).

In a study of patients with ulcerative colitis, those who had been treated surgically and responded to an Internet invitation to fill in SF-36 and bowel disease questionnaires turned out to be younger and in worse health than post-surgery patients drawn from a surgical clinic (Soetikno R M, Mrad R, Pao V, Lenert L A 1997 Quality-of-life research on the Internet: feasibility and potential biases in patients with ulcerative colitis. Journal of the American Medical Informatics Association 4: 426). The respondents tended to be well-off and well-educated. Most were prepared to release their medical records to verify the diagnosis (Soetikno R M, Provenzale D, Lenert L A 1997 Studying ulcerative colitis over the World Wide Web. American Journal of Gastroenterology 92: 457).

Technical advice on Internet surveys is provided by Batinic B 1997 (How to make an internet based survey? www.psychol.uni-giessen.de/~Batinic/survey/faq_soft.htm) and by Watt J H (Using the Internet for quantitative survey research. URL: www.SwiftInteractive.com/white-p1.htm), who rhapsodizes about their speed and low cost, and says 'If you haven't done Internet survey research—you will.' See note 3, p. 279 (use of the Internet for pretests of questionnaires).

7 Control groups

Controls are never needed in studies in which hypotheses are not tested, and are sometimes superfluous in studies that do test hypotheses. In Bradford Hill's words, 'If we survey the deaths of infants in the first month of life and find that so many are caused by dropping the baby on its head on the kitchen floor I am not myself convinced that we need controls to convince us that it is a bad habit. If, on the other hand, so many of the deaths are found to be of infants whose mothers had influenza during pregnancy then I should shriek for controls before I was satisfied that the two events were related'.[1] The fact that 79% of patients receiving lithotripsy treatment for kidney stones in Wyoming chose country-western music when asked what they would like to hear during the procedure[2] does not convincingly indicate that country-western music is associated with kidney stones, in the absence of a comparison with people without kidney stones.

The term 'control' is used with various connotations in epidemiologic studies.[3] In the present context, it refers to a group (or its members) with which study subjects are compared; the controls generally differ from the study subjects in their exposure to a postulated aetiological factor (in a cohort study), in their disease experience (in a case-control study), or in their exposure to an experimental treatment or programme (in a trial).

Controls should be selected from the same study population as the study subjects with whom they are compared, or (failing this) from a similar study population. In any type of controlled study, and however the controls are selected, the analysis should include a comparison of all the possibly relevant characteristics of the study and control groups, to see whether there are differences that may explain the findings of the study.

Use is sometimes made of *matched controls*; that is, controls chosen in such a way that with regard to selected characteristics they are the same as, or similar to, the study subjects or groups with whom they are compared.

This chapter will deal with matching, and then with the selection of controls for cohort studies and trials. The use of controls in trials will be discussed more fully in Chapters 32 (clinical trials) and 33 (programme trials). The selection of controls in case-control studies will be considered in Chapter 9. Cross-sectional and cohort studies of total populations have built-in controls.

MATCHING

If there are differences between the characteristics of study and control groups, they may sometimes obscure or distort ('confound') the associations being studied. For example, one of the reasons for the 12-year delay in ending the iatrogenic epidemic of retrolental dysplasia, a blinding disease of premature infants caused by high-dose oxygen therapy, was that the cases were compared with controls who were mainly full-term. Because of the difference in maturity status there were more congenital, placental and prenatal disorders in the cases than in the controls, leading to the conclusion that retrolental dysplasia was the result of anoxia during intrauterine development.[4]

One way of avoiding or reducing such differences, so as to ensure similarity with respect to possible confounding factors that may distort the findings, is to match the control group with the study group. If the groups are large enough, the differences can instead be handled by appropriate computations during the analysis of the findings (see p. 314).

Matching reduces the confounding effect (less well in case-control than in follow-up studies; see p. 112) and (under certain conditions) adds to the precision with which the association under study is estimated.[5]

Matching can be done in two ways:

1. Each control may be selected so as to be similar to a specific member of the study group (*individual matching* or, if one control is chosen per case, *pair-matching*). This may be done by formulating matching criteria and then seeking suitable controls

for each subject. A large pool of potential controls may be needed if there are more than two or three matching variables and a very close match is demanded on each variable. Individual matching may also be achieved by selecting a spouse, sibling, friend, neighbour[6] or fellow-worker, a child born on the same day in the same hospital, a patient in the same hospital ward, etc.

2. The controls may be so selected that, as a group, they are in specified respects (e.g. age and sex) similar to the study group (*group matching*). For *frequency matching* the potential controls are divided into strata (say age–sex groups) and an appropriate number of individuals is then selected from each stratum, so that the frequency distributions are similar in the study and control groups. *Mean matching* ('balancing') tries to produce groups with similar mean values.

The control and study groups need not be equal in size; if individual matching is used, two or more controls can be selected for each subject. There may be good reasons for having unequal groups.[7]

Whatever method is used, clear-cut rules[8] should be laid down, in order to ensure objectivity when deciding whether a match is sufficiently close and when choosing between two or more candidates who meet the matching criteria.

Matching should not be undertaken when it is unnecessary, since it has disadvantages:

1. It complicates the selection of controls, and may be costly. The study may suffer delay if large numbers of potential controls have to be screened, or if a pool of potential controls is not immediately available (e.g. if the controls are patients suffering from a specific condition, and it is necessary to wait for the appearance of a suitable candidate).

2. It may lead to the exclusion of subjects if enough suitable controls cannot be found. If there are numerous matching variables, many subjects may be 'wasted' in this way, and the study group may become less representative of the reference population.

3. A confounding variable that has been controlled by matching can no longer be studied as an independent variable. If cases and controls are matched for age it becomes impossible to study the relationship of the disease to age: a comparison of the ages of the cases and controls will provide information only on the effectiveness of the matching procedure. Also, it becomes difficult to reach useful conclusions on associations with variables that are closely linked with age. Note, however, that the effect of age as a *modi-*

fier (see p. 310) of other relationships can still be examined, i.e. it is possible to see whether an association—between, say, drinking and coronary heart disease—is consistent in different age groups.

4. The groups may inadvertently be made so similar that the difference that the investigation was designed to seek may be falsely reduced or masked ('matched out') in the crude data; this is sometimes called *overmatching*.

5. Unnecessary matching (i.e. in the absence of a strong confounding effect) may impair the precision with which the association can be measured.[5] This is also sometimes called 'overmatching'.

Matching is useful if three conditions are met (the first two are prerequisites for a strong confounding effect):

1. There is likely to be a marked disparity between the groups if the characteristic is not 'held constant' by matching.

2. The characteristic is believed to be strongly associated with whatever is being compared in the groups (e.g. disease incidence in a prospective study, or exposure to a causal factor in a case-control study).

3. The groups are so small (e.g. because of the cost of studying large groups), or there are so many potential confounders, or the confounders have so many categories, that the handling of confounding effects during the analysis may be unfeasible or inefficient.

CONTROLS IN COHORT STUDIES

In a cohort study of the association between a suspected causal factor and a disease, the ideal control group for the cohort exposed to the factor is a group that would have the same disease rate as the exposed group, if the factor was unassociated with the disease. The closest approximation to this ideal is achieved in a cohort study of a total population (or a representative sample of a total population), where inclusion in the study is not influenced by exposure to the factor. Such a study has built-in controls (an *internal comparison group*). A well-known example is the cohort study of British physicians by Doll and Hill, which provided one of the first clear demonstrations of the effect of smoking on lung cancer mortality.[9] In cohort studies of total populations the amount or duration of exposure (number of cigarettes per day, duration of smoking, etc.) can often be taken into account, instead of simplistically using two groups, 'exposed' and 'nonexposed'; this permits examination of the dose–response relationship (see p. 319).

If an *external comparison group* of unexposed people is used, the controls should if possible be selected from the same population as the exposed group; if the exposed people are members of a special population (e.g. workers in a factory) the controls should be drawn from the same special population. Failing this, the comparison population should be one that is as similar as possible to the population of which the exposed persons are members, with respect to factors (other than the exposure) that may influence the risk of incurring the disease.

Since it may not be possible to find a completely satisfactory control group, it is frequently decided to use two or more groups drawn from different sources, and to see whether the various comparisons yield similar conclusions. In a study of workers exposed to a specific occupational hazard, for example, one comparison might be with disease incidence in the general population—a comparison that is probably biased by the 'healthy worker effect' (see p. 75). Another might be with workers in some other industry. Sometimes both internal and external comparison groups are used.

The choice of control groups is sometimes constrained by the need to ensure that the same methods of investigation, especially for case detection, are applied as in the exposed group or groups. It is advisable to gather information—for both exposed and non-exposed subjects—about all factors that may affect the risk of the disease, so that their influence can be taken into account when the findings are analyzed and interpreted.

The need to define 'non-exposure' may sometimes lead the investigator to give closer thought to the meaning of 'exposure', and to formulate the research hypothesis more precisely. What control group is required in a cohort study of the effect of smoking? This depends on the definition of smoking. Are 'non-smokers' people who have never smoked at all, or those who have never smoked regularly, or those who do not smoke at present, or those who have not smoked for a given number of years, or those who have not smoked (say) at least 20 cigarettes a day for a continuous period of at least 10 years?

CONTROLS IN EXPERIMENTS

'I was a 90 lb weakling, and look at me now!' is not convincing evidence of the effectiveness of a course of treatment, as the change may well have been due to processes of adolescence or other factors quite unrelated to the treatment. To be reasonably convincing, 'before–after' studies of this sort (without external controls) must be replicated, or extended in time so as to see what happens when the treatment is withdrawn.

In most experiments separate control groups are used. The findings in the experimental group are compared with those in a control group not exposed to the experimental procedure. Infant mortality dropped after the introduction of a programme; but what happened in other (similar) regions? This approach is often the best available method of evaluating a programme or procedure. In the absence of an external control group we run the risk that we may think that a change is a specific effect of the intervention that we are testing, when actually it is not.[10] The main circumstances that may confuse the issue are:

1. *Changes that are due to other causes.* People may recover from illnesses for reasons quite unconnected with the care they receive. Changes happen because people age, they mature, they adapt to disability, they become integrated into new social settings, and external events and changes exert their influence on them. Food prices may alter, foodstuffs low in calories or saturated fats may become readily available, there may be a publicity campaign about cigarette smoking, a new medical service may be started, a war may break out or come to an end, etc.

2. *Non-specific effects caused by the intervention or the experiment.* The administration of a treatment may produce a *placebo effect* or a *nocebo effect*[11] (from the Latin for 'to please' and 'to injure', respectively) that expresses the subject's belief or expectancy concerning its consequences. The placebo effect of a drug or procedure is cognate to a *caring effect*[12] resulting from the subjects' belief that they are receiving care. If the subjects know that they are participating in an experiment, this awareness may in itself produce changes (the *guinea pig effect*). This is part of the possible influence of the experimental situation as a whole—the examinations and other procedures, the feedback of investigation findings, the special relations with investigators, etc.—that is sometimes called the *Hawthorne effect.* This name comes from a study of industrial efficiency at the Hawthorne Plant in Chicago in the 1920s,[13] which showed that work output increased when experimental changes were made to working conditions, even when these were worsened. Production rose

both when illumination was improved and when it was reduced to the brightness of a moonlit night. In a study of smoking by schoolchildren, the Hawthorne effect was considered as a reason for the relatively low rates observed in schools that had been surveyed repeatedly.[14]

3. *Artifacts.* The change may not be real, but only an expression of a change in methods of measurement—in diagnostic criteria or techniques, in the completeness of recording or notification, in laboratory procedures, etc.[15]

4. *Regression towards the mean.*[15] Even if the methods have not altered, an artifact may arise if measurements are very unreliable or if the characteristics they measure are very unstable. If such measurements are repeated in the same subjects, the second value will tend to be lower than the first if the initial value was high, and vice versa. A study sample selected on the grounds of initially high values of blood pressure will tend to have lower blood pressures when examined a second time, and this may be interpreted as an effect of treatment. There are various ways of overcoming this problem, one of the simplest being to use a suitable control group that is selected in the same way as the intervention group.

Depending on circumstances and the detailed objectives of the study, a control group may be exposed to an alternative treatment or programme, to no intervention whatever, or to placebo treatment. In therapeutic trials the controls are commonly given the usual standard treatment for their disease.

The groups that are compared should be similar, apart from their exposure to the experimental treatment. A story is told of a sea captain who tested a seasickness remedy during a voyage, and was very enthusiastic about the results: 'Practically every one of the controls was ill, and not one of the subjects had any trouble. Really wonderful stuff'. A sceptic asked how he had chosen the controls and subjects. 'Oh, I gave the stuff to my seamen and used the passengers as controls'.[16] Similarly, trials in which a vaccine was administered to volunteers (who may be a very select group) and in which the subsequent incidence of the disease was compared with that in a general population have led to erroneous conclusions. Experiments of this sort are similar to surveys in which different populations are compared, in that all the possibly relevant characteristics of the groups should be studied, and a careful search made for differences that may explain the findings of the study.

Various experimental and quasi-experimental designs, and methods of allocating subjects to experimental and control groups, will be discussed in Chapters 32 and 33.

NOTES AND REFERENCES

1. Hill A B 1962 Statistical methods in clinical and preventive medicine. Livingstone, Edinburgh, p. 365.
2. Childs S J 1997 Editorial: new etiology of urinary calculi. Infections in Urology 10(3): 69.
3. Last J M, Abramson J H, Friedman G D, Porta M, Spasoff R A, Thuriaux M 1995 A dictionary of epidemiology, 3rd edn. Oxford University Press, New York.
4. Jacobson R M, Feinstein A R 1992 Oxygen as a cause of blindness in premature infants: 'autopsy' of a decade of errors in clinical epidemiologic research. Journal of Clinical Epidemiology 45: 1265.
5. For references and more detailed discussions of the effects of matching, see Rothman K J, Greenland S 1998 (Modern epidemiology, 2nd edn. Lippincott-Raven, Philadelphia, pp 147–161) or Costanza M C 1995 (Matching. Preventive Medicine 24: 425).
6. As an example of the use of neighbourhood controls, in a study in Toronto 'five age-matched controls were obtained for each case. They were also matched by neighbourhood and by type of dwelling (house or apartment) in the expectation that this would lead to reasonably close socioeconomic matching. Controls were obtained by door-to-door calls, which started at the fourth door to the right of the case and proceeded systematically round the residential block or through the apartment building'. No one was found at home in two-thirds of the dwellings visited. To get an idea of whether this produced bias in the selection of controls and hence influenced the findings, a separate analysis was subsequently done, in which cases were compared with only 'those controls who were enrolled immediately after the case (or another control) had been interviewed—i.e. controls obtained without an intervening failure'. Clarke E A, Anderson T W 1979 Does screening by 'Pap' smears help prevent cervical cancer? A case-control study. Lancet ii: 1.
   In urban areas of North Carolina, a door-to-door search for neighbourhood controls matched by sex, age and race and with no history of heart attack or angina pectoris, in which the interviewer proceeded in ever-widening circles around the home of the index case, required an average of 98 minutes (94 km of travel) for each successfully matched case: Ryu J E, Thompson C J, Crouse J R 1989 Selection of neighborhood controls for a study of coronary heart disease. American Journal of Epidemiology 129: 407.
7. There may be *more than one control per subject*. If there is a constraint on the number of subjects, this increases the efficiency of the study. This may be especially important in a clinical trial where treatment is inconvenient, costly or potentially hazardous. Enlarging the control group compensates for the small number of subjects. The additional benefit is small if the ratio is increased beyond three or four; but a higher ratio may be indicated on economic grounds if the treatment is very expensive. See note 5.
8. *Individual matching* requires the prior formulation of a set of matching criteria. For each variable, it may be decided that the control must be in the same category as the case (e.g. the same 5-year age group: 30–34, 35–39, etc.; this is sometimes called *category, within-class* or *stratified matching*), or must have a defined degree of similarity (e.g. an age within 2 years of the case's; this is *caliper matching*).

Matching may be made easier (and less exact) by reducing the number of matching variables or relaxing the requirements. For example, an age disparity of up to 10 years may be regarded as acceptable. Alternatively, it may be decided that a close match will be sought, but a less close match (using a less strict criterion) will be accepted if necessary. A method sometimes used is *'nearest available' matching*, i.e. selecting the potential control who is nearest (say, in age) to the case. This method has the advantage that matches can always be found, but it is less effective than other methods in the control of confounding.

Clear rules must be laid down, stating the procedures and priorities. If one potential control is closely matched in age and less closely in educational level, and another is closely matched in education and less closely in age, which will be chosen? Standard procedures should also be laid down to cover instances where there are two or more potential controls who satisfy the criteria equally. It may be decided to select the one who is closest to the case in respect of a given matching variable (age), or the one who best meets one or more additional matching criteria, which are applied only in such instances. Use may also be made of random numbers.

For a detailed discussion of the above and other matching methods, see Anderson S, Auquier A, Hauck W W et al 1980 (Statistical methods for comparative studies: techniques for bias reduction. Wiley, New York, Ch 6).

9. Doll R, Peto R 1976 Mortality in relation to smoking: 20 years' observations on male British doctors. British Medical Journal 2: 1525.

10. Illustrations of misleading conclusions yielded by uncontrolled trials are cited by Ederer F 1975 (American Journal of Ophthalmology 79: 758), who cites Professor Hugo Muench of Harvard University's second law: 'Results can always be improved by omitting controls'.

11. *Placebo effects* are expressions of the patient's belief or expectancy that the treatment is beneficial; they may reflect the belief or expectancy of the healer, and the relationship between healer and patient may be a crucial factor.

A poser: Which was the placebo group in a trial in which preoperative patients were divided into two groups: A. (experimental)—visited for five minutes by the anaesthetist, who carefully explained what pain might be expected and tried to establish a warm and sympathetic relationship; B. (control)—cursorily visited by the anaesthetist? The patients in group A subsequently needed far less pain medication, and their hospital stay was 2.6 days shorter (Egbert L D, Battit G E, Welch C E, Bartlett M I 1964 Reduction of postoperative pain by encouragement and instruction of patients. New England Journal of Medicine 270: 825).

Another poser: Which is the placebo group in a randomized trial that compares patients who receive a homoeopathic remedy, the preparation of which involves repeated dilution in a solvent (to the extent that a dose may contain an infinitesimal amount of the agent, or maybe none) with patients who receive only the solvent? For the results of such trials, see Linde K, Clausius N, Ramirez G, Melchart D, Eitel F, Hedges L V, Jonas W B 1997 (Are the clinical effects of homoeopathy placebo effects? A meta-analysis of placebo-controlled trials. Lancet 350: 834). According to Vandenbroucke J P 1997 (Homoeopathy trials: going nowhere. Lancet 350: 824), 'a randomized trial of "solvent only" versus "infinite dilutions" is a game of chance between two placebos'.

Nocebo effects are occasioned by anxiety, fear, mistrust or doubt, and expectations of sickness. They may find expression in the reporting of side-effects of treatments. In clinical trials they are unlikely to reach the extreme of voodoo death. See Kaada B 1989 (Nocebo—the antipode to placebo. Nordisk Medecin 104: 192); Benson H 1997 (The nocebo effect: history and physiology. Preventive Medicine 26: 612) and Hahn R A 1997 (The nocebo

phenomenon: concept, evidence, and implications for public health.
Preventive Medicine 26: 607).

12. *Caring effects* are described by Hart J T, Dieppe P 1996 (Caring effects.
Lancet 347: 1606), who cite a randomized control trial in which patients
with chronic arthritis who were phoned twice a week showed significant
improvements in pain and physical and psychological disability, although
they did not use more drugs or other therapies than controls; Weinberger M,
Tierney W M, Booher P, Katz P 1989 (Can the provision of information to
patients with osteoarthritis improve functional status? A randomized
controlled trial. Arthritis and Rheumatism 36: 243); Weinberger M, Tierney
W M, Cowper E A, Katz B P, Booher P A 1993 (Cost effectiveness of
increased telephone contact for patients with osteoarthritis: a randomized
controlled trial. Arthritis and Rheumatism 36: 243).

13. Roethlisberger F J, Dickson W J 1939 Management and the worker.
Harvard University Press, Cambridge, Mass.

14. Murray M, Swan A V, Kiryluk S, Clarke G C 1988 The Hawthorne effect in
the measurement of adolescent smoking. Journal of Epidemiology and
Community Health 42: 304.

15. The term *regression toward the mean* comes from a 19th century finding that
although tall parents tended to have tall children, the children tended to be
less tall than their parents; the children of short parents tended to be taller
than their parents. The principle is that 'if all the flies in a closed room are on
the ceiling at eight o'clock in the morning, more flies will be below the ceiling
than above the ceiling at some time during the next 24-hr period'; Schor S
1969 (The mystic statistic: the floor-and-ceiling effect.) Journal of the
American Medical Association 207: 120

    Ways of preventing spurious conclusions, say in a study of the effect of
treatment on people with high cholesterol levels, include (1) comparing the
changes in treated and control groups that were selected in exactly the same
way; (2) using two or more initial measurements (e.g. one when deciding
whether the level is high enough to warrant inclusion in the trial, and another
for use as the baseline for measuring change; or basing the decision on a
mean of two or more measurements); and (3) statistical solutions.

    The effect of regression to the mean can be estimated in the analysis, e.g.
by DIFFER, a statistical program in the PEPI package (see note 7, p. 292).

16. Wilson E B Jr 1952 An introduction to scientific research. McGraw-Hill,
New York, p. 42.

8 Sampling

It is often decided to study only a part, or sample, of the study population (the 'sampled' or 'parent' population). Samples may be chosen of, for example, residents of a neighbourhood, people with (or without) a given disease, or people exposed (or not exposed) to a suspected causal factor. The decision to sample may be forced on the investigator by his lack of resources. The procedure may make for better use of available resources; because of the restricted number of individuals to be studied, it is possible to investigate each of them more fully than might otherwise have been possible, and to make greater efforts to ensure that information is in fact obtained from each individual. Frequently it is decided to have the best of both worlds, by obtaining easily acquired types of information about the total study population, but limiting certain parts of the study, which require more intensive investigations, to one or more samples.

Provided that certain conditions are met, there is no difficulty in applying the results yielded by a sample to the parent population from which it has been selected, with a degree of precision that meets the investigator's requirements. Statistical techniques are available that make it possible to state with what precision and confidence such inferences may be made. The conditions to be met are:

1. The sample must be *well chosen*, so as to be representative of the parent population. Otherwise there will be *selection bias*.
2. The sample must be *sufficiently large*. If a number of representative samples drawn from the same parent population are

investigated, it can be expected that, by chance, there will be differences between the findings in each sample; this problem of *sampling variation* is minimized if the sample is large.
3. There must be *adequate coverage* of the sample. Unless information is in fact obtained about all or almost all members of the sample, the individuals studied may not be representative of the study population; here too there may be *selection bias*.

Mere size is not enough. A sample that is badly chosen or inadequately covered remains a biased one, however big it may be. This was strikingly shown by the notorious poll conducted by the Literary Digest in 1936 which, although based on 2 000 000 ballots, dismally failed to predict Roosevelt's landslide victory in the presidential election. These ballots constituted 20% of the 10 000 000 that had been sent out to an unrepresentative sample comprising Literary Digest and telephone subscribers.

This chapter deals with sampling methods and sample size, followed by remarks on substitutions and random numbers.

SAMPLING METHODS

A sample chosen in a haphazard fashion, or because it is 'handy', is unlikely to be a representative one. Such samples have been termed 'chunks' or 'accidental' or 'incidental' samples, or 'samples of convenience'.[1] Their use has no place in community medicine research, except possibly in exploratory and other surveys where the investigator is doing no more than obtaining a 'feel' of the situation, and in some qualitative studies (see pp 166 and 348).

The recommended method is *probability sampling*, the distinctive feature of which is that each individual unit in the total population (each *sampling unit*) has a known probability of being selected. Generalizations can be made to the 'parent' population with a measurable precision and confidence (see p. 296).

First, however, a word on the nonprobability sampling methods that are sometimes used—quota, purposive and snowball sampling. In *quota sampling* the general composition of the sample, e.g. in terms of age, sex and social class, is decided in advance; quotas, or required numbers, are determined for, say, men and women of different ages and social classes, and the only requirement is that the right number of people be somehow found to fill these quotas. The disadvantage of this method is that the persons chosen may not be representative of the total population in each category, and generalizations made from the findings may be incorrect. *Purposive samples* are those selected because the investigator presumes that they are typical of the study population. In a study of general practices, for example, what is believed to be a representative cross-section of practices may be selected; subsequent generalizations from the findings may or may not be valid. In some qualitative studies (see p. 166) subjects are purposively selected not in order to represent the study population, but in such a way that they will express a wide range of the beliefs, practices or experiences under study. In *snowball sampling*[2] (*chain referral sampling*) people who meet the criteria for inclusion in the study are asked to name others who meet these criteria. This may be a useful way of identifying hard-to-find individuals, e.g. those with deviant or illegal behaviour, or homeless people. But the sample, say of drug abusers, will not necessarily be representative of all drug abusers.

We will discuss four types of probability sampling (random, systematic, cluster and stratified), and two-stage and multistage sampling.

It is important to set up the sampling rules in advance and to avoid any possibility that selection may be influenced by whim or convenience. The interviewers in a household survey, for example, should be told in advance which homes to visit. If inclusion in the sample depends on information that is collected during the visit, the interviewer should be given precise instructions for making the choice.[3]

Random sampling

Random sampling (or 'simple random sampling') is a technique whereby each sampling unit has the same probability of being selected—the laws of chance alone decide which of the individual units in the parent (or 'target') population will be selected. To avoid confusion with the colloquial meaning of the word 'random', i.e. 'haphazard' or 'without a conscious bias', the term 'strict random sampling' is sometimes preferred.

The basic procedure is:

1. To prepare a *sampling frame*. This is usually a list showing all the units from which the sample is to be selected, arranged in any order. For example, it might be a list of the registered patients

in a particular practice. The preparation of a sampling frame may sometimes require considerable effort; it is seldom easy, for example, to obtain an up-to-date list of the elderly people living in a neighbourhood. In a country or city that maintains a population register, this may constitute a sampling frame; but such registers are often out-of-date, especially with regard to addresses; moreover, with the increase in concern for the individual's right to privacy, registers of this kind are becoming less accessible to investigators. Voters' lists, telephone directories, or lists of people with driving licences may be used, but these may tend to leave out some categories of people.[4] If the frame is an incomplete and biased representation of the study population, the sample too will inevitably be biased, however strictly the rules of random sampling are applied.

2. To decide on the size of the sample (see pp 96–99).
3. To select the required number of units at random, by drawing lots or using random numbers. The use of random numbers is explained on pages 99–100. When one matched control has to be chosen randomly from a small group of suitable candidates, it is often simplest to draw lots or (if there are up to six candidates) to throw a die.

The ratio 'number of units in sample/number of units in sampling frame' is referred to as the *sampling ratio* or *sampling fraction*. It is usually expressed either in the form '1 in n' (e.g. '1 in 3', '1 in 4', etc.) or as a percentage or proportion.

Random sampling does not ensure that the characteristics of the sample and the population will coincide exactly; chance differences will exist: but by the use of appropriate statistical methods[5] it is possible to calculate the probability that these divergences lie within given limits (see p. 296).

Random sampling may be applied not only to the selection of subjects from a population, but to the selection of times or locations. In the latter instance, areas or the co-ordinates of points are used as the sampling units; the sampling frame may be a map rather than a list.

In a region where nearly everyone has a telephone at home, *random digit dialling* (i.e. phoning numbers selected at random) is a convenient way of selecting a sample, either for telephone interviews or for subsequent home interviews or other investigations. Phone numbers are kept in the sample only if they turn out to be for residential addresses. If there is no reply the call is repeated a number of times, at different times and on different weekdays. A two-stage procedure may be used, whereby a sample of households is first selected by random digit dialling and information is then obtained about the members of the household, the subsequent selection of subjects being determined by age, sex, or other eligibility criteria, or by using a random or systematic selection rule, such as the choice of the member with the latest birthdate in the year. The detailed procedure[6] is designed in a way that reduces the proportion of wasted calls; unlisted numbers are not excluded. Random digit dialling may be very time-consuming,[7] especially if there are many answering machines.

High success rates have been reported; in some studies in the United States, information on household composition was obtained for over 90% of the residential numbers phoned, and over 80% of the eligible subjects were subsequently interviewed. Samples selected by random digit dialling have been reported to be reasonably representative of the general population; but the possible selective exclusion of underprivileged population groups may be important in some studies.

Systematic sampling

Instead of selecting randomly, a predetermined system may be used. The usual technique requires a list, not necessarily numbered, of all the sampling units. Having decided on the size of the required sample, the investigator calculates the sampling ratio, expressed as '1 in n', rounds n off to the nearest whole number, and uses this figure (k) as a *sampling interval*. Every kth item in the list is then selected, starting with an item (from the first to the kth) selected at random. This technique is often easier than simple random sampling.

Such a sample can be considered as essentially equivalent to a random sample, provided that the list is not arranged according to some system or cyclical pattern. If a 1 in 30 systematic sample is selected from a list of persons arranged according to decreasing age, there may be an appreciable age difference between a sample where the first member selected was the first on the list, and one where the first person selected was the 30th. If the list is one of dwelling units, listed in such a way that ground-floor and upper-floor dwellings alternate, then a 1 in 2 systematic sample (or any systematic sample using an even number as the sampling interval) will contain either ground-floor dwellings only, or upper-floor dwellings only.

Other methods of systematic sampling may be used, not requir-ing prior listing of the sampling units. For example, it may be decided to select every third patient admitted to a hospital, or every patient whose personal identity number, social security number, hospital registration number, or birthdate (day of the month) ends with a predetermined and randomly selected digit or digits. These methods are usually chosen because of their convenience.

Cluster sampling

In cluster sampling, a simple random sample is selected not of individual subjects, but of groups or clusters of individuals. That is, the sampling units are clusters, and the sampling frame is a list of these clusters. The clusters may be villages, apartment buildings, classes of schoolchildren, housing units, households or families (note that these latter terms are not synonymous),[8] etc.

This is often a convenient method, especially when at the outset there is no sampling frame showing all the individual subjects; it is, of course, also more convenient to investigate people living in a relatively small number of households or villages, rather than the same number of persons, randomly selected, in more scattered places of residence.

The technique has the disadvantage, however, that if the clusters contain similar persons ('high intraclass correlation'), it is difficult to estimate the precision with which generalizations may be made to the parent population. If attitudes to contraception are studied by questioning a simple random sample comprising 200 individuals, it is easy to state the precision with which the findings may be applied to the total population. On the other hand, if 40 families containing 200 individuals are selected, and if attitudes on contraception tend to 'run in families', then in effect only 40, not 200 entities have been studied. Moreover, if a quarter of these families each contain 10 or more individuals, these large families will contribute an undue proportion—at least half—of the individuals in the sample (and a relationship may be assumed between family size and views on contraception).

Other things being equal, a large number of small clusters is preferable to a small number of large clusters.

Stratified sampling

To use this method, the population (the sampling frame) is first divided into subgroups or *strata* according to one or more characteristics, e.g. sex and age groups, and random or systematic sampling is then performed independently in each stratum (*stratified random sampling, stratified systematic sampling*).

This procedure has the advantage that there is less sampling variation than with simple random or systematic sampling. It eliminates sampling variation with respect to the properties used in stratifying, and if the strata are more uniform than the total population with respect to other attributes, it reduces sampling variation with respect to other properties also. The greater the differences between the strata and the less the differences within the strata, the greater is the gain due to stratification.

The same sampling ratio may be used in all strata. This is called *proportional allocation*, since the number of individuals chosen in each stratum is proportional to the size of the stratum. Alternatively, different sampling ratios may be used in different strata (*disproportionate stratified sampling*). This permits heavier sampling in subgroups with few members, so as to provide acceptable estimates, not only for the population as a whole, but also for each of its subgroups. In a clinical trial, for example, this can ensure that the sample will contain enough elderly subjects for separate study —the effectiveness and safety of treatments often differ in younger and older people.

Estimates for the total population are prepared by combining the data for the various strata. If varying sampling fractions were used, an appropriate weighting procedure is required. If a uniform sampling fraction was used, the sample is *self-weighting* and can for some purposes be treated as if it were a simple random or systematic sample. The use of varying sampling ratios greatly adds to the complexity of the analysis and should not be decided upon lightly. There is of course no objection to the use of different sampling ratios if the strata are to be kept separate throughout the analysis— e.g. if people of different religions are to be studied as separate groups.

Two-stage and multistage sampling

In two-stage sampling, the population is divided into a set of first-stage sampling units ('primary sampling units'), and a sample of these units is selected by simple random, stratified or systematic sampling. Individuals are then chosen from each of these primary units, using any method of sampling. The sample may be biased if very few first-stage units are selected.

The first-stage units may be census tracts, villages, classes of schoolchildren, households, or other aggregations. They may be time periods, e.g. if samples are chosen of patients who attend a clinic on randomly chosen days. This method has the same advantages as cluster sampling—less travel by interviewers, fewer school teachers to negotiate with, no need for a sampling frame showing all individuals in the population, etc. Two-stage cluster sampling (the selection of clusters within the chosen first-stage sampling units) will be discussed in Chapter 31.

The analysis is simplified if 'self-weighting' procedures are used. These ensure that each individual has an equal chance of entering the sample (the 'equal probability of selection method', or *'epsem'* sampling).[9] One method is to select primary units with a probability proportional to their size (*PPS* sampling), and then choose an equal number of individuals from each primary unit; for an example, see page 345.

Multistage sampling is used in large-scale surveys. A sample of first-stage sampling units is chosen, each of the selected units is divided into second-stage units, samples of second-stage units are selected, and so on. Different methods (simple random, stratified, systematic or cluster sampling) may be used at any stage.

SUBSTITUTIONS

It usually happens that after a sample has been selected it is found that some of the selected subjects cannot be investigated. People may have died or moved away, may refuse, or may be unavailable for a variety of other reasons. It is tempting to replace such subjects with other randomly selected subjects. This is an acceptable (although usually unnecessary) procedure, provided that it is remembered that if the omissions produce a sample bias, substitutions will not remove this bias. The outcome will merely be a large biased sample instead of a small biased sample. What is important, if there are more than a few omissions, is to examine the possible bias by determining the reasons for omission and, if possible, studying the demographic and other characteristics of the subjects omitted; the relevance of this bias to the study findings can then be appraised.

SAMPLE SIZE

If numbers are too small it may be impossible to make sufficiently precise and confident generalizations about the situation in the parent population, or to obtain statistical significance (see p. 307) when associations are tested. It may thus be impossible to achieve the study's objectives. On the other hand, it is wasteful to study more subjects than these objectives require. Moreover, if numbers are large enough *any* difference, however small, will be statistically significant, and there may hence be a tendency to ascribe false importance to trivial differences. ('Samples which are too small can prove nothing; samples which are too large can prove anything.')[10]

'How big should my sample be?' has been likened to the question 'How much money should I take when I go on vacation?'[11] (How long a vacation? Doing what? Where? With whom?) Calculations of sample size require both decisions and surmises.

For example, suppose a simple random sample is to be used to provide a confidence interval of a given width for the prevalence of a disease, indicating the range within which it is probable (with a given degree of confidence, usually 95%) that the true prevalence lies. To calculate the size of the sample needed for this purpose, the following must be plugged into the formula or the computer program:

1. A reasonably close estimate of the actual prevalence. (If in complete doubt, 50% can be used; this maximizes the sample size and hence errs on the safe side.)
2. The maximum acceptable difference between the estimated prevalence (based on the sample) and the actual prevalence; this 'acceptable margin of error' is half the confidence interval.
3. The required confidence level (usually 95%).
4. Also, optionally, the size of the population; this is relatively unimportant—its effect on the calculated sample size (the *finite population correction*)[12] is usually very small.

To calculate the sizes of the random samples required for a comparison of two groups, e.g. to test whether there is a significant difference between the rates of a disease in two groups in a trial or analytic survey, the requirements are:

1. A reasonably close estimate of the actual rate in one group.
2. The magnitude of the difference (or odds, rate or risk ratio) to be detected.
3. The relative size of the two samples.
4. The required significance level (e.g. 5%).
5. The required power of the test for detecting the difference (e.g. 90%), or the required precision (the width required for the confidence interval).

Computation of sample sizes can be done by using formulae, tables, nomograms, or computer programs.[13] The computed size should be increased to allow for the loss of members of the sample;[13] a larger sample will be needed if separate analyses of subgroups are intended.

Consideration must be given to practical constraints. A large sample may be difficult or impossible to find, or there may be an insufficiency of resources or time. A balance may have to be struck between the cost and the usefulness of the sample. The larger the sample, the less the sampling variation, i.e. the less the likelihood that the sample will be a misleading one. As a very rough guide, the usefulness of a sample is proportional not to its absolute size but to the square root of its size. To double the usefulness of a sample, its size must be increased fourfold; above a sample size of about 200, the absolute size of the sample must be augmented considerably to make an appreciable difference to its usefulness. This means that it may be necessary to balance increased cost (largely determined by the size of the sample) against increased usefulness (largely determined by the square root of its size). A 'sensitivity analysis'[14] may be helpful—a series of calculations of sample size, based on different assumptions and requirements.

Samples that are to be compared with one another, e.g. in case-control studies and clinical trials, are usually kept approximately equal in size, since (for a given total sample size) this provides the most precise results (i.e. a measure of association that has a narrow confidence interval). But equal groups are by no means essential, and there may be good reasons for having unequal ones.[15] The relative size of the groups must be taken into account when calculating sample size.

In some therapeutic and prophylactic trials in which the subjects enter the investigation serially, as they become available, no initial decision is made about the sample size. Instead, rules are set up in advance whereby at any stage it can be decided, on the basis of the findings to date, whether enough subjects have been studied to give a sufficiently definite answer, so that the trial can be stopped. This procedure is termed *sequential analysis*.[16]

A basic difficulty in calculations of sample size, whether they are done in advance or by the sequential method, is that the result depends on the attribute that is to be measured or compared. Samples of very different sizes are needed to study differences between two groups in their blood lipid levels, in their incidence of coronary heart disease, or in their mortality rates. It is seldom that a study is conducted to investigate only a single characteristic, and the real question often becomes not 'How many subjects do I need?' but 'With such-and-such a sample size (determined by practical considerations), about what variables and about what associations can I expect to get useful findings?—and in these circumstances, is the study worth doing?'

Cluster samples present a special case.[17] The required sample size is generally larger than for a simple random sample in the same study population, for the same maximum acceptable difference and confidence level.

The *power* of a test—its ability to demonstrate a difference if it exists, for given sample sizes—can be appraised by the same basic formulae as for calculating sample size, but used in reverse, i.e. a sample size is entered instead of power, and power is calculated instead of a sample size.

RANDOM NUMBERS

Tables of random numbers (digits arranged in a random order) are to be found in most statistics textbooks, or can be provided by a computer.[18] A short specimen (provided as an illustration, and *not* for use) is shown here (Table 8.1), and a table for actual use is provided in Appendix B (p. 407).

Table 8.1 Random numbers

Rows	Columns		
	1–4	5–8	9–12
1	96 22	74 70	80 46
2	82 14	73 36	41 54
3	21 47	59 93	48 40
4	89 31	62 79	45 73
5	63 29	90 61	86 39
6	71 68	93 94	08 72
7	05 06	96 63	58 24
8	06 32	57 11	81 59
9	91 15	38 54	73 30
10	54 60	28 35	32 94

To use a table of random numbers in selecting a sample, a number must first be allocated to each sampling unit (e.g. from 1 to the total number of sampling units). Successive random numbers are then read from the table, and the sampling units whose numbers coincide with these random numbers are chosen. This is continued until enough units have been selected. Numbers not appearing in the list of sampling units are ignored, and numbers that reappear after they have already been selected are generally also ignored. The starting-point is chosen at random, e.g. by shutting one's eyes and using a pin.

As an example, if five units are to be chosen out of nine, numbered from 1 to 9, one could start say at the '8' in row 4 of Table 8.1, and read off numbers 8, 9, 3, 1 and 6 (moving horizontally). Or one could move vertically and select the units numbered 8, 6, 7, 9 and 5; the two zeros would be ignored, as there are no subjects numbered '0'. To choose a sample from 86 units, we would use pairs of digits. Moving horizontally from the same starting-point, we would select the units numbered 89 (ignored), 31, 62, etc. To choose a sample from between 100 and 999 sampling units, we would use sets of three digits (893, 162, 794, 573, 632, and so on). With between 1000 and 9999 sampling units, we would use sets of four digits (8931, 6279, etc.).

Sometimes many numbers have to be discarded and the process may become very tedious. For example, with 195 units to choose from, if we started from the same '8' in row 4 and moved horizontally, we would find only two helpful numbers among the first 16 we looked at: 162 in row 4 and 050 (or 50) in row 7. In such instances short-cut methods may be used.[19]

NOTES AND REFERENCES

1. Riegelman R K, Hirsch R P 1989 (Studying a study and testing a test, 3rd edn. Little, Brown, Boston, p. 222) point out that, in a sense, all present-day or past samples are convenience samples 'when we desire to extrapolate research observations to patients seen in the future. Time ... cannot be randomly sampled'.
2. Faugier J, Sargeant M 1997 Sampling hard to reach populations. Journal of Advanced Nursing 26: 790.
3. Specimen instructions for interviewers: 'Ask if any children aged under 15 years live in the home. If 'yes', carry on with the interview if there is an 'A' in the sealed envelope'; this requires a prior allocation of the required proportion of As, in accordance with the sampling fraction; the envelopes should be well shuffled.
4. See Smith W, Mitchell P, Attebo K, Leeder S 1997 (Selection bias from sampling frames: telephone directory and electoral roll compared with door-to-door population census: results from the Blue Mountains Eye Study. Australian and New Zealand Journal of Public Health 21: 127).
    A New York study that used driver's licence files as a sampling frame for the selection of controls found differences (e.g. in age, income and alcohol consumption) between cases of breast cancer with and without licences (Bowlin S J, Leske M C, Varma A, Nasca P, Wienstein J A, Caplan L 1997

Breast cancer risk and alcohol consumption: results from a large case-control study. International Journal of Epidemiology 26: 915).

5. For a detailed exposition of the statistical aspects of sampling and the handling of sample data, see Cochran W G 1977 (Sampling techniques, 3rd edn. John Wiley, New York).

6. *Random digit dialling* is usually done by the procedure described by Waksberg J 1978 (Sampling methods for random digit dialing. Journal of the American Statistical Association 73: 40). See Corey C R, Freeman H E 1990 (Use of telephone interviewing in health care research. Health Services Research 25: 129); Olson S H, Kelsey J L, Pearson T A, Levin B 1992 (Evaluation of random digit dialing as a method of control selection in case-control studies. American Journal of Epidemiology 135: 210); and Perneger T V, Myers T L, Klag M J, Whelton P K 1993 (Effectiveness of the Waksberg telephone sampling method for the selection of population controls. American Journal of Epidemiology 138: 574).

In a study in Washington requiring blood tests, potential subjects were chosen by random digit dialling. The response rate was 83% in this phase, 81% in the next phase (a telephone interview) and 67% in the third phase (blood-taking). The overall rate was thus $(83 \times 81 \times 67)\%$, or only 45%, illustrating the effect of offering repeated opportunities for non-response (Brown I M, Tollerud D J, Pottern L M, Clark J W, Kase R, Blattner W A, Hoover R N 1989 Biochemical epidemiology in community-based studies: practical lessons from a study of T-cell subsets. Journal of Clinical Epidemiology 42: 561).

7. Kingery J W 1989 Sampling strategies for surveys of older adults. In: Fowler F J (ed) Health survey research methods. National Center for Health Services Research and Health Care Technology Assessment, Rockville, Md.

8. One research institute used the following operational definitions: 'A *household unit* is a room or group of rooms occupied or vacant and intended for occupancy as separate living quarters. In practice, living quarters are considered separate and therefore a housing unit when the occupants live and eat apart from any other group in the building, and there is either direct access from the outside or through a common hall, or complete kitchen facilities for the exclusive use of the occupants, regardless of whether or not they are used'. (The definition then goes on to explain what is meant by 'living apart', 'eating apart', 'direct access', etc.) A *household* is everyone who resides in a housing unit at the time the interviewer speaks to a household member and learns who lives there, including those who have places of residence both there and elsewhere. The household also includes people absent at the time of contact, if a place of residence is held for them in the housing unit and 'no place of residence is held for them elsewhere'. 'A *family unit* consists of household members who are related to each other by blood, marriage, or adoption. A person unrelated to other occupants in the housing unit—or living alone—constitutes a family unit with only one member.' If there is more than one family unit in the household, the 'primary family unit' is the one that owns or rents the home. 'If families share ownership or rent equally, the one whose head is closest to age 45 is usually considered to be the primary family.' (Survey Research Center, Institute for Social Research 1976 Interviewer's manual. University of Michigan, Ann Arbor, pp 39, 91, 94.)

9. *Epsem* sampling, which is based on probability proportional to size in the first stage, and selection of the same number of individuals from each chosen unit in the second stage, is convenient if there are not too many primary units. It is described by Yeoman K A 1970 (Statistics for the social scientist: 2. Applied statistics. Penguin Books, Harmondsworth, pp 131–132).

If there are many primary units (e.g. households) it is easier to divide them into strata according to their size, and use a different sampling fraction for each stratum, the sampling fractions being proportional to the size of the units. If a single member of each selected household is required, use may be made of a simple method described by Cochran W G 1977 (see note 5), pp 364–465.

An alternative to the 'proportional-to-size' selection of primary units is selection by simple random or systematic sampling, and the use of a uniform sampling ratio in the second stage.

10. Sackett D L 1979 Bias in analytic research. Journal of Chronic Diseases 32: 51.
11. Moses L E 1985 Statistical concepts fundamental to investigations. New England Journal of Medicine 14: 890.
12. The *finite population correction*, the factor introduced into the calculation to allow for the effect of the size of the parent population, is one minus the sampling fraction. If the sampling fraction is low this factor is close to unity, and the correction has a negligible influence and may be omitted (Armitage P, Berry C 1994 Statistical methods in medical research, 3rd edn. Blackwell Scientific Publications, Oxford, pp 83–84).
13. *Calculations of sample size.* To estimate a proportion from a simple random sample, the required sample size is

$$z^2 p \; (1-p)/d^2$$

where z = 1.96 for 95% confidence, 1.645 for 90% confidence
p = estimated proportion in study population
d = acceptable margin of error.

If the finite population correction is used, the required sample size is

$$Nz^2 p(1-p)/[d^2(N-1) + z^2 \; p(1-p)]$$

where N = size of the study population.

For other sample size formulae, refer to a statistics text, e.g. Altman D G 1991 (Practical statistics for medical research. Chapman & Hall, London, pp 455–460); Armitage P, Berry C 1994 (Statistical methods in medical research. Blackwell Scientific Publications, Oxford, pp. 195–206); Daniel W W 1995 (Biostatistics: a foundation for analysis in the health sciences, 6th edn. John Wiley, New York, pp 259–261); McNeil D 1996 (Epidemiological research methods. John Wiley, New York, pp 265–281); or Selvin S 1996 (Statistical analysis of epidemiologic data, 2nd edn. Oxford University Press, New York, pp 83–102). Formulae for use with a wide variety of statistical tests are given by Lachin J M 1981 (Introduction to sample size determination and power analysis for clinical trials. Controlled Clinical Trials 2: 93). For sample sizes when comparing several groups in a trial, see Fleiss J L 1986 (The design and analysis of clinical experiments, John Wiley, pp 371–376). For comparison of unequal groups, see Fleiss J L 1981 (Statistical methods for rates and proportions, 2nd edn. John Wiley, pp 46–47).

For tables showing sample sizes for a comparison of two proportions, see Fleiss J L 1981 (Ch. 3); or Schlesselman J J 1982 (Case-control studies: design, conduct, analysis. Oxford University Press, New York, Appendix A). For a nomogram, see Altmann D G 1991 (p. 486).

Numerous computer programs are available. In the PEPI package (see note 7, p. 292), SAMPLE computes sample size for estimating a proportion from a random or cluster sample and a mean from a random sample, SAMPLES computes sample sizes for comparisons based on simple and stratified independent samples and matched samples, and POWR estimates the power of various tests. SAMPLES can base the calculation on the required power or the width required for the confidence interval.

Compensating for losses. Allowance can be made for losses from the study sample (nonresponse, dropouts etc.)—but of course without compensating for possible selection bias—by multiplying the computed sample size by 10 000/(100-R)2, where R is the expected percentage of losses (Lachin J M 1981 [see note 13]).

14. Laird N M, Weinstein M C, Stason W B 1979 Sample size estimation: a sensitivity analysis in the context of a clinical trial for treatment of mild hypertension. American Journal of Epidemiology 109: 408.

15. See note 7, page 86.

16. Armitage P 1975 Sequential medical trials, 2nd edn. Blackwell, Oxford.

17. The required size of a *cluster sample* depends not only on the factors influencing the required size of a simple random sample, but also on the cluster size and the evenness or unevenness of the distribution of the disease or characteristic (does it occur more in some clusters than in others?).

    When a cluster sample has been used in a study, it is customary to compute and report the *design effect*, which is the ratio of the required sizes for cluster and random samples. Design effects of 2 or 3 are not uncommon, and the value may be much higher if the distribution of the disease is very uneven. The simplest way to estimate sample size for a cluster-sample survey is to calculate the required size of a simple random sample and then multiply this by the design effect reported in a previous cluster-sample survey of the same disease in a similar population, using a similar cluster size, or in a previous round of the same survey. If different studies yielded different design effects, it is prudent to use the highest value.

    The larger the cluster size, the larger the design effect. If a design effect D_1 is based on a cluster size b_1 and you wish to estimate the sample size required for a cluster size b_2, the required design effect D_2 is approximately:

$$D_2 = 1 + (D_1 - 1)(b_2 - 1)/(b_1 - 1)$$

    Methods of estimating the design effect are described by Bennett S, Woods T, Liyanage W M, Smith D L 1991 (A simplified general method for cluster-sample surveys of health in developing countries. World Health Statistics Quarterly 44: 98) and Katz J, Zeger S L 1994 (Estimation of design effects in cluster surveys. Annals of Epidemiology 4: 295). For comparisons of cluster samples, see Kerry S M, Bland J M 1998 (Sample size in cluster randomization. British Medical Journal 316: 549). For stratified cluster randomization, see Donner A 1992 (Sample size requirements for stratified cluster randomization designs. Statistics in Medicine 11: 743).

18. Computer programmes that generate random numbers (such as RANDOM in the PEPI package: see note 7, p. 292) actually produce *pseudorandom numbers*, generally using algorithms whose capacity to produce sequences of numbers that are to all intents and purposes random have been thoroughly tested.

19. Short cuts can be taken when using a table of random numbers to choose a sample. For example, if there are between 101 and 200 sampling units to choose from, read the successive three-digit numbers, and subtract the largest possible multiple of 200 from every number above 200 (also, read 000 as 200). Using the example in the text (p. 99), the sampling units selected would then be 93 (893 minus 800), 162, 194 (794 minus 600), 173 (573 minus 400), 32, 190, 18, 39, etc. If there are between 201 and 300 sampling units, subtract a multiple of 300 from numbers above 300, discarding numbers above 900. If there are between 301 and 400 sampling units, subtract 400 from numbers above 400, discarding numbers above 800. And if there are between 401 and 500, subtract 500 from numbers above 500 (take 000 as 500).

9 Selecting cases and controls for case-control studies

Selecting cases and controls for case-control studies[1] is not always as easy as it seems. Inappropriate selection of subjects is an important reason for the conflicting results these studies often produce, and for doubts about the applicability of their findings.

The usual procedure is to identify cases and then select controls. Exceptionally, an investigator may start with a data set that can be used as the control data, and then seek suitable cases for comparison ('control-initiated' studies).[2]

SELECTING CASES FOR A CASE-CONTROL STUDY

Five interrelated decisions are required:

1. What is the definition of a case?
2. Which cases will be eligible for inclusion in the study?
3. From what source will they be drawn?
4. How will they be chosen from this source?
5. How many cases are required?

A case-control study is generally performed in order to reach conclusions that are applicable not only to the specific individuals studied or the specific study population from which they are drawn, but to a reference population. The cases must therefore be suitable representatives of this reference population, and this must be kept in mind when making the above decisions.

A clear operational definition (see Ch. 11) of the disease (or other health condition) under consideration is essential. The cases may be new ones developing during a defined period (incident cases), or existing (prevalent) cases. If possible, incident cases should be used. The time lapse since exposure to the suspected causal factors is then shorter, so that it may be easier to obtain correct information about this exposure and its duration and time relationship to the onset of the disease. Also, the use of new cases avoids *prevalence–incidence bias*: if prevalent cases are used, patients who recover rapidly are likely to be under-represented, and those who die soon after onset (e.g. sudden deaths from coronary heart disease) will not be represented at all, so that if a difference is detected between cases and controls in their exposure to some factor, it may be difficult to infer that the factor is a cause of the disease rather than a determinant of recovery or survival. Prevalent cases are sometimes the only choice, for example in studies of chronic conditions with ill-defined onset times, congenital anomalies diagnosed at or after birth, and under-use or over-use of health services. If a condition is rare, incident cases may be too few to permit a useful comparison.

Eligibility criteria (inclusion and exclusion criteria) are determined mainly by the investigator's concept of the reference population, e.g. a wish to apply the findings to elderly people, fertile women, or truck drivers. Subjects are sometimes excluded on the grounds that they could not have been exposed to the 'causal' factor under study; for example, postmenopausal women and those who were sterilized many years previously might be excluded from a case-control study of the short-term effects of 'the pill'—and men certainly would be. Such decisions will reduce the cost of the study, unless it is difficult to identify ineligible subjects, but other advantages have been questioned.[3] Among other reasons for limiting eligibility, it may be decided to restrict the study to a certain category of case in order to avoid effects that might be confused with the effects of the factor under study; for example, a study might be restricted to non-smokers to avoid effects connected with smoking (see *confounding*, p. 311).

Eligibility criteria should preferably be decided in advance, even if they can be applied only after the collection of data. Care must obviously be taken not to exclude cases because of characteristics or behaviour that may be consequences of the exposure under study.

Two alternative strategies can be used for case identification. First, the cases can be sought in a defined population, e.g. the residents of a defined neighbourhood or region, the registered patients of a general practice, members of a prepaid health care plan, the children in a school, a group of factory workers or, for a nested case-control study, the people included in a cohort study. The aim would be to identify all, or a representative sample of, the eligible cases in this *population base* (*source population, study base*). A preselected source population of this kind may be termed a *primary study base*. In a study in which individuals move into or out of the source population, and this is taken into account by using person-time measures (e.g. person-years), the study base is a population-time base rather than a population base.

The other strategy is to use any convenient source of eligible cases, such as a hospital or general practice, and then try to define the population base from which the cases are drawn (a *secondary study base*). Sometimes this is easy; if the cases in a food-poisoning outbreak turn out to have attended a wedding party, for example, it is obvious that the party-goers as a whole constitute the population base for a case-control study to identify the offending foods. Usually it is more difficult, and only a vague definition of the population base is feasible. In a study of hospital patients, for example, the population base may be visualized as comprising those people who, if they had the disease being studied, would be admitted to the hospital or hospitals under consideration. A tertiary-care referral hospital that also provides general care for surrounding neighbourhoods may have patients who come from different population bases with different referral patterns, and it might be decided that a case-control study should be limited to patients from close by.[4] It is important to define the population base, however vaguely, both because the controls should be drawn from the same base and because the characteristics of the base will determine to whom the results can be generalized.

The identification of cases in the population base is sometimes complete or reasonably complete, e.g. if use is made of a case-finding survey, a cancer register, or information accumulated by a community health service that provides ongoing care for a defined population, or if the disease is one that always, or almost always, leads to hospitalization.

If case identification is incomplete, the investigator should have an idea of what the major selective factors are. Disease cases drawn from clinical sources, for example, may not be representative of all people with the disease, since there may be under-representation of those with mild symptoms and of people with a low availability or use of medical services. Cases drawn from a hospital or consultative clinic may not be typical of all cases under clinical care, and cases drawn from a teaching hospital may not be representative of all hospital cases (*referral filter bias*); also, the study may be affected by Berksonian bias (see p. 74). If the cases are drawn from other 'special populations' (see p. 73) this too will of course affect the ability to generalize.

Cases may be identified by case-finding procedures using examination, interviews or questionnaires, or from documentary sources such as clinical records, cancer and other special registers and death certificates. Whatever method is used, the cases should be chosen in an unbiased way (see *selection bias*, p. 298), e.g. by taking all consecutive eligible cases diagnosed in a given period or by selecting a random sample (see Ch. 8) representing all eligible cases identified.

Practical problems (the availability of cases, the accessibility of disease registers and other records, etc.) often influence the selection of cases. These and other constraints may necessitate reservations when the findings are interpreted.

The required number of cases is determined by the methods described in Chapter 8 (see p. 97). If cases are difficult to find, this can to an extent be compensated for by increasing the number of controls (see below).

SELECTING CONTROLS FOR A CASE-CONTROL STUDY

The main decisions to be made are:

1. Who can be a control?
2. How will controls be found?
3. How many controls are needed?
4. Should the controls be matched?

A case-control study typically compares the exposure of cases and controls to a factor suspected of being a cause of a disease (or other outcome). The purpose of the controls is to provide an estimate of what the exposure status of the cases would be if the factor was not associated with the disease. They should represent people who, if they had the disease in question, could have become cases in the study. The main requirements are that at the time of selection the controls should be free of the disease (confirmation of which may require special procedures), and that they should (ideally) come from the same study base as the cases. The controls should be representative of disease-free people in the study base (rather than of 'all disease-free people').

Any eligibility criteria applied to the cases (apart from the presence and characteristics of the disease) should be applied to the controls also. Exposure to the suspected cause must of course play no part in the selection of controls. A person who develops the disease after being selected as a control and is then selected as a case should be included in the study both as a control and as a case.[5]

If the study base is well defined and the study includes all or a representative sample of the cases in this base, it should be easy to find suitable controls by taking a representative sample of (or all) the individuals without the disease in the study base. If the study has a population-time base, in which people are members (and are hence prospective controls) for different periods, it may be decided to use a sampling procedure that takes account of duration of membership in the base[6] (this does not apply to a *case-cohort study*, whose controls represent all members of the cohort at the start of follow-up, irrespective of their duration of membership).[5] Interest is confined to the control's exposure status at or before the time of selection. Control selection may be difficult if the population base is very dynamic; in a case-control study of risk factors for injury while driving tractors, for example, it may be difficult to obtain information about the time spent on tractors by prospective controls.[7]

It may be hard to find suitable controls if the study base is vaguely defined or difficult to sample. Use is then usually made of population controls, friends or neighbours etc., or hospital or clinic controls. Each of these methods presents its own problems. Some studies are based on no more than a hope, well-founded or poorly-founded, that the controls resemble members of the study base. 'If only we lived in an epidemiologist's utopia ...', laments an epidemiologist, 'Alas, we do not live in such a place but must instead struggle on in a world of imperfect information and limited resources ... The literature on myriad threats to the validity of case-control studies conducted under real-world circumstances will no doubt continue to grow.'[8]

Population controls (community controls) may be selected by any sampling method (see Ch. 8), including random digit dialling. The obvious advantages of population controls must be weighed against the disadvantages, which include cost, inconvenience and the probability of a high nonresponse rate. Moreover, if the cases are drawn from a hospital a representative population sample may not reflect the true study base, because not everyone would land up in this hospital if they had the disease. Also, it may be difficult to ensure that the controls will be investigated in the same way as the hospital cases, and the controls may differ from hospital patients in their motivation to recall and report past events.

Use may also be made of controls identified through their relationship with the cases, e.g. friends, neighbours, spouses, siblings, fellow-workers or classmates. Such controls may tend to resemble the cases in their circumstances, lifestyles or (for blood relatives) genetic characteristics. This similarity may be an advantage, since the reduction of irrelevant differences between cases and controls may make it easier to test the study hypothesis. But it may also blur the very difference sought by the study; friends may, for example, tend to have similar smoking habits. The use of friends as controls presents particular difficulties; not only may there be reluctance to name friends, but particularly sociable or prestigious people are most likely to be named, which may cause bias if these characteristics are related to the variables under study. Selecting the control at random from a list of friends may reduce this bias, but cannot remove it. People living nearby may be useful controls for hospital cases, even if they would not go to the same hospital if they had the disease; but there may be important bias if the factors influencing hospitalization are strongly associated with the variables under study.

The use of hospital or clinic controls (patients with other diseases) for comparison with hospital or clinic cases is convenient, and it may be possible to assume that they are drawn from the same catchment population and are subject to the same selective factors as the cases. It should be remembered, however, that the probability of reaching a specific institution may vary for different diseases, depending on the reputation of its specialists, the availability of other services, etc. To minimize this problem, diseases that are similar are sometimes used, e.g. cancer controls for cancer cases. The problem is avoided if cases and controls have the same clinical picture, e.g. in a study of women referred for breast biopsies of suspicious nodules, in which those found to have breast cancer (cases) are compared with those not found to have cancer or precancerous conditions (controls).[9]

The main disadvantages of controls who have other diseases is that they are obviously a selected group, not necessarily representative of people without the disease under study. If the analysis reveals (or fails to reveal) interesting differences between the cases and controls, this may have more to do with the epidemiology of the diseases of the control patients than with the disease under study. This problem is reduced if patients with diseases known or suspected to be associated with the postulated causal factor are not used as controls—patients with lung cancer would not be good controls in a study of smoking and cervical cancer. Also, it may be wise to use a variety of diseases rather than a single disease. Patients admitted because of traffic accidents or for elective surgery are sometimes used as controls, in the probably unjustified hope that they represent the population base. Other controls sometimes used because of their easy accessibility include blood donors and hospital visitors.[10]

To avoid bias in the choice of hospital controls, systematic methods are sometimes used, e.g. the first eligible patient admitted after the study case, or the eligible patient closest in age in the same hospital ward. The best hope for avoiding Berkson's bias is to use controls who have a disease that has the same probability of hospitalization as the disease under study; the direction of the bias depends on whether the probability of hospitalization is higher for the disease under study or for the comparison condition. It is usually found that drawing controls from all hospital patients who are free of the disease under study underestimates the association between the disease and the causal factor, and use of population controls overestimates it.[11]

When deciding on a control group, attention must of course be paid to the feasibility of obtaining information comparable to that collected about the study group. An issue sometimes raised in studies where information about dead cases is obtained from proxy informants (relatives or friends) is whether dead controls (who died of other causes) should be sought, so as to ensure comparability. This procedure may, however, introduce its own biases, and it is usually preferable to use live controls and obtain the information about them from proxy informants.[12]

It is seldom easy to find a source of controls that is both convenient and free of possible bias. Each instance must be considered on its merits, and a careful choice made of the lesser of the alternative evils. It is often best to use two or more control groups (of different kinds), and to see whether different comparisons yield the same conclusion; discrepancies may throw light on the study's biases.

The number of controls per case is based on statistical requirements (see p. 97) and practical considerations. For a given total sample size, equal numbers of cases and controls yield the most precise results. If there are few cases the study's power and precision can be boosted by using more controls (after 4 controls per case, there is generally little extra benefit). If controls are individually matched, analytic methods can cope with any number (or a variable number) of controls per case.

Matching (see Ch. 7) per se does *not* prevent confounding in a case-control study; on the contrary, it introduces a bias by diminishing the difference between the total groups of cases and controls in their exposure to the postulated causal factor. However, the pay-off is that if an appropriate technique to control confounding is used in the analysis (e.g. stratification, see p. 314) this bias is removed and the results are then generally more precise than they would be if the controls were not matched.[13] If a variable is matched it becomes impossible to examine its association with the disease, but it remains possible to see whether it modifies the association between the exposure and the disease. Matching may be counterproductive if the controls are matched for variables that do not affect risk.

NOTES AND REFERENCES

1. The selection of subjects for case-control studies is considered in more detail by Lasky T, Stolley P D 1994 (Selection of cases and controls. Epidemiologic Reviews 16: 6); Wacholder S, McLaughlin J K, Silverman D T, Mandel J S 1992 (Selection of controls in case-control studies I. Principles. American Journal of Epidemiology 135: 1019); Wacholder S, Silverman D T, McLaughlin J K, Mandel J S 1992 (Selection of controls in case-control studies II. Types of controls. American Journal of Epidemiology 135: 1029); Wacholder S, Silverman D T, McLaughlin J K, Mandel J S 1992 (Selection of controls in case-control studies III. Design options. American Journal of Epidemiology 135: 1042); and Rothman K J, Greenland S 1998 (Modern epidemiology, 2nd edn. Lippincott-Raven, pp 93–114).
2. Greenland S 1985 Control-initiated case-control studies. International Journal of Epidemiology 14: 130.
3. For a debate on the exclusion of subjects with no opportunity for exposure, see Poole C 1986 (Exposure opportunity in case-control studies. American Journal of Epidemiology 123: 352); Schlesselman J J, Stadel B V 1987 (Exposure opportunity in epidemiologic studies. American Journal of Epidemiology 125: 174); and Poole C 1987 (Critical appraisal of the exposure-potential restriction rule. American Journal of Epidemiology 125: 179).
4. A study of patients treated for lymphoma in a Jerusalem teaching hospital showed differences between Jerusalem residents and patients referred from other regions, with respect to age, country of birth, religion, histologic type, and form of treatment (Paltiel O, Ronen I, Polliack A, Epstein L 1998 Two-way referral bias: evidence from a clinical audit of lymphoma in a teaching hospital. Journal of Clinical Epidemiology 51: 93).
   The possible bias caused by the inclusion of referred patients in a case-control study in such a hospital is explained diagrammatically by Morabia A

1997 (Case-control studies in clinical research. Preventive Medicine 26: 674).

5. Rothman K J, Greenland S 1998 (see note 1), pp 97–98, 108–110.

6. A simple way of allowing for variable duration of membership in the study base (*density sampling*) might be by stratified random sampling (using a uniform sampling fraction) after stratifying the prospective controls by their duration of membership in the base.

   A more elaborate method is *risk-set sampling*: each case's controls are selected from the *risk set* of people in the source population who are at risk of becoming a case at the time the case is diagnosed (Rothman K J, Greenland S 1998 [see note 1], pp 97–98).

7. Mittelman M A, Maldonado G, Gerberich S G, Smith G S, Sorock G S 1997 Alternative approaches to analytical designs in occupational injury epidemiology. American Journal of Industrial Medicine 32: 129.

8. Thompson W D 1990 Nonrandom yet unbiased. Epidemiology 1: 262.

9. For an example, see Cade J, Thomas E, Vail A 1998 (Case-control study of breast cancer in south east England: nutritional factors. Journal of Epidemiology and Community Health 52: 105).

10. Hospital visitors have been used as convenient substitutes for community controls in a number of studies: see Rathbone B, Martin D, Stephens J, Thompson J R, Samani N J 1996 (Helicobacter pylori seropositivity in subjects with acute myocardial infarction. Heart 76: 308); Perez-Padilla R, Regalado J, Vedal S, Pare P, Chapela R, Sansores R, Selman M 1996 (Exposure to biomass smoke and chronic airway disease in Mexican women. A case-control study. American Journal of Respiratory and Critical Care Medicine 154: 701); Sankaranarayanan R, Varghese C, Duffy S W, Padmakumary G, Day N E, Nair M K 1994 (A case-control study of diet and lung cancer in Kerala, south India. International Journal of Cancer 58: 644); Narendranathan M, Cheriyan A 1994 (Lack of association between cassava consumption and tropical pancreatitis syndrome. Journal of Gastroenterology and Hepatology 9: 282); and Armenian H K, Lakkis N G, Sibai A M, Halabi S S 1988 (Hospital visitors as controls. American Journal of Epidemiology 127: 404).

    A study in the Philippines found that hospital visitors and neighbourhood controls were similar with respect to numerous social and behavioural characteristics; visitors of the cases studied were not chosen (Ngelangel C A 1989 Hospital visitor-companions as a source of controls for case-control studies in the Philippines. International Journal of Epidemiology 18: S50).

11. These conclusions about *Berkson's bias* are based on algebraic analyses by Feinstein A R, Walter S D, Horwitz R I 1986 (An analysis of Berkson's bias in case-control studies. Journal of Chronic Diseases 39: 495) and Peritz E 1984 (Berkson's bias revisited. Journal of Chronic Diseases 37: 909).

12. There does not seem to be strong justification for using dead controls for dead cases (Gordis L 1982 American Journal of Epidemiology 115: 1).

    The study base consists of living subjects, and people who die represent a special sample from that base (Wacholder S, McLaughlin J K, Silverman D T, Mandel J S 1992; see note 1). In a study that used both living and dead controls, more smoking, drinking and diseases were reported for dead than living controls—'it appears that exposures associated with premature death are overrepresented in dead controls'; this difference appeared to be real, and not attributable to the obtaining of information from next of kin (McLaughlin J K, Blot W J, Mehl E S, Mandel J S 1985. American Journal of Epidemiology 121: 131, 122: 485).

13. For a more detailed discussion of the pros and cons of matching in case-control studies, see Rothman K J, Greenland S 1998 (see note 1), pp 150–160.

10 The variables

The characteristics that are measured are referred to as variables, whether they are measured numerically (e.g. age or height) or in terms of categories (e.g. sex or the presence or absence of a disease).

When an association between two variables is studied the variables may be referred to as *dependent* and *independent*. The variable we try to 'hang on' to another variable is termed the *dependent variable*. For example, in a study of prevalence of a disease in different age and sex groups, the presence of the disease may be referred to as the dependent variable, and age and sex as independent variables. On the other hand, if we study the frequency of a given symptom among persons with different diseases, the type of disease is the independent variable. If we want to know whether transcendental meditation affects the blood pressure, blood pressure is the dependent variable. Whenever we consider a causal association the outcome (the postulated effect) is the dependent variable.[1] In a therapeutic trial, the treatment is the independent variable and the measure of outcome is the dependent variable.

A variable based on two or more other variables may be termed a *composite variable*. Adiposity, for example, may be measured in terms of a 'body mass index' (Quetelet's index) calculated by dividing the person's weight by the square of his height; the units used—grams and centimetres or pounds and inches—must of course be specified. Dental caries may be measured by a DMF index, calculated by adding the number of permanent teeth that are decayed (D), the number that are missing (M), and the number that have been filled (F).

Incidence and prevalence rates, sex ratios, and all other *rates*[2] and ratios are composite variables, since they are based on separate numerator and denominator information.

During the planning of the study it is necessary to select and clarify the variables that will be measured.

SELECTION OF VARIABLES

The variables to be studied are selected on the basis of their relevance to the objectives of the investigation. If the study objectives have been formulated in writing, as previously recommended (see p. 48), the key variables will have been specifically mentioned in the objectives; the more specific the formulation of objectives, the greater the number of variables that will have been included.

There may also be variables that have not been mentioned but require to be measured if the study is to attain its aims. In selecting these additional variables, it is helpful to start with a list of all the characteristics (other than the independent variables that have already been specified) that are known or suspected to affect or cause the characteristics (dependent variables) that the investigator wants to study. Each of these variables can then be considered in turn, to decide whether it should be included in the study on any of the following five grounds:

1. It is important enough to warrant study as an *independent variable* in its own right. Its omission was an oversight.
2. It is a possible *confounding factor*, i.e. it may obscure the relationship between some other independent variable and the dependent variable, or have other deceptive effects on that relationship. It may produce an association that has little meaning in itself (see p. 312). The variable can confound the picture only if it is associated with the other independent variable as well as with the dependent one. In a study of the relationship between work accidents and age, we may decide to take the type of occupation into account, since older workers may have fewer accidents merely because they are in safer jobs. Confounding effects can arise only if the confounding variable (occupation) both influences the dependent variable (accidents) and is associated with the independent variable (age). It may be decided to eliminate the effect of possible confounders by using matching (see p. 80), but this does not obviate the need to measure them. In a trial,

subjects may be randomly allocated to experimental and control groups in order to neutralize the effect of possible confounders (see p. 311), but these variables should still be measured so that the effectiveness of the randomization procedure can be checked.

3. It may be a *modifier variable* (see p. 310), i.e. it may modify the relationship between some other independent variable and the dependent variable (or, in a trial, it may modify the effect of the treatment). It specifies the conditions for the relationship. Are older workers especially prone to accidents only in their first year of employment? Or does their special proneness (or immunity) vary in different departments of the factory? To know this, we must add 'length of employment' and 'department' to our list of variables.

4. It may be an *intervening cause* (see p. 316) that will explain a causal mechanism. Can a difference in the use of protective equipment explain the relationship between age and accidents?

5. It has a strong enough *influence* on the dependent variable to warrant its inclusion, without necessarily meeting the above criteria. If variables that strongly affect the dependent variable are included in the statistical analysis of associations (even for this reason only), this may (under certain conditions) appreciably increase the precision with which the effects of other independent variables—i.e. those of interest to the investigator—can be estimated, and increase the statistical significance of these effects. In a study of the effects of smoking or a disease on pulmonary function, for example, it would probably be decided to include sex, age, height, and the presence of a cold or cough, all of which may affect the test results.

Apart from variables with an obvious relevance to the study objectives, consideration should be given to the following four types of variables:

1. *Universal* variables. These are variables which are so often of relevance in investigations of groups or populations, that their inclusion should always be considered. They should not be automatically included, but should be automatically considered for inclusion. A suggested basic list of these variables is:

   - Sex
   - Age
   - Parity
   - Ethnic group

- Religion
- Marital status
- Social class, and attributes that may be used as indicators of social class or as variables in their own right, e.g. occupation, education, income, and household crowding index
- Place of residence (e.g. region, urban/rural)
- Geographical mobility (e.g. nativity, date of immigration).

This list may of course require modification to suit the investigator's specific interests and the reality of the populations in which he works. In certain communities it may be necessary to replace social class, for example, by some other measure of social stratification, or to add 'race' (which refers primarily to a group's relative homogeneity with respect to biological inheritance, whereas 'ethnic group' refers primarily to its shared history, social and cultural tradition, and way of life).

2. Measures of *time*. Apart from obviously relevant measurements (such as the date of onset in any study of disease incidence), in a follow-up survey or clinical trial it may be necessary to record the dates on which the subject entered and left the study. This is essential information for both the analytic techniques commonly employed in studies with varying observation periods: the use of 'person-years of observation'[3] as a denominator for the calculation of rates, and the life table method.[4]

3. *Ecologic (contextual)* measures. In a study based on individuals, consider the inclusion of relevant environmental and group variables. These may be *environmental measures* (e.g. the air pollution level, the degree of exposure to chemicals in the workplace, or the prevalence of disease-carrying mosquitoes in the neighbourhood), *aggregate measures* summarizing the status of individuals (e.g. the prevalence of tuberculosis in the place of residence), or other *(global)* measures, such as the level of poverty or crime in the region of residence, or the availability of specific screening or other health care facilities.[5]

4. Variables that delineate the *study population* (see p. 71) or populations. The characteristics of the study population may indicate the extent to which generalizations may be made from the findings. If groups are to be compared, their demographic and other similarities and dissimilarities should be known; if a sample is to be used, its characteristics should be compared with those of the parent population; if there are many non-respondents, they (or a sample of them) should be compared with respon-

dents. Measures of the attributes of the study population or populations should be included for these purposes. These may be attributes with a bearing on the study topic, or may be quite unrelated ones, introduced solely as checks on the adequacy of the matching, sampling or allocation procedures.

NUMBER OF VARIABLES

How many variables should be studied? The only answer, and not a very helpful one, is 'as many as necessary and as few as possible'. One thing is clear: the initial list is usually too long, and will have to be pruned to facilitate the collection and processing of the data. Bradford Hill tells of a plan submitted to him for a proposed inquiry into the causes of prematurity:

> It ran to a trifle of 180 questions, which covered a catholic range. For instance, it seemed that the author was confident that some person or persons—undefined in the draft I saw—could accurately inform her for each of the woman's previous confinements of the time interval between birth of the child and the placenta; the incidence of congenital malformations in her blood relations; whether she wore high- or low-heeled shoes; how often she took a hot bath; the state of health of the father at the time of conception; and the frequency of sexual intercourse, which was engagingly included under the subheading 'social amenities'. This, in my view, is not the scientific method; it is mere wishful thinking, mere hoping that *some* rabbit may come out if only the hat be made big enough.[6]

CLARIFYING THE VARIABLES

Once the variables have been selected, each of them should be clarified. There are two aspects to be considered. First, an operational definition must be formulated, clearly defining the variable in terms of objectively measurable facts, and stating, if necessary, how these facts are to be obtained (see Chs 11 and 12). Secondly, the scale of measurement to be used in data collection should be specified (Chs 13 and 14).

An example is given showing part of the list of variables to be measured in a survey of illnesses among hospitalized infants (Table 10.1). Whether the record should take this or another format is a matter of taste; but the information it contains should certainly be recorded somewhere. It will be noted that the list contains two variables, age and social class, on which no direct data are obtained. In this study, age is a composite variable based on the date of birth and date of admission, and social class is inferred from the father's occupation. The construction of the list in this way serves as a reminder of the basic data that must be collected.

If the investigation is concerned with more than one study population, more than one list of variables may be needed; but the

Table 10.1 Selected variables in a survey of illnesses among infants

Variable	Definition	Scale
Date of birth	Infant's date of birth, as recorded in hospital records	Full date (day, month, year)
Date of admission	Date of infant's admission to hospital, as recorded in hospital records	Full date (day, month, year)
Age	Infant's age at admission to hospital, calculated from date of birth and date of admission	Completed months (0 to 11) (99 if unknown)
Mother's age	Age at birth of infant, as stated by mother	1. Under 20 years 2. 20–24 years 3. 25–29 years 4. 30–34 years 5. 35–39 years 6. 40 years or more 9. No information
Father's occupation	Father's usual occupation, as stated by mother	Detailed occupation
Social class	Father's occupational grade, using British Registrar-General's grading scheme (see p. 124)	1. Social class I 2. Social class II 3. Social class III 4. Social class IV 5. Social class V 9. Unclassifiable
Reason for admission to hospital	Final diagnosis, according to hospital records; if two or more, the one stated by hospital physician to have been the principal reason for admission	Detailed categories in International Classification of Diseases (10th revision)
Haemoglobin	In capillary blood, measured by [specified] method within 24 hours of admission	g per 100 ml, rounded off downwards to nearest g
Mother's satisfaction with hospital	Response to specific question put to mother within week after infant's discharge or death	1. Very satisfied 2. Satisfied on the whole 3. Somewhat dissatisfied 4. Very dissatisfied 9. Don't know, or no answer

full details about each variable need not be obsessively inserted in each list.

COMPLEX VARIABLES

Some variables are too complex to be easily measured as single entities, and are best broken up into component aspects that can be regarded as separate variables and measured separately.

If we wish to investigate the 'attitude to abortions', for example, we would be well advised to obtain separate measures of the attitudes to abortions performed for medical, economic and psychological reasons, to those carried out by medical practitioners and by unqualified persons, to those performed on married and unmarried women, etc. It may afterwards be possible to combine these separate measures into a single integrated measure of 'attitude to abortions' (now a composite variable).

Similarly, if we wish to study electrocardiogram (ECG) findings we may, instead of making a global and probably subjective appraisal of the ECG pattern, give separate consideration to a series of different measurable aspects, Q and QS patterns, S-T junction and segment depression, etc. This approach is the basis of the Minnesota code for the classification of ECG findings, which is widely used in epidemiological studies.[7] Different combinations of ECG findings may afterwards be used to provide electrocardiographic diagnoses of myocardial infarction and other disorders (composite variables). In longitudinal studies in which ECG examinations are repeated, electrocardiographic diagnoses may be based on the combined findings of serial Minnesota codes.

NOTES AND REFERENCES

1. By the definition used in the text, chronic bronchitis is the dependent variable in a study of the effect of smoking on the occurrence of chronic bronchitis, even if a case-control study is used. The term may also be used differently: in a study that compares the smoking habits of cases (bronchitics) and controls, a statistician might regard smoking habits as the dependent variable in the statistical analysis, the postulated effect (disease) being the independent variable; if a regression analysis is used, the variable predicted by the regression equation is called the dependent variable.
2. A *rate* expresses the frequency of an event or characteristic. It is generally calculated by dividing the number of events (e.g. deaths or disease onsets) by the total of the periods during which individual members are in the study population (expressed in person-years or other person-time units—see note 3) or by dividing the number of persons with a characteristic (e.g. a disease) by the 'population at risk' (the total number of persons in the group or

population), and then multiplying by 100, 1000, or another convenient figure. There is an increasing tendency to use the term 'rate' only for 'true' rates whose denominators are person-time units, and to use other terms (e.g. 'proportion') for other measures.

The importance of *denominator data* cannot be overstressed (see p. 71). It has been said that in the same way as a clinician keeps a stethoscope handy, an epidemiologist should always carry a denominator in his back pocket. If the numerator is confined to a specific category, e.g. males, the denominator should be similarly restricted (sex-specific rates, age-specific rates, etc.).

Prevalence tells what proportion of individuals have a disease or other attribute at a given time. It is a measure of what *exists. Incidence* refers to what *happens* (e.g. disease onsets or deaths) during a specified period. Incidence may be expressed as a *cumulative incidence ('risk')*—the proportion of initially disease-free individuals who develop the disease during a stated period—or as a *person-time incidence rate* ('incidence density', 'mortality density'). For clarification, see any recent epidemiology textbook.

Standardized and other *adjusted rates* are estimates of what the rate *would* be under specified conditions, e.g. if the age or sex composition of the study population conformed with a specified standard, or if the groups under comparison were similar with respect to defined independent variables. *Crude rates* are rates (for a whole population) that have not been adjusted.

3. To calculate *person-years* (or person-months, etc.) of observation, it is necessary to know the length of each subject's period of observation, from the start of follow-up until its end (i.e. until occurrence of the 'endpoint' event under study: death, loss of contact, conclusion of the study, or withdrawal from follow-up for some other reason). The sum total of these periods can be used as a person-time denominator for an incidence or mortality rate. It has been called 'candidate time' (Miettinen OS 1985 Theoretical epidemiology: principles of occurrence research in medicine. Wiley, New York, p. 319).

A member of an Internet discussion group ('list') on epidemiological methods (which you can join by sending an e-mail message 'SUBSCRIBE EPIDEMIO-L < your first and last name >' to LISTPROC@CC. UMONTREAL. CA) thanked other members for explaining how to compute the incidence rates he wanted, then added: 'P.S. It was cows, not persons!' ('Individual-time' rather than 'person-time'?).

4. The analysis of *survival* (non-occurrence of a defined endpoint event, such as the onset of a disease or complication, or death) is discussed by (among others) Selvin S 1996 (Statistical analysis of epidemiologic data, 2nd edn. Oxford University Press, New York, Chs 10–12).

5. Morgenstern H 1998 Ecologic studies. In: Rothman K J, Greenland S 1998 Modern epidemiology, 2nd edn. Lippincott-Raven, Philadelphia, pp 459–480.

6. Hill A B 1962 Statistical methods in clinical and preventive medicine. Livingstone, Edinburgh, p. 360.

7. Prineas R J, Crow R C, Blackburn H 1982 The Minnesota code manual of electrocardiographic findings: standards and procedures for measurement and classification. John Wright PSG, Boston.

The use of serial readings is described by (among others) Crow R S, Prineas R J, Hannan P J, Grandits G, Blackburn H 1997 (Prognostic associations of Minnesota Code serial electrocardiographic change classification with coronary heart disease mortality in the Multiple Risk Factor Intervention Trial. American Journal of Cardiology 80: 13).

11 Defining the variables

Each of the variables measured in a study should be clearly and explicitly defined. Unless this is done, there can be no assurance that, if the study were performed by a different investigator, or repeated by the same investigator, similar findings would be obtained.

The same term may have more than one meaning, even in day-to-day usage; there are no hard and fast, universally accepted, 'correct' definitions. The investigator must choose a definition that will be useful for the purposes of the study. Like Humpty Dumpty, the investigator can say, 'when *I* use a word, it means just what I choose it to mean—neither more nor less'.

There are two kinds of definition—conceptual and operational.

The *conceptual definition* defines the variable as we conceive it. This definition is often akin to a dictionary definition. For example, 'obesity' may be variously defined as: 'excessive fatness'; or as 'over-weight'; or as 'a bodily condition which is socially regarded as constituting excessive fatness'. In effect, the conceptual definition is a definition of the characteristic we would like to measure.

In contrast, the *operational definition* (or 'working definition') defines the characteristic we will actually measure. It is phrased in terms of objectively observable facts, and is sufficiently clear and explicit to avoid ambiguity. Where necessary, it states the method by which the facts are obtained. 'Obesity', for example, might be operationally defined in different surveys as:

> a weight, based on weighing in underclothes and without shoes, which exceeds, by 10 per cent or more, the mean weight of persons of the subject's sex, age and height (in a specified population at a specified time)

or as

> a skinfold thickness of 25 mm or more, measured with a Harpenden
> skinfold caliper at the back of the right upper arm, midway between
> the tip of the acromial process and the tip of the olecranon process
> (this level being located with the forearm flexed at 90°), with the arm
> hanging freely and the skinfold being lifted parallel to the long axis of
> the arm

or as

> a positive response to the question 'Are you definitely over-weight?'

or as

> a positive response to the question 'Does your husband/wife think you
> are too fat?'

It is often helpful, but it is not always essential, to formulate the
conceptual definition of a variable. On the other hand, it is always
necessary to formulate the operational definition.

In doing this, the investigator is heavily influenced not only by
the need to come as close as possible to the conceptual definition, but
also by considerations of practicability. In most research on blood
pressure, the characteristic in which the investigator is interested is
the pressure within the arteries; as intra-arterial measurements are
usually not feasible, blood pressure is usually defined in terms of
measurements made externally with a sphygmomanometer. This
operationally defined blood pressure may be markedly different
from the intra-arterial pressure, particularly in fat subjects.

Similarly, social class may be operationally defined in terms of
the classification of occupations (summarized in Table 11.1) used
by the British Registrar-General; in the case of children, the father's
occupation is often used, and in the case of married women, the
husband's. Social class, so defined, does not necessarily corre-
spond with the researcher's conception of social class, which may
have to do with prestige or wealth or power or social connections
or knowledge or living conditions or lifestyle.[1] But in a particular
investigation this definition (or some other simple definition, such
as educational level) may be a practical one to use, while the information the researcher really wants may be difficult or impossible to
obtain.

In other words, the investigator is playing what has been called
a 'substitution game'. He is substituting what he *can* measure—a
proxy variable—for what he *would like* to measure. Discrepancies
may be unavoidable, but the investigator should at least be aware

Table 11.1 Social class: classification of occupations	
Social class	Occupations (selected list)
I. Upper and middle	Higher professional, e.g. medicine, engineering, architecture, authors, scientists Large employers Directors of business
II. Intermediate	Lower professional, e.g. teachers, pharmacists, social workers Owners of small businesses and managers Farmers
III. Skilled workers and clerical workers*	Artisans, clerks, foremen, supervisors
IV. Intermediate	Semi-skilled workers, e.g. factory operatives Agricultural labourers
V. Unskilled workers	Labourers, etc. Domestic servants Casual workers

*May be divided into IIIN—nonmanual skilled workers, and IIIM—manual skilled workers

of them. If they are perforce large, he may need to reconsider whether it is worth his while measuring the variable at all, and even whether his whole investigation is worthwhile.

As an example, suppose we wish to perform a survey to test the hypothesis that drivers whose emotional health is disturbed have a higher risk of being involved in road accidents. Clearly, 'emotional health' will be difficult to define in operational terms. The defining of 'accidents', on the other hand, seems an easier nut to crack; after all, everyone knows what an accident is. In actual fact, the task is not so easy. Do we want to include all mishaps occurring on the road, including 'near misses', or only those which result in damage? If the latter, are we to include any damage, whether to vehicles, lamp-posts, cats, dogs, etc., or only injury to human beings? If we confine the study to accidents causing injuries to humans, will we include mild and transient injuries, such as temporary emotional shock, or only more severe ones?—and if the latter, what precisely do we mean by 'more severe'? Whatever definition of 'accident' we are considering, is it a practical one? Will we be able to get the required information? Maybe we will have to fall back on accidents reported to the police or insurance companies (which are not necessarily representative samples of accidents), or even confine ourselves to fatal accidents. In the latter instance our case ascertainment may be fairly complete, but we will be investigating only the tip of the iceberg, and ignoring the main bulk of accidents. Maybe accidents defined in different ways have different associations with emotional health.[2] Can we find a definition that meets our need, or should we give the whole thing up as a bad job?

In the light of what has been said above it is clearly impossible to suggest a list of 'recommended' definitions. Instead, we will draw attention to a number of questions that may arise when definitions are sought for certain frequently used variables.

1. *Occupation*—Present or usual occupation? Occupation for which subject was trained (profession or trade), or work actually performed? If retired or unemployed, will previous occupation be used?
2. *Education*—Number of years of education, or last grade attained, or type of educational institution last attended, or age at completion of full-time education?
3. *Income*—Personal income, family income, or average family income per member? Income from all sources, or only from gainful employment? Total (gross) earnings, or net earnings, after subtraction of income tax and social security payments and other 'deductions at source'? Is income 'in kind', e.g. free lodgings or self-grown vegetables or crops, included?
4. *Crowding index* (mean number of persons per room in housing unit)—What rooms are excluded (bathrooms, showers, toilets, kitchens, store-rooms, rooms used for business purposes, entrance halls)? Are children taken as wholes or halves in the computation?
5. *Social class*[1]—Based on occupation, education, crowding index, income, neighbourhood of residence, home amenities, or subject's self-perception? Based on one of these, or a combination? If based on occupation, will women be graded by their own or their husbands' occupations? If the latter, how will unmarried women, widows and divorcees be graded? Will all members of the household be graded according to the occupation of the head of the household? And if so, how is 'head of the household'[3] defined? What occupational classification is suitable for use in the specific community being studied?
6. *Ethnic group*[4]—In terms of 'race' (see p. 118), country of birth, father's country of birth, mother's country of birth, tribe, religion, or subject's self-perception?

7. *Marital status*—In terms of legal status (single, married, widowed, divorced; and, in some communities, 'common law marriages' and 'separated'); or in terms of stability of union, e.g. stable union, casual union? Present status, or total marital experience ('second marriage', etc.)?

8. *Parity*—Total number of previous pregnancies, or only those terminating in still or live births, or number of children delivered?

9. *Date of onset of disease*—Date when first symptoms were noticed, or date when first diagnosed, or date of notification?

10. *Presence of chronic disease*[5]—Based on duration since onset? If so, what duration makes it chronic?—3 months, 6 months, a year? Based on presence of certain diseases that are defined as chronic whatever their duration? If so, what diseases? Do they include dental caries, myopia, obesity? Are chronic symptoms enough (cough, constipation)? What about conditions that come and go, e.g. frequently recurrent sore throats?

11. *Disability*—Capacity to function, or actual performance? Difficulty in performance, or need for assistance?[6] Appraised by self, by family, or by examiner? What functions are considered?—ability to get around alone, or perform physical activities,[7] or carry out major activity (work, housework, schoolwork—but what is a pensioner's 'major activity'?), or see, hear, carry out activities of daily living? Emphasis on impairments (physical and mental abnormalities) or disability (reduced capacity to function) or handicap (reduced capacity to fulfil a social role)? Long-term disability only, or temporary disability also (days of work-loss or school absence, days in bed, days with restricted activity on account of illness or injury)? Measured as percentage disability, using rating scales established for entitlement to benefits (workmen's compensation, etc.)? Emphasis on effect on quality of life, for use in computation of quality-adjusted life-years?[8]

12. *Overall or general health*—Appraised by physician, nurse, or self?[9]—and if by self, appraisal in comparison with others of same age and sex? Physical, mental, social, or comprehensive health? Based only on presence or absence of specific diseases? Subjective wellbeing? Functional capacity? Positive aspects of health?

13. *Quality of life*[10]—'Health-related quality of life' (personal experience more specifically related to health or health care) or (more generally) overall life satisfaction, living standards, goal

achievement, social utility? Related to a specific health problem and its care, or 'generic'? Appraised in relation to a specific group (e.g. elderly, children)?[11] A global appraisal, or measures of different dimensions (physical, emotional and social function, role performance, pain, etc.)? Assessed by whom?[12] Subjective wellbeing as well as functional status?

14. *Physician visit*—Including telephone consultations? What if the service was provided by a nurse or other person acting on the doctor's instructions? If a patient comes for a certificate or to collect a letter, is this a visit? Can a visit be paid in absentia— if a mother comes to consult a doctor about her child, is the visit ascribed to the mother or the child? If she consults the doctor about herself, and the doctor uses the opportunity to discuss her son's health, or to prescribe treatment for him, is the visit ascribed to the son also?

15. *Hospitalization*—Is hospitalization for childbirth included? Is the hospital stay of a well newborn baby included? Is overnight stay essential? Is overnight stay in a casualty ward included? What institutions qualify as hospitals?

16. *Breast-feeding*—Is a single breast-feeding enough to label an infant as 'breast-fed'? When is a child 'exclusively breast-fed' and when 'partially breast-fed'?—does *any* bottle-feeding, even with small quantities of liquid, make the child 'partially' breast-fed? Is a child who receives minimal supplementary ('token') breast-feeding to be regarded as breast-fed?[13]

If it is hoped to obtain information which can be directly compared with the findings of other studies, care must be taken to use the operational definitions used in the other studies. For a few variables, such as 'underlying cause of death'[14] and 'neonatal death', internationally recommended and generally accepted definitions are available.

Finally, it must be noted that there are some variables for which, paradoxically, detailed operational definitions can be formulated only after the findings have been analyzed. These are composite variables based on combinations of a number of separate items, using rules that are determined only after the actual interrelationship between the items has been examined (see pp 152–155).

NOTES AND REFERENCES

1. *Measures of social class* are reviewed by Krieger N, Williams D R, Moss N E 1997 (Measuring social class in US public health research: concepts,

methodologies and guidelines. Annual Review of Public Health 18: 401) and Berkman L F, Macintyre S 1997 (The measurement of social class in health studies: old measures and new formulations. IARC Scientific Publications 138: 51). Also, see a set of papers on 'Measuring social inequalities in health', introduced by Krieger N, Moss N 1996 (Accounting for the public's health: an introduction to selected papers from a U.S. conference on 'measuring social inequalities in health'. International Journal of Health Services 26: 383). For a brief discussion, see Susser M, Warren W, Hopper K 1985 (Sociology in medicine, 3rd edn. Oxford University Press, New York). Also, see Abramson J H, Gofin R, Habib J, Pridan H, Gofin J 1982 (Indicators of social class: a comparative appraisal of measures for use in epidemiological studies. Social Science and Medicine 16: 1739).

The British Registrar-General's classification is sometimes called the *OPCS classification* (Office of Population Censuses and Surveys 1980 Classification of occupations. HMSO, London). For a comprehensive review of occupation-based measures, see Hauser R M, Warren J R 1997 (Socioeconomic indexes for occupations: a review, update, and critique. In: Raftery A E, ed. 1997 Sociological methodology 1997. American Sociological Association and Basil Blackwell, Cambridge, Mass., pp 177–298); also available on the Internet (www.ssc.wisc.edu/cde/cdewp/1996papers.htm).

In many populations, *neighbourhood of residence* may be a simple and useful measure of social class, one advantage being that it is as easily applicable to women as to men. In Scotland, for example, coronary heart disease in both sexes bears similar relationships to occupation-based social class and to a 'deprivation index' based on features of the area (postal-code sector) of residence, namely the prevalence of unemployment, household crowding, semiskilled or unskilled labour, and nonownership of a car (Woodward M 1996 Small area statistics as markers for personal social status in the Scottish heart health study. Journal of Epidemiology and Community Health 50: 570). See Carstairs V 1995 (Deprivation indices: their interpretation and use in relation to health. Journal of Epidemiology and Community Health 49 [suppl 2]: S3).

A combination of criteria may be more useful than a single criterion. A cohort study in Britain, for example, showed wider mortality differentials when house and car ownership were taken in conjunction with occupation-based social class than when the latter was used alone (Wannamethee S G, Shaper A G 1997 Socioeconomic status within social class and mortality: a prospective study in middle-aged British men. International Journal of Epidemiology 26: 532).

2. In a national study in Britain, the definition of 'childhood accident' was found to be a crucial factor in determining results. Accidents 'resulting in an injury for which the child was admitted to hospital' were associated with large family size, whereas accidents 'resulting in an injury which warranted medical attention' were not (Stewart-Brown S, Peters T J, Golding J, Bijur P 1986 Case definition in childhood accident studies: a vital factor in determining results. International Journal of Epidemiology 15: 352).

3. Identification of the *head of the household* or *head of the family* usually presents no problem. If in doubt, members of the household or family can be asked whom they regard as the head. Alternatively, detailed operational definitions may be devised—'Do not expect your informant to know our definition of a family head. Determine it yourself on the basis of these criteria ...' (Survey Research Center, Institute for Social Research 1976 Interviewer's manual. University of Michigan, Ann Arbor, pp 94–95).

4. Distinctive features of an *ethnic group* include shared origins and history, traditions, language and other components of culture, and a sense of identity and group membership. It may be best determined by self-assessment. See

Senior P A, Bhopal R 1994 (Ethnicity as a variable in epidemiologic research. British Medical Journal 309: 327) and Bhopal R 1997 (Is research into ethnicity and health racist, unsound, or important science? British Medical Journal 314: 1751).

A focus on ethnicity may be useful in the appraisal of the health, health care and needs of definable sectors of the population, and (potentially) may lead to exploration of social, economic, environmental and behavioural influences that account for many differences in health. See Muntaner C, Nieto F J, O'Campo P 1996 (The bell curve: on race, social class, and epidemiologic research. American Journal of Epidemiology 144: 531).

5. In a well-known survey of *chronic disease* in the USA, the initial working definition was: 'Chronic disease comprises all impairments or deviations from normal which have *one or more* of the following characteristics: are permanent, leave residual disability; are caused by nonreversible pathological alteration; require special training of the patient for rehabilitation; may be expected to require a long period of supervision, observation or care'. This was found to be too vague and to include too many trivial disorders. In practice the examining physicians recorded all chronic conditions they detected, but conditions were disregarded if they were not 'medically disabling', i.e. if it was thought they did not affect the patient's wellbeing or interfere with his activities and were unlikely to do so. The report states: 'It is difficult to state concisely and specifically what conditions are included in these data on "chronic diseases". In the final analysis, the definition is the list of 47 diagnostic categories, plus two "all other" groups, for which data are presented'. These hold-all 'other diagnoses' groups included a quarter of all cases (Commission on Chronic Illness 1959 Chronic Illness in the United States, Vol III. Chronic illness in a rural area: the Hunterdon study. pp 149–151); and 1957 Vol IV. Chronic illness in a large city: the Baltimore study. pp 49–50; 513–520. Harvard University Press, Cambridge, Mass.).

In the United States Health Interview Survey a condition was considered chronic if it was reported to have been first noticed more than 3 months previously, or if it was in a list of 34 conditions that were always considered chronic. These were phrased in lay terms, e.g. 'heart trouble' and 'repeated trouble with back or spine'. (National Center for Health Statistics 1975 health interview survey procedure 1957–1974. Vital and Health Statistics series 1, no 11. Department of Health, Education, and Welfare, Washington, pp 127–128).

6. Some measures of disability in activities of daily living focus on difficulty in performance, others on the need for assistance by another person. Obviously, many people have difficulty without requiring assistance; in one study, 13% of elderly people reported trouble getting into or out of bed, but only 3% needed assistance. A focus on difficulty is appropriate in studies of the effects of illnesses, impairments, or care, whereas a need for assistance is especially relevant in studies concerned with planning or costing of services (Jette A M 1994 How measurement techniques influence estimates of disability in older populations. Social Science and Medicine 38: 937).

7. Abramson J H, Ritter M, Gofin J, Kark J D 1992 A simplified index of physical health for use in epidemiological studies. Journal of Clinical Epidemiology 45: 651.

8. See note 12, page 65.

9. Numerous studies have shown that negative self-appraisals of health are predictive of subsequent mortality (Idler E L, Benyamini Y 1997 Self-rated health and mortality: a review of twenty-seven community studies. Journal of Health and Social Behavior 38: 21).

10. Measures of *quality of life*, which have proliferated in recent years, are reviewed at length by Bowling A 1997 (Measuring health: a review of quality

of life measurement scales. Open University Press, Buckingham) and briefly by Carr A J, Thompson P W, Kirwan J R 1996 (Quality of life measures. British Journal of Rheumatology 35: 275). Core elements are summarized by Muldoon M F, Barger S D, Flory J D, Manuck S B 1998 (What are quality of life measurements measuring? British Medical Journal 316: 542). Also, see Guyatt G H, Feeny D H, Patrick D L 1993 (Measuring health-related quality of life. Annals of Internal Medicine 118: 622); Fitzpatrick R, Fletcher A, Gore S, Jones D, Spiegelhalter D, Cox D 1992 (Quality of life measures in health care I: Applications and issues in assessment. British Medical Journal 305: 1074); Fletcher A, Gore S, Jones D, Fitzpatrick R, Spiegelhalter D, Cox D 1992 (Quality of life measures in health care II: Design, analysis and interpretation. British Medical Journal 305: 1145); and Spiegelhalter D, Gore S M, Fitzpatrick R, Fletcher A, Jones D R, Cox D R 1992 (Quality of life measures in health care III: Resource allocation. British Medical Journal 305: 1205).

Cultural factors should not be ignored. When asked about the effects of their symptoms on the quality of life, French patients considered all sexual aspects of life more important than English patients did (Calais D S F, Marquis P, Deschaseaux P, Gineste J L, Cauquil J, Patrick D L 1997 Relative importance of sexuality and quality of life in patients with prostatic symptoms: results of an international study. European Urology 31: 272).

11. Quality of life in specific age groups: see Pal D K 1996 (Quality of life assessment in children: a review of conceptual and methodological issues in multidimensional health status measures. Journal of Epidemiology and Community Health 50: 391); and Kutner N G, Ory M G, Baker D I, Schechtman K B, Hornbrook M C, Mulrow C D 1992 (Measuring the quality of life of the elderly in health promotion intervention clinical trials. Public Health Reports 107: 530).

12. Doctors and patients may disagree about the quality of life. Patients with multiple sclerosis, for example, are less concerned than their doctors about their physical disability; their ratings of physical disability do not correlate with their quality-of-life appraisals (Rothwell P M, McDowell Z, Wong C K, Dorman PJ 1997 Doctors and patients don't agree: cross sectional study of patients' and doctors' perceptions and assessments of disability in multiple sclerosis. British Medical Journal 314: 1580). In a study in which cardiac outpatients, family members and medical staff were asked what they considered were important elements in the patients' quality of life, the patients, in contrast to family and staff, chose aspects that reflected the positive aspects of life (Woodend A K, Nair R C, Tang A S 1997 Definition of life quality from a patient versus health care professional perspective. International Journal of Rehabilitation Research 20: 71). Yet subjects were asked to make their own ratings in only 13 of 75 quality-of-life studies reviewed by Gill T M, Feinstein A R 1994 (A critical appraisal of the quality of quality-of-life measurements. Journal of the American Medical Association 272: 619).

13. Labbok M H, Belsey M, Coffin C J 1997 A call for consistency in defining breast-feeding. American Journal of Public Health 87: 1060.

14. World Health Organization 1992 International statistical classification of diseases and related health problems: tenth revision, vol 1. World Health Organization, Geneva, p. 1235.

12 Definitions of diseases

It is as important to establish clear operational definitions for diseases as for other variables. This is a far from easy task. Clinicians tend to establish a diagnosis by making a clinical judgement of the extent to which the picture presented by the patient conforms with their *concept* of the disease in question. Use is seldom made of rigid diagnostic rules. That is, the diagnosis tends to be based on a conceptual rather than on an explicit operational definition. Inevitably, doctors often disagree.

In a survey or trial, unless clear working definitions are used the findings will not be reproducible, nor will it be easy to apply the conclusions in clinical or other real-life situations. If we have formulated and used an operational definition of rheumatic fever, we can report how many cases of rheumatic fever we have found, with the assurance that another investigator, using the same definition, would have obtained similar findings. This is the basis of good research. Our rigid rules may mean the inclusion of cases who some clinicians think do not have the disease, as well as the exclusion of patients who some clinicians think do have the disease, or who they believe should be given the benefit of the doubt and treated as if they had the disease, in order to prevent complications. Such discrepancies, although we should try to minimize them by choosing a satisfactory definition, need not concern us. The clinicians' decisions (or some of them) may be best for their patients, but when we report our findings concerning rheumatic fever, we know and can explain exactly what we mean by the term.

Unfortunately, few diseases have satisfactory and widely accepted operational definitions. The definitions provided in medical text-books are usually conceptual ones. Here is one example:[1]

> A *common cold* is an acute, self-limited, infectious disorder characterized by nasal obstruction and/or discharge and frequently accompanied by sneezing, sore throat, and nonproductive cough.

It is obvious that this definition does not aim to provide rules for diagnosing a cold. No method is mentioned for determining the infectious nature of the disorder, and the phrase about sneezing, sore throat and cough is equivocal—are these manifestations essential for the diagnosis?

OPERATIONAL DEFINITIONS

By contrast, operational definitions of diseases, like those of other variables, should be phrased in terms of objectively observable facts, and should be sufficiently clear and explicit to avoid ambiguity. Operational definitions of this sort are formulated in terms of *diagnostic criteria*; that is, the definition constitutes a set of rules for the diagnosis of the disease, based on the presence or absence of specified criteria.

These criteria may be *manifestations* or *causal experiences*.[2] Manifestational criteria include physical findings, symptoms, behaviour, the course of the illness, the response to specific therapy, etc. 'Causal' criteria are types of experience begun at a time preceding the illness, and often loosely called 'the cause' of the illness, e.g. difficult birth, an accident, exposure to lead, or contact with a case of measles. For a specific disease, either manifestational or experiential criteria, or both, may be used.

The diagnostic criteria of a disease are chosen from those manifestations and experiences which are relatively frequent among persons whom clinicians diagnose as suffering from the disease, by comparison with their frequency among well persons and among patients with other diseases. Certain of these manifestations and experiences are selected as diagnostic criteria, and rules are established for the diagnosis of the disease. For example, the disease may be diagnosed:

1. only when all the criteria are present or
2. only when a sufficient number of them are present or
3. only when specific combinations of criteria are present or
4. only when certain specific criteria (or specific combinations) are

present, and certain other additional conditions are met (e.g. a sufficient number of 'minor' criteria are present) or

5. only when a score, obtained by adding defined weights allocated to each of the criteria, reaches a specified level; such a weighting system makes it possible to attach more diagnostic importance to some criteria than to others or
6. only when one of the above conditions is met, and in addition the presence of certain defined other diseases can be excluded.

As an illustration, a diagnosis of an initial attack of rheumatic fever can be made (with 'a very high probability') in the presence of any two of the following major manifestions or the presence of any one major manifestation and any two minor manifestations, provided (in all instances) that there is also supporting evidence of preceding group A streptococcal infection:[3]

Major manifestations
- Carditis
- Polyarthritis
- Chorea
- Erythema marginatum
- Subcutaneous nodules

Minor manifestations
- Arthralgia
- Fever
- Elevated acute phase reactants
  — Erythrocyte sedimentation rate
  — C-reactive protein
- Prolonged PR interval

Evidence of antecedent group A streptococcal infection
- Positive throat culture or rapid streptococcal antigen test
- Elevated or rising streptococcal antibody titre

The rules may sometimes be validated by a comparison with diagnoses established by a 'better' set of criteria, i.e. an operational definition which, prima facie or because it incorporates more sophisticated or accurate tests (but is too elaborate or expensive for general use), appears to approach closer to the conceptual definition of the disease. Usually, the decision on the usefulness of the rules is based solely on the degree to which the diagnoses they establish conform with those made on the basis of clinical judgements. Despite the obvious limitations of this method it is frequently the only practicable one.

Depending on the purpose of the study, a more or less specific definition should be used. If the aim is to identify persons who almost certainly have the disease, a highly specific definition is required, using criteria that may fail to identify many people who clinicians say have the disease. On the other hand, if the aim is to detect all persons who have the disease, even at the expense of falsely including many who do not have it, less stringent criteria are required.

The operational definition should not only distinguish the disease from other diseases, but should also serve to delimit it along its own biological gradient. If the disease is poliomyelitis, it may be wished to include only the relatively few persons with persistent paralysis, or the larger number with transient paralysis, or the considerably larger number who take ill but have no paralysis, or the even larger number who have subclinical infections.

The choice of the criteria to be used is heavily influenced by the methods by which the data are to be collected. Very different criteria may be used in a study based solely on interviews, one in which clinical examinations are performed, and one utilizing bio-chemical, microbiological, radiological and other diagnostic tests. The definitive criterion of acute rheumatic fever is finding Aschoff bodies in a microscopic study of heart muscle,[4] and this is obviously of limited applicability, as is a definition of chronic bronchitis that specifies 'chronic inflammatory, fibrotic and atrophic changes in the bronchial structures'. At the other extreme, no medical training is required to diagnose chronic bronchitis if it is defined as 'the production of phlegm from the chest at least twice a day on most days for a least three months each year for two or more years',[5] the data being obtained by the use of a standard questionnaire.

The use of standard definitions is especially important in multicentre trials and other studies conducted in a number of co-operating general practices or other health services, in studies that compare the occurrence of diseases in different regions or countries, and in studies of time trends. A change in diagnostic criteria—insistence on demonstration of the malaria parasite in the blood—caused an 11-fold reduction in the annual number of cases of malaria in the United States between 1946 and 1949.[6]

We have stated that few diseases have satisfactory and widely accepted working definitions. Paradoxically, difficulties frequently arise not because of a lack, but because of a surfeit of operational definitions. Different investigators use different definitions, and their findings are difficult to compare. A comparison of six different commonly used sets of diagnostic criteria for dementia showed that the prevalence of this disorder in the same large sample of elderly people in Canada varied from 3 to 29%, depending on which set of criteria was used—only 1% had dementia according to all six sets of criteria;[7] and the prevalence of benign prostatic hyperplasia in a community sample of men ranged, according to different definitions, from 4 to 19%.[8]

For some diseases, standardized criteria have been proposed by expert committees. Use of these criteria facilitates comparisons. Even then there may be difficulties, since there may be differences in the way the criteria are understood or applied. Moreover, experts tend to change their recommendations from time to time: a comparison of 'old' and 'new' World Health Organization criteria for definite myocardial infarction, for example, showed that only 82% of the cases who met the old criteria also met the new criteria; the new definition required Minnesota coding of the ECGs (see p. 121) rather than subjective appraisal.[9]

To come back to the common cold, the textbook we have cited[1] provides two operational definitions:

1. *Suggestive.* A constellation of acute upper respiratory symptoms with a predominance of sneezing, nasal obstruction, and discharge suggests a diagnosis of a common cold.
2. *Definitive.* For decisions on clinical care, presence of the common cold syndrome and absence of a history of hayfever or exposure to noxious substances may be considered as providing a definitive diagnosis. Although not necessary for optimal care, isolation of one of the causative viruses from a person with the common cold syndrome would solidify the diagnosis.

The purpose of the first definition is unclear, since it does not apparently provide a sufficient basis for decisions on care. The second is more useful, but not completely unambiguous; the 'common cold syndrome' presumably refers to the constellation mentioned in the first definition, but what does 'a predominance of sneezing, nasal obstruction, and discharge' mean—must all three be present?—can a cold be diagnosed in the absence of sneezing, or in the absence of nasal obstruction? Note that the isolation of a relevant virus is not an essential criterion.

In an investigation based on questions put weekly to a population sample, a common cold might be defined as 'a report of a stuffy or running nose'. The diagnosis may not be completely valid, as some cases of allergic rhinitis may be included, and some people with running noses may not report them, but the definition has the advantages that it is unequivocal and eminently practical. A different definition might of course be used if virological tests were warranted by the study's purpose and resources.

SIDE-STEPPING THE ISSUE

In many (or even most) investigations, the need to formulate diagnostic criteria is side-stepped, and diseases are operationally defined in terms of reports of their presence. That is, the process of diagnosis is left to someone else (usually a doctor, sometimes the patient, a relative, teacher, etc.), and a report of the disease is taken as evidence of its presence; e.g. 'haemorrhoids' may be operationally defined as:

a recorded diagnosis of 'haemorrhoids' or 'piles' (in a specified clinical record)

or as

a positive response to the question 'Did a doctor ever tell you you had haemorrhoids or piles?'

or as

a positive response to the question 'Do you have piles?'

The use of second-hand diagnostic information of this sort, not based on defined criteria, has obvious limitations. It is often the only practicable approach, however, and should by no means be rejected, particularly if the information is obtained from well equipped clinical services with a high standard of medical practice. If this 'imperfect' method is the only practical method, it should be used, provided that consideration is given to the effects this 'imperfection' may have on the findings, and that (if necessary) caution is used in interpreting the findings.

NOTES AND REFERENCES

1. Couch R B 1996 In: Hurst J W (ed) 1996 Medicine for the practicing physician, 4th edn. Appleton & Lange, Stamford, Conn., pp 479–481.
2. MacMahon B, Pugh T F 1970 Epidemiology: principles and methods. Little, Brown, Boston, Mass., pp 47–54.
3. These are the Jones criteria (Special Writing Group of the Committee on Rheumatic Fever, Endocarditis, and Kawasaki Disease of the Council on

Cardiovascular Disease in the Young of the American Heart Association 1992 Guidelines for the diagnosis of rheumatic fever: Jones criteria, 1992 update. Journal of the American Medical Association 268: 2069).

4. Schlant R C 1996 In: Hurst J W (ed) 1996 (see note 1) pp 1255–1258.
5. Fletcher C M 1963 Some problems of diagnostic standardization using clinical methods, with special reference to chronic bronchitis. In: Pemberton J (ed) Epidemiology: reports on research and teaching. Oxford University Press, Oxford, p. 253.
6. Mainland D 1964 Elementary medical statistics, 2nd edn. W B Saunders, Philadelphia, pp 131–132.
7. The following six sets of diagnostic criteria were compared in this study: DSM-III (Diagnostic and statistical manual of mental disorders, 3rd edn); DSM-III-R (ditto, 3rd edn, revised); DSM-IV (ditto, 4th edn); CAMDEX (Cambridge Examination for Mental Disorders of the Elderly); ICD-9 (International classification of diseases, 9th edn); and ICD-10 (ditto, 10th edn). The respective results for the prevalence of dementia in the same 1879 men and women were: 29.1%, 17.3%, 13.7%, 4.9%, 5.0% and 3.1%. The main reasons for the disparities were different requirements concerning long-term memory, abstract thinking and other executive functions, work and activities of daily living, and duration of symptoms (Erkinjuntti T, Ostbye T, Steenhuis R, Hachinski V 1997 The effect of different diagnostic criteria on the prevalence of dementia. New England Journal of Medicine 337: 1667).
8. Bosch J L, Hop W C, Kirkels W J, Schroder F H 1995 Natural history of benign prostatic hyperplasia: appropriate case definition and estimation of its prevalence in the community. Urology 46(3 suppl A): 34.
9. Beaglehole R, Stewart A W, Butler M 1987 Comparability of old and new World Health Organization criteria for definite myocardial infarction. International Journal of Epidemiology 16: 373.

13 Scales of measurement

As part of the process of clarifying each of the variables to be studied, its scale of measurement should be specified. This chapter will discuss the types of scale and the criteria of a satisfactory scale, and will briefly describe the International Classification of Diseases and some other commonly used classifications.

TYPES OF SCALE

The scale of measurement may be *categorical* (consisting of two or more mutually exclusive categories) or *metric* (noncategorical: interval and ratio scales).

A categorical scale consists of mutually exclusive categories (classes). If these do not fall into a natural order, the scale is *nominal*. Numbers may be used to identify the categories, but these are 'code numbers' with no quantitative significance. Examples are:

1. *Marital status*: single, married, widowed, divorced.
2. *Religion*: Christian, Jewish, Muslim, Buddhist, freethinker, other.
3. *Type of anaemia*: 1, iron deficiency anaemia; 2, other deficiency anaemias; 3, hereditary haemolytic anaemias; 4, acquired haemolytic anaemias; 5, aplastic anaemia; 6, other anaemias.

If the categories fall into what is regarded as a natural order, the scale is *ordinal*. The scale shows ranks, or positions on a ladder; each class shows the same situational relationship to the class that follows it. If numbers are used, they indicate the positions of the categories in the series. Examples are:

1. *Social class*: I, II, III, IV, V.
2. *Years of education*: 0, 1–5, 6–9, 10–12, more than 12.
3. *Severity of a disease*: mild, moderate, severe.
4. *Limitation of activity*: 0, none; 1, limited activity but not home-bound; 2, home-bound but not bed-bound; 3, bed-bound.

An ordinal scale is 'stronger' than a nominal one, in the sense that it provides more information. Where there is a choice, use of an ordinal scale is preferable.

A scale may be a mixed nominal and ordinal one, i.e. some but not all of the categories may be ranked. A scale including a number of ranked categories and also a category of 'unclassifiable' is of this sort—the scale as a whole is nominal, but it is ordinal if the 'unclassifiable' class is excluded.[1]

A scale with only two categories is a *dichotomy* (or *binary scale*).[2] Many statistical procedures are applicable to dichotomies but not to scales with three or more categories. Numbers may be used as code numbers, or to indicate the presence or absence of an attribute (1 and 0 respectively). Examples are:

1. *Agreement with a statement*: agree, disagree.
2. *Sex*: 1, male; 2, female.
3. *Presence of a disease*: 0, absent; 1, present.
4. *Occurrence of headaches*: 0, no; 1, yes.

Interval and ratio scales (*noncategorical, metric* or *dimensional* scales) use numbers that indicate the quantity of what is being measured. They have two features: firstly, equal differences between any pairs of numbers in the scale mean equal differences in the attribute being measured, i.e. the difference between any two values reflects the magnitude of the difference in the attribute—the difference in temperature between 22 and 26°C is the same as that between 32 and 36°C; this makes the scale an *interval scale*. Secondly, in some of these scales, zero indicates absence of the attribute, as a consequence of which the ratio between any two values indicates the ratio between the amounts of the attribute—an income of $1000 is twice as high as an income of $500; this additional feature makes the scale a *ratio scale*. Most noncategorical scales have both these features; exceptional ones, like the Centigrade scale for temperature, are interval but not ratio scales—0° does not mean 'absence of heat', and 20° is therefore not 'twice as hot' as 10°. Examples of ratio scales are:

1. *Weight:* measured in kilograms or pounds.
2. *Mortality rate:* number of deaths per 1000 persons at risk.
3. *Feminine beauty:* measured in milli-helens.[3]

An interval or ratio scale provides more information than an ordinal one, and is to be preferred when there is a choice.

Interval and ratio scales may be *continuous* or *discrete*. The scale is continuous if an infinite number of values is possible along a continuum, e.g. when measuring height or cholesterol concentration. It is discrete if only certain values along the scale are possible—a woman's parity, for example, cannot be 2.35.

An interval or ratio scale may be 'collapsed' into broader categories by grouping values together, e.g.

Income (in monetary units): 0–49, 50–99, 100–149, etc.

If equal *class intervals* are used, as in this example, the scale can still often be treated as an interval one, taking the midpoints (25, 75, 125, etc.) as the values of the successive classes. Strictly speaking, however, it may now be an ordinal scale, since the individual values may not be uniformly spread within the classes, and the intervals between the average incomes of people in adjacent classes may hence not be equal. The scale is degraded to an ordinal scale if an 'open-ended' category is used (for instance, a top income group of '500 or more'). An accurate mean value cannot be calculated from such a scale. Similarly, the scale becomes an ordinal one if the class intervals vary, e.g. 0–49, 50–199, 200–399, etc.

The selection of a scale for measuring a variable is partly determined by the variable itself and the methods available for measuring it. Marital status, type of work, and type of anaemia cannot be measured by interval or ratio scales. For most variables, however, alternative methods of measurement are available.

Clearly, decisions concerning scales of measurement may influence the methods by which data will be collected. If it is decided to measure the frequency or severity of headaches (ordinal scales) instead of merely determining whether the subject suffers from headaches (using a 'yes–no' nominal scale), different questions are required. The categories are often printed in the questionnaires or examination schedules (see pp 262–265).

Different statistical procedures are appropriate for different kinds of scale. The scale used when the data are collected, however, is not necessarily the one that will be used throughout the analysis. Observations concerning a variable measured by one kind of scale may be analyzed by a procedure suited to another kind of scale, in accordance with the research hypothesis and the purpose of the analysis. Age (measured by an interval scale) may indeed be treated as an interval scale variable, e.g. when calculating a mean age or examining a correlation between age and some other variable. But for some purposes it may be appropriate to use a nominal scale, merely dividing the subjects into different age groups, and not assuming a monotonic relationship (i.e. a consistent increase or decrease in the other variable when people in younger and older categories are compared). Ethnic group is measured by a nominal scale; but it may be treated as an ordinal scale variable by arranging the categories in a specific sequence, in an analysis designed to see whether its categories have an ordered relationship with another variable.

During the planning phase, thought should be given to the scales that will be used when the data are analyzed. At this stage it is often helpful to construct *skeleton* or *dummy tables*, i.e. tables without figures or containing fictional figures respectively, incorporating the variables under consideration. If there are categories, they should be specified in the column or row headings. At this stage it is not essential to decide precisely how the finer categories will be 'collapsed' into broader categories for the purposes of analysis. It is often desirable to defer such decisions, since they may be difficult to make without knowing the actual distribution of the values. If doubt exists about the way a variable will be treated in the analysis, care should be taken to collect data in such a way as to leave the options open.

CRITERIA OF A SATISFACTORY SCALE

A satisfactory scale of measurement is one that meets the following seven requirements.

Requirements

1. Appropriate
2. Practicable
3. Sufficiently powerful
4. Clearly defined components
5. Sufficient categories
6. Comprehensive
7. Mutually exclusive

---

1. It is *appropriate* for use in the study, keeping in mind the conceptual definition of the variable and the objectives of the study. Occupations, for instance, may be classified in different ways, depending on whether the purpose is to use occupation as a measure of social class, of habitual physical activity, or of exposure to specific physical and chemical hazards. Similarly, different classifications may be used for the region of birth of immigrants, depending on whether the variable is to be used as an indicator of environmental conditions in childhood, of ethnic group, or of genetic attributes. In measuring birth weights, it may be decided to use categories extending evenly along the whole weight spectrum, or, if the specific subject of inquiry is the effect of low birth weight, to use narrow categories for babies of low birth weight and broad categories for heavier babies.

2. It is a *practicable* scale—one that is geared to the methods that will be used in collecting the information. For example, if the data are to be obtained from records that list marital status as 'single', 'married', 'widowed' and 'divorced', there is no point in deciding upon a more elaborate scale of measurement, e.g. including 'married once', 'married more than once', etc. Account should be taken of the precision of the methods to be used in collecting the data. Can accurate ages be obtained in terms of years and months, or only in terms of years? If people tend to 'round off' their ages ('I am 40 years old', '50 years old', etc.), a scale showing each year separately will have only spurious precision (see p. 190). Will it be possible to get detailed data on income or the number of cigarettes smoked per day, or is it only possible to use broad categories? Is the balance to be used for weighing sufficiently discriminatory to warrant measurements in tenths of kilograms, or should whole kilograms be used? Is there any point in recording liver enlargement in centimetres, if tests have shown a negligible correlation between measurements made by different physicians on the same patients?

3. The scale is *powerful* enough to satisfy the objectives of the study. If there is a choice, an ordinal scale should be used rather than a nominal one, and an interval or ratio scale rather than a categorical one. An analysis using the whole spectrum of haemoglobin levels is likely to be more informative than one using a dichotomy, such as 'below 12 g per 100 ml' and '12 or more g per 100 ml'. In measuring an attitude an ordinal scale should

be used, based on the provision of graded alternative responses
to a question or on a score derived from the responses to a series
of questions, rather than a simple dichotomy such as 'agree–
disagree' or 'important–unimportant'.

4. The components are *clearly defined*. Wherever necessary, operational definitions should be formulated not only for the variable,
but for the categories. This applies especially to nominal and
ordinal scales. If cases of a disease are to be classified as 'active'
and 'healed', or patients with a malignant neoplasm according
to the stage of the disorder, these categories need careful definition. In the case of numerical measurements decisions may
be needed on the number of decimal places to be used, and
on how values are to be rounded off—downwards, or to the
nearest number. It is usually preferable to round off downwards,
so that the category '73 kg', for example, includes all weights
between 73.0 and 73.9 kg; if this is done it must be remembered
that the average value of the weights in this category will be
73.5 kg.

5. The scale contains *sufficient categories*. While the number of
categories should not be multiplied unnecessarily, the compres-
sion of data into too few categories may lead to a loss of useful
information. For example, if immigrants from North Africa have
a particularly high rate of mortality from cerebrovascular disease,
this fact may become less obvious or may be completely masked
if they are included in a broader category of 'immigrants from
Africa and Asia'. Often 'articulated' scales are used—scales containing categories that 'branch', like the bones of the limbs—
i.e. categories which are divided into subcategories and, if
necessary, sub-subcategories; the use of such a scale leaves
the options open for a later decision as to the use of broad or
narrow categories. With numerical data it is often similarly
advisable to collect the information in a detailed form and to
decide later whether to use the full scale or a 'collapsed' one (or
both). With numerical data the use of too few categories may
prevent the calculation of an accurate mean.

6. The scale is *collectively exhaustive (comprehensive)*. It provides a
niche for the classification of every subject. This may necessitate
the inclusion of one or more of the following categories:

- *Other*.
- *Not applicable*, e.g. information on the duration of marriage
  may be collected only from people who are at present mar-

ried; in this case the scale used may be 'under 5 years', '5–9.9 years', '10–19.9 years', '20–29.9 years', '30–39.9 years', '40 years and more', and 'not applicable'.

- *Unknown* (it may sometimes be desirable to subdivide this category, e.g. to distinguish between subjects who did not know the answer to a question and those with information lacking for other reasons: the question was not asked, the response was illegible, a page of the completed questionnaire was mislaid, etc.).

7. The categories are *mutually exclusive*. Each item of information should fit into only one place along the scale. For example, a scale including both '70 to 80' and '80 to 90' is generally unacceptable, as '80' could fit into either of these categories. Similarly, if a scale includes 'married' and 'remarried', a remarried person could fit into either category. If a scale for measuring the conditions producing disability includes the categories 'blindness' and 'deafness', either a clear rule should be formulated whereby persons who are both blind and deaf are assigned to one of these categories, or the scale should include the categories 'blind, not deaf', 'deaf, not blind' and 'blind and deaf'. In the Minnesota code for ECG findings (see p. 121), where different codable items may coexist in the same scale of measurement (e.g. that for T wave items), only one is coded, the order of precedence being clearly stated.

INTERNATIONAL CLASSIFICATION OF DISEASES

The International Classification of Diseases (ICD), published by WHO[4] and now in its tenth revision (ICD-10), is widely used as a nominal scale for the categorization of diseases. Each disease category is given a three-character code (a letter and two numerals), and almost all categories are divided into subcategories.

Since our principles of nosology are far from rational the arrangement of the ICD is arbitrary. Some diseases are classified by their aetiology ('infectious and parasitic diseases'), some by their site ('diseases of the respiratory system'), some by a pathological feature ('neoplasms'), some by age at onset ('certain conditions originating in the perinatal period'), etc. Neoplasms are subclassified by their sites, but an optional supplementary morphological classification is provided. Injuries are classified in two ways, by their nature and by their external causes. Codes are provided for factors (other than illness) that may bring a person into contact with a health service or influence health status (e.g. immunization, contraceptive management, living alone, extreme poverty). Special short lists are provided for the tabulation of mortality and morbidity.

Some diseases have dual codes—a mandatory dagger code (marked with a †) for classifying the underlying general disease, and an optional asterisk code (*) for classifying it according to its manifestation in a particular organ or site. If *both* codes are used, the categories of the classification are not mutually exclusive.

'Glossary descriptions' are provided for mental disorders and some other conditions. These descriptions fall far short of ideal operational definitions.

Coding is best left to experienced coders. One can do it oneself, but care must be taken. To code a disease, it is first looked up in the index, which is published as a separate volume. The index includes diagnostic terms that are not specifically stated in the classification itself. After using the index, reference should be made to the appropriate item in the classification, since this may contain a note leading to a modification of the code number. The conventions used in the classification must be clearly understood if the book is to be used effectively.[5] Before drawing inferences from tabulations based on the ICD it is wise to examine the details of the classification, so as to be sure of what is and what is not included in the various categories.

Adaptations of the ICD include an American 'clinical modification' (ICD-9-CM),[6] which is more detailed than the ICD; it divides the ICD's categories into more specific subcategories.

CLASSIFICATIONS FOR USE IN PRIMARY CARE

The International Classification of Health Problems in Primary Care (ICHPPC) is a classification designed primarily to permit a general or family practitioner to code diagnoses or other problems at the time of the patient encounter.[7] It includes diseases (classified more simply than in the ICD), important signs and symptoms, social and family problems, forms of preventive care, and administrative procedures.

A newer version (ICHPPC-2-Defined), which is an adaptation of the ninth revision of the ICD, contains definitions of most of the rubrics. These were designed as 'the briefest possible definitions which would reduce variability in coding', and stipulate criteria that *must* be fulfilled if miscoding is to be avoided. As examples, a diagnosis is coded as 'acute upper respiratory infection' (a category that includes colds, nasopharyngitis, pharyngitis and rhinitis) only if two criteria are met: (1) evidence of acute inflammation of the nasal or pharyngeal mucosa and (2) absence of criteria for more specifically defined acute respiratory infections listed in the classification. A diagnosis of 'anxiety disorder, anxiety state' requires both of the following: (1) 'generalized and persistent anxiety or anxious mood, which cannot be associated with, or is disproportionately large in response to, a specific psycho-social stressor, stimulus, or event' and (2) 'no evidence of other psychological disorders'. For the rubric 'problems with aged parents or in-laws' the criterion (surprise! surprise!) is 'a problem experienced by an adult (age 18 or over) with his parents or in-laws'.

The authors stress that the definitions are not intended to serve as a guide to diagnosis. Their purpose is to reduce chances of miscoding *after* a diagnosis has been made, and not to reduce diagnostic error.

The International Classification of Primary Care (ICPC)[8] permits patients' encounters to be classified not only according to the physician's diagnosis or assessment of the health problem (using the ICHPPC codes), but also according to the reason for the encounter as expressed by the patient, and the nature of the diagnostic and therapeutic interventions undertaken in the process of care. One or more of these axes may be used. The patient's reason for encounter (which may need clarification by the care provider) may be a symptom, a disease, getting a prescription, test result or certificate, etc. The 'process' components include various diagnostic, preventive, therapeutic and administrative procedures, and referrals. The ICPC is consistent with the use of problem-oriented clinical records, which use the SOAP acronym: S = subjective (the patient's reason for the encounter), O = objective signs, A = assessment (diagnosis) and P = plan (the process of care or intervention); but objective signs are not classified by the ICPC. The authors suggest use of the ICPC as a basis for an information system based on disease episodes (from onset to resolution) for which there may be more than one encounter.

The International Classification of Impairments, Disabilities and Handicaps (ICIDH)[9] may be found useful in studies concerned with disability and rehabilitation.

NOTES AND REFERENCES

1. As an example, the categories of *Katz's index of IDL* are: Independent in: A, continence, transferring (bed–chair), going to toilet, dressing, bathing; B, all but one of these functions; C, all but bathing and one additional function; D, all but bathing, dressing and one additional function; E, all but bathing, dressing, going to toilet, transferring, and one additional function; F, dependent in all six functions; other: dependent in at least two functions, but not classifiable as C, D, E or F (Katz S, Ford A B, Moskowitz R W, Jackson B A, Jaffe M W 1963 Studies of illness in the aged: the Index of ADL: a standardized measure of biological and psychosocial function. Journal of the American Medical Association 185: 914).

2. *Dichotomies* can be treated not only as nominal, but also as ordinal, interval, or (in some instances) ratio scales. Many statistical procedures are applicable to dichotomies but not to nominal scales that have three or more categories. Dichotomies and other nominal scales can usefully be regarded as different types of scales.

3. A milli-helen is 'the quantity of beauty required to launch exactly one ship'. Dickinson R E 1958 The Observer (letter, Feb. 23rd).

4. World Health Organization 1992–1994. International statistical classification of diseases and related health problems: tenth revision, vols 1, 2 and 3. World Health Organization, Geneva.

5. The ICD uses round brackets (...) to enclose words or phrases whose presence or absence does not matter. Square brackets [...] enclose alternative wordings or explanatory phrases. Terms preceding a colon are incomplete, and must be completed by one of the modifiers that follow the colon. 'NOS' stands for 'not otherwise specified' (i.e. without qualification). 'How to use the ICD' is explained in vol 2 of the classification (see note 4), pp 18–29.

6. ICD-9-CM 1998: International classification of diseases, 9th revision: clinical modification. Practice Management Information Corporation, 1997.
   ICD-9-CM can be downloaded from ftp://ftp.cdc.gov/pub/Health_Statistics/NCHS/Publications/
   The final draft of the new U.S. coding system for procedures, ICD-10-PCS, is available at www.hcfa.gov/stats/icd10/icd10.htm

7. World Organization of National Colleges, Academies and Academic Associations of General Practitioners/Family Physicians (WONCA). Classification Committee 1983 ICHPPC-2-Defined, 3rd edn. Oxford University Press, Oxford.

8. Lamberts H, Wood M (eds) 1987 ICPC: International Classification of Primary Care. Oxford University Press, Oxford. Hofmans-Okkes I M, Lamberts H 1996 The International Classification of Primary Care (ICPC): new applications in research and computer-based patient records in family practice. Family Practice 13: 294.

9. World Health Organization 1980 International classification of impairments, disabilities and handicaps (ICIDH). WHO, Geneva. See Dekker J 1995 (Application of the ICIDH in survey research on rehabilitation: the emergence of the functional diagnosis. Disability and Rehabilitation 17: 195) and Duckworth D 1995 (Measuring disability: the role of the ICIDH. Disability and Rehabilitation 17: 338).

14 Composite scales

Variables based on two or more other variables may be termed *composite variables*. Examples are: (1) caloric intake, which is calculated from the intake of a variety of foodstuffs, (2) the presence or stage of a disease, which may be based on a set of symptoms and clinical signs, (3) an attitude, when measured by the responses to a series of separate questions, and (4) overall health, based on separate measures of physical and mental health. Scales used for measuring composite variables may be termed *composite scales*.

The manner in which the component data are brought together into a composite scale is usually decided upon in advance, using rules that enter into the operational definition of the composite variable. There are also techniques (e.g. Guttman scaling, factor analysis) that require the collection and analysis of the component data to see how they 'hang together', before deciding how to combine them.

The scale may be based on *combinations of categories*. For instance, hypertension may be defined as a systolic blood pressure of 160 mmHg or more and/or a diastolic pressure of 95 mmHg or more, and the absence of hypertension as a systolic pressure below 140 mmHg together with a diastolic pressure below 90 mmHg. If other combinations of systolic and diastolic pressures are placed in an intermediate or 'borderline' group, this provides a composite scale of the ordinal type. The scale might be elaborated by adding 'and/or receiving specific treatment for hypertension' to the definition of hypertension, and adding 'and not under treatment' to the definitions of the other categories. A composite scale of the nominal type is sometimes referred to as a *typology*.

Formulae are used for composite variables that express relationships between other variables. Examples are: the length of gestation, usually estimated from the date of onset of the last menstrual period and the date at which pregnancy ended; average family income per head; adiposity indices based on weight and height; and all rates.[1]

Use is often made of *combination scores* computed from the separate scores allotted to a set of component variables. Combining several variables in this way generally carries advantages over reliance on any single component variable (but if the components are heterogeneous, one or more of them may be more useful for some purposes than the combination score). The simplest technique is to add up the component scores, using the raw or weighted scores; appropriate weights are sometimes determined by rather complicated procedures.

This chapter will review Guttman scaling and combination scores in more detail, and then provide guidelines for the construction of a composite scale.

GUTTMAN SCALE

One way of combining component items into a composite scale is to see whether the results conform with a *Guttman scale* (*scalogram*),[2,3] i.e. a 'hierarchy', and then use the Guttman scale type as a score. As a simple example, consider the following three 'yes–no' questions:

1. 'Do you weigh more than 50 kg?'
2. 'Do you weigh more than 75 kg?'
3. 'Do you weigh more than 100 kg?'

The only four possible combinations of correct replies (to questions 1, 2 and 3 respectively) are 'no–no–no', 'yes–no–no', 'yes–yes–no', and 'yes–yes–yes'; these are four 'scale types' that constitute an ordinal scale. Question 2 cannot be answered 'yes' unless question 1 is also answered 'yes', and question 3 cannot be answered 'yes' unless both questions 1 and 2 are also answered 'yes'. All the responses should conform with the above scale types—there should be no deviant responses. The scale types might be numbered 0 to 3—i.e. (in this instance) the number of 'yes' responses, and they then provide an ordinal measure of weight. If analysis of the findings of a study reveals a set of variables that are acceptably 'scalable' in this way, each scale type expresses a position along the dimension that is measured. If a few responses do not fall into scale types they can be assigned to the closest scale type by the use of preset rules.

Guttman scales have been used for attitudes, dietary habits, clinical manifestations of a disease, and other attributes. Among British students, for example, a Guttman scale for 'meat avoidance' could be constructed from questions about the eating of poultry, beef, lamb and pork; but (contrary to previous assumptions) the eating of fish did not fit into the scale.[4] In a study of schoolchildren, the scale types for 'risk behaviours' were: none; alcohol; alcohol and cigarettes; alcohol, cigarettes and sex; alcohol, cigarettes, sex and drugs.[5]

The number attached to a scale type not only constitutes a measure, it also provides qualitative information. For example, in a community survey the reported ability to perform six activities constituted an excellent Guttman scale.[6] The activities were: 1, light work in the home (e.g. washing dishes); 2, walking in the vicinity of the house; 3, moderate work in the home (e.g. moving a chair or table); 4, walking uphill or upstairs; 5, running a short distance; and 6, active sports. The scale types were: 0, can do none of these activities; 1, can do activity 1 only; 2 can do activities 1 and 2 only; and so on. A scale type (score) of 3 tells us that the subject can do light or moderate work in the home and take a walk in the vicinity of the house, but no more vigorous activities.

The building blocks in developing the scale need not be separate items. They can also be combinations (connected by 'or', 'and/or', or 'and') of 'yes–no' items, combinations (connected by 'or') of possible responses to multiple-category items, etc. As a result, there may be different ways of constructing a hierarchy from the same variables. While the categories of Katz's index of independence in daily living[7] constitute a Guttman scale, an analysis of all the possible permutations revealed four hierarchies that were at least as good, and 103 that satisfied the minimum for scalability.[8]

COMBINATION SCORES

The simplest combination score is the number of positive responses to a set of 'yes–no' items (every 'yes' is taken as 1 and every 'no' as 0). This method is often used for scoring questionnaires like the Cornell Medical Index (CMI),[9] which comprises questions about the presence of symptoms, illnesses, etc. Similarly, the diagnosis of rheumatoid arthritis can be based on the number of diagnostic criteria that are fulfilled.[10] Note that 'number of symptoms' scores are not always acceptable, and they should not be used uncritically.[11]

If there are graded alternative responses to the items, with pre-set scores, the scores for all the items can be added. For example, a series of questions about attitudes, with the format 'How strongly do you agree or disagree with the following statement?' might have possible responses of '1, strongly agree; 2, agree; 3, undecided; 4, disagree; 5, strongly disagree'. Scales of this kind are called *Likert-type*.[12] A commonly used Likert-type scale is the *Apgar score* used to appraise the status of newborn infants. This is the sum of the points (0, 1 or 2) allotted for each of five items: heart rate (over 100 beats per minute, 2 points; slower, 1 point; no beat, 0), respiratory effort, muscle tone, response to stimulation by a catheter in the nostril, and skin colour. An internationally used Prostate Symptom Score is based on seven symptoms, each with a 0 to 5 score expressing its frequency.[13] Likert scales are used in the SF-36 (Medical Outcomes Study 36-item Short Form Health Survey) questionnaire, which has achieved considerable popularity in recent years.[14]

Arbitrary weights are sometimes given to the items before their scores are added, based on the importance attributed to each item by the investigator or by a group of experts (see Ch. 20). For instance, in a study of the quality of medical care, scores were given for the quality of records, the quality of diagnostic management and the quality of treatment and follow-up. These three scores were then combined, using weights of 30%, 40% and 30% respectively.[15]

The component items may also be given scores based on or validated by a careful analysis of data collected in the current or a previous study. For example, a detailed study of patients in a metabolic laboratory was used to authenticate a 'clinical diagnostic index of thyrotoxicosis', with scores (based on 'diagnostic significance') for various clinical signs and symptoms (e.g. preference for cold, +5; palpable thyroid, +3; increase in weight, −13) and a recommendation that a total of 20 or more could be taken to indicate the presence of thyrotoxicosis.[16]

A variety of statistical methods (not necessarily simple) can be used to determine item scores. Among the more complicated procedures are *Rasch (item response theory) methods*[17] and *factor analysis*. Rasch methods may be used to appraise whether the items form a hierarchy, whether they measure a single dimension, whether they are appropriately spaced along this dimension, and reproducibility. Factor analysis reports the fundamental dimensions that underlie the data collected for a group of variables (labelling them 'factor 1', 'factor 2', etc.), as well as stating what weights should be attached to the items in order to measure each dimension. The investigator then determines (some would say, divines) what characteristic is measured by each factor, and gives it a name. This kind of analysis is most convincing if the findings are replicated in different samples. The measurement of *health locus-of-control* can be cited to demonstrate its use. Sets of questions were devised in order to grade people according to their belief that their health was under their own control (internal locus-of-control) or determined by external factors. But factor analysis revealed that there were also other dimensions, including beliefs in control by health providers and by others, and belief in the role of chance.[18]

A combination scale often used for attitudes is based on a set of 'agree–disagree' or 'true–false' questions concerning statements that represent different points along the dimension to be measured.[19] The statements may be selected in such a way that each respondent may be *a priori* expected to agree with only one or two of them and disagree with the others (*Thurstone-type differential scale*), or in such a way that agreement may be expected with all statements up to (or after) a particular point in the series (*cumulative scale*), as in the Guttman model). The selection and scoring of the questions are usually based on the judgements of a population sample or a panel of experts.

Various manipulations may be applied to the component scores or the combination score, however these are obtained. For example, scores may be converted to percentages, or standardized according to the findings in a standard population.

CONSTRUCTING A COMPOSITE SCALE

Creating a satisfactory composite scale for general use can be a difficult and laborious process. But for an investigator who wants only to produce a combination score based on 'yes–no' or Likert-scored items, to serve the purposes of a specific study in a specific population, the task may not be overwhelming.

Here are simple guidelines.[20] When following these, take account of the purpose of the scale—is it 'discrimination' (i.e. to compare individuals or groups with different intensities of a characteristic), measurement of change, or prediction of a future event or status? If possible the scale should be tested in a sample of the study population rather than in the whole study population; if numbers permit, separate tests should be performed in subgroups (men and women, age groups, etc.).

1. Start with what seems to be an appropriate list of component items (questions, symptoms, etc.). The items should be relevant ones (see 'face validity', p. 189), and should cover all important facets (see 'content validity', p. 190). If the purpose of the scale is discrimination between individuals or groups, try to include items that express different intensities or quantities of the characteristic. If the purpose is to measure change, the items should represent changeable characteristics and offer a sufficient number of graded response alternatives. If the aim is prediction, all important predictors should be included. Decide on the scoring of the items: 1/0 ('yes–no') or a Likert scale.

2. Collect data, in a pretest or the study proper.

3. Examine the distribution of the combination scores. Is there enough variation to make the scale useful? If the aim is to detect change, is there a concentration at the worst score (a *floor effect*) or the best score (a *ceiling effect*), which might prevent the detection of deterioration or improvement?

4. Examine the relationships between the items.[3] This may provide a basis for the deletion of items. This examination is relatively unimportant if the scale measures a heterogeneous attribute, such as the presence of a disease with diverse unrelated manifestions, or to predict a future event—good predictors do not necessarily have to be present at the same time.

   a. Measure the correlations between items and between each item and the total score of the other items. Negatively correlated items have no place in the same scale.[21] On the other hand, if the aim is discrimination very highly correlated items may not be helpful, since they may be measuring almost exactly the same thing; medium correlations suggest that the items reflect diversity with respect to the characteristic being measured.

   b. Compute *Cronbach's alpha coefficient*,[22] which measures the scale's internal consistency; its value depends on the average correlation between items and on the number of items. A value of 0.7 or higher is generally regarded as satisfactory, indicating that the items may be measures of much the same attribute; but a value in excess of 0.8 is preferable.[23] *Alpha* may be regarded as an indicator of reliability (see Ch. 16).

   c. If possible, determine whether the findings are consistent with the assumption that the scale measures a single attribute, e.g. by testing for Guttman scalability[2] (easily done for 'yes–no' items, more difficult for multiple-response items). If so, this is probably the best scale to use, although there is no guarantee that what the scale measures is indeed what the investigator wants to measure.

   d. Make any required modifications to the scale, and retest. If the scale is internally consistent but contains an unwieldly number of items, it may be worth dropping some; the items to be kept should be ones that examine different facets, rather than those that maximize internal consistency.

5. If possible, test the scale's reliability (see Ch. 16) and validity, with and without modifications. Validity tests should take account of the purpose of the scale (see Ch. 17). Any composite score based on decisions (possibly arbitrary) about the inclusion and weighting of items is open to criticism unless such tests are done—and yet only 25% of clinical trials published in 1986–1995 and using quality of life as an outcome measure reported the reliability of the quality-of-life measure, and only 23% gave information on its validity![24]

6. When the scale is ready, test it in a different sample, so as not to be misled by chance 'quirks' in the initial sample.

The construction of a good composite scale is never easy. However, it is comforting that if the items measure a single dimension and have a clear-cut ranking of their categories, *how* they are brought together into a composite scale is not always of great consequence. This was shown in a survey of disability in London, where information was obtained about the capacity to perform various activities. Four separate composite scales were developed, including a Guttman scale and an additive scale in which each activity, and the degree of disability in performing it, was given an arbitrary score based on the criteria used by local social workers for defining handicap. The scores yielded by the different methods turned out to be highly correlated with one another.[25]

NOTES AND REFERENCES

1. See note 2, page 121.

2. The essence of a *Guttman scale* (*scalogram*) is a set of unambiguous and hierarchical questions. Contrast the questions about weight in the text with the following three, which would elicit 'helter-skelter' nonscalable replies: 1. 'Are you taller than a table?'; 2. 'Are you taller than the head of a pony?'; 3. 'Are you taller than a good-sized bookcase?' (Ford R N 1954 A rapid scoring procedure for scaling attitude questions In: Riley M W, Riley J W Jr, Toby J 1954 Sociological studies in scale analysis. Rutgers University Press, New Brunswick, pp 273–305).

   The main criteria of *scalability* are (1) that the *coefficient of reproducibility* (the proportion of nonerroneous responses) must be at least 90%, and (2) that the *coefficient of scalability* (which allows for the possibility of chance compliance with a Guttman scale) should be well above 60%. It has also been suggested that the frequency of no single deviant ('nonscale') type should exceed 5% of the number of respondents, that erroneous responses to any item should not exceed 15%, and that over half the positive responses and over half the negative responses to each item should be nonerroneous (Ford 1954, pp 294–295). For these purposes, an erroneous response to an item may be defined as one that differs from the response to be expected in a perfect scale type with the same number of 'yes' responses; a more elaborate method of counting errors (for specific items) is suggested by Ford 1954 (pp 285–290).

   The coefficient of scalability may be defined as the difference between the coefficient of reproducibility and the *coefficient of reproducibility by chance* (*CRC*), expressed as a proportion of (1–CRC). CRC is calculated by estimating the probability of each perfect scale type (by multiplying the appropriate marginal probabilities, based on the total numbers of 'yes' and 'no' responses to each item) and then summing the probabilities of all perfect scale types (Riley 1963, vol 1, pp 476–477, see below).

   If the scale is satisfactory, respondents falling into nonscale types can be assigned to the closest scale type, i.e. the one requiring correction of the smallest number of erroneous responses. Ford 1954 (pp 290–291) provides rules for use if there are alternative 'closest scale types'. Assignment is sometimes made to the scale type with the same number of 'yes' responses.

   The *Guttman scale* technique is described in detail by Gorden R L 1997 (Unidimensional scaling of social variables: concepts and procedures. Free Press, New York) and Stouffer S A, Guttman L, Suchman E A, Lazarsfeld P F, Star S A, Clausen J A 1966 (Measurement and prediction. Wiley, New York) and briefly by Goode W J, Hatt P K 1952 (Methods of social research, McGraw-Hill, New York, pp 285–295) and Riley M W 1963 (Sociological research, vol 1, pp 470–488 and vol 2, pp 97–99. Harcourt Brace and World, New York).

3. The SCALE programme in the PEPI package (see note 7, p. 292) can appraise scalability and measure correlations and Cronbach's *alpha* for a set of 'yes–no' items.

4. Santos M L, Booth D A 1996 Influences on meat avoidance among British students. Appetite 27: 197.

5. Palti H, Halevy A, Epstein Y, Knishkowy B, Meir M, Adler B 1995 Concerns and risk behaviors and the association between them among high-school students in Jerusalem. Journal of Adolescent Health 17: 51.

6. Abramson J H, Ritter M, Gofin J, Kark J D 1992 A simplified index of physical health for use in epidemiological studies. Journal of Clinical Epidemiology 45: 651.

7. See note 1, page 150.

8. Lazaridis E N, Rudberg M A, Furner S E, Cassel C K 1994 Do activities of daily living have a hierarchical structure? An analysis using the Longitudinal Study of Aging. Journal of Gerontology 49: M47.

9. Brodman K, Erdman A J Jr, Wolff H G 1956 Cornell Medical Index

questionnaire (manual). Cornell University Medical College, New York. Abramson J H 1966 The Cornell Medical Index as an epidemiological tool. American Journal of Public Health 56: 287.

10. Arnett F C, Edworthy S M, Bloch D A et al 1988 The American Rheumatism Association 1987 revised criteria for the classification of rheumatoid arthritis. Arthritis and Rheumatism 31: 315.

11. An analysis (using a Rasch model) of 20 common symptoms reported by a sample of elderly people provided strong evidence against the hypothesis that the number of symptoms measured a single dimension. Some of the symptoms were negatively correlated with one another (Dean K, Edwardson S 1996 Additive scoring of reported symptoms: validity and item bias problems in morbidity scales. European Journal of Public Health 6: 275).

12. For further details of *Likert-type scales*, see Gorden R L 1997 ([see note 2], pp 38–40) or Selltiz C, Wrightsman I S, Cook S W 1976 (Research methods in social relations, 3rd edn. Holt, Rinehart & Winston, New York, pp 418–421). On the Internet, try trochim.human.cornell.edu/kb/scallik.htm

    The scores allotted to the alternatives are usually decided arbitrarily, but may be based on the judgements of respondents who are asked to rate each alternative along a graphic (visual analogue) scale; for an example, see Bullinger M 1995 (German translation and psychometric testing of the SF-36 Health Survey: Preliminary results from the IQOLA Project. Social Science and Medicine 41: 1359).

13. Barry M J, Fowler F J Jr, O'Leary M P, Bruskewitz R C, Holtgrewe H L, Cockett A T 1992 The American Urological Association symptom index for benign prostatic hyperplasia: The Measurement Committee of the American Urological Association. Journal of Urology 148: 1549.

14. Ware J E Jr, Snow K K, Kosinski M A, Gandek B 1993 SF-36 Health Survey manual and interpretation guide. The Health Institute, New England Medical Center, Boston. On the Internet, visit www.sf36.com for a specimen questionnaire and up-to-date information (including details of the latest version).

15. Morehead M A 1967 The medical audit as an operational tool. American Journal of Public Health 57: 1643

16. Crooks J, Murray I P C, Wayne E J 1959 Statistical methods applied to the clinical diagnosis of thyrotoxicosis. Quarterly Journal of Medicine 28: 211.

17. For examples of the use of Rasch methods, see note 11 and Haley S M, McHorney C A, Ware J E Jr 1994 (Evaluation of the MOS SF-36 Physical Functioning Scale (PF-10): 1. Unidimensionality and reproducibility of the Rasch item scale. Journal of Clinical Epidemiology 47: 671).

18. Lau R R, Ware J E Jr 1981 Refinements in the measurement of health-specific locus-of-control beliefs. Medical Care 19: 1147. Ware J E Jr 1984 Methodological considerations in the selection of health status assessment procedures. In: Wenger N K, Mattson M E, Furberg C D, Elinson J (eds) Assessment of quality of life in clinical trials of cardiovascular therapies. LeJacq Publishing, New York, pp 87–111.

    Differences of opinion about the dimensions of locus-of-control persist (Talbot F, Nouwen A, Gauthier J 1996 Is health locus of control a 3-factor or a 2-factor construct? Journal of Clinical Psychology 52: 559. Raja S N, Williams S, McGee R 1994 Multidimensional health locus of control beliefs and psychological health for a sample of mothers. Social Science and Medicine 39: 213).

19. For further details on *Thurstone-type and cumulative scales* see Gorden R L 1997 ([see note 2], pp 35–38) or Selltiz et al ([see note 12], pp 413–417, 421–422). A demonstration of the construction of a Thurstone scale can be sought on the Internet: trochim.human.cornell.edu/kb/scalthur.htm

    Thurstone's method of paired comparisons, one of the procedures for deriving scores from the judgements of respondents, is explained by McKenna S P, Hunt S M, McEwen J 1981 (Weighting the seriousness of perceived sleep problems using Thurstone's method of paired comparisons. International Journal of Epidemiology 10: 93). Unfortunately these judgements, and hence the scores, may vary in different populations (Bucquet D, Condon S, Ritchie K 1990 The French version of the Nottingham Health Profile: a comparison of item weights with those of the source version. Social Science and Medicine 30: 829; Prieto L, Alonso J, Viladrich M C, Anto J M 1996 Scaling the Spanish version of the Nottingham Health Profile: evidence of limited value of item weights. Journal of Clinical Epidemiology 49: 31); and a different procedure, using the same judgements, may yield different scores (Kind P 1982 A comparison of two models for scaling health indicators. International Journal of Epidemiology 11: 271).

If the scale is based on the opinions of judges, it may be possible to treat it as an interval scale (*Thurstone-type equal-appearing interval scale*).

20. Kirshner B, Guyatt G 1985 A methodological framework for assessing health indices. Journal of Chronic Diseases 38: 27.
21. If it is believed that negatively correlated items are alternative manifestations of a singular underlying characteristic—like headache and diffuse aches in the study by Dean and Edwardson 1996 (see note 11)—it may be worth combining them into a single 'and/or' component of the scale, and retesting.
22. Cronbach L J 1951 Coefficient alpha and the internal structure of tests. Psychometrika 16: 297. Guilford J P, Fruchter B 1978 Fundamental statistics in psychology and education, 6th edn. McGraw-Hill, Auckland, pp 427–428.
23. Carmines E G, Zeller R A 1979 Reliability and validity assessment. Sage Publications, Beverly Hills.
24. Kong S X, Gandhi S K 1997 Methodologic assessments of quality of life measures in clinical trials. Annals of Pharmacotherapy 31: 830.
25. Bebbington A C 1977 Scaling indices of disablement. British Journal of Preventive and Social Medicine 31: 122.

15 Methods of collecting data

During the planning phase of the study it is necessary to decide on the methods to be used for collecting information. The methods of collecting information may be broadly classified as follows:

1. *Observation*, i.e. the use of techniques varying from simple visual observation to those requiring special skills, e.g. clinical examinations, or sophisticated equipment or facilities, such as imaging procedures and biochemical and microbiological examinations.
2. *Interviews and self-administered questionnaires* (see Chs 18 and 19).
3. *The use of documentary sources*—clinical records and other personal records, death certificates, published mortality statistics, census publications, etc. (see Ch. 21). Data derived from these sources are called *secondary*, as opposed to the *primary data* (based on observation, interviews or questionnaires) first recorded by the investigators.

There are usually alternative methods of collecting the desired data. Information about hypertension, for example, may be obtained by measuring blood pressure (observation), by asking the subjects whether a doctor has ever told them they have 'high blood pressure' (interview), or by referring to medical records (documents). Furthermore, observational measurements of blood pressure may be made sitting or lying, with or without a prior rest period, by intra-arterial pressure measurements, ordinary indirect sphygmomanometry, an electronic gadget, etc. Diet may be studied by weighing the food eaten, by asking questions, or by using written records in which the subject has noted the amounts

and types of foodstuffs eaten. If questions are asked, they may refer
to the food eaten in the last 24 hours or in the last 48 hours, or the
frequency with which different food items are usually consumed,
etc. Exposure to tobacco smoke can be studied by asking questions
about the smoking habits of the subjects or the people with whom
they live or work. It can also be studied by measuring the concentration of carbon monoxide in expired air or of thiocyanate or
cotinine in the saliva or other body fluids or (for passive smoking)
nicotine in the hair.[1] If attitudes, feelings, values or motivations are
to be measured, they will usually be inferred from the responses to
questions, a large variety of which can be devised; sometimes they
may be inferred from observations or documentary records of
actions, or from the responses to projective tests (in which the
subject is required to react to a picture or other stimulus).

Different methods may yield very different information. The
prevalence of chronic diseases, for example, may be studied by
interviews, or by conducting examinations or using existing clinical records. Most comparisons have shown very little correspondence between information obtained from interview surveys and
that obtained by medical examinations. There is usually considerable under-reporting of chronic diseases in interviews. Laymen are
not physicians, and cannot be expected to supply the same information. They differ in what they know, and they differ in their
language and concepts ('kidney trouble' is by no means the same
thing as 'renal disease'). On the other hand, neither are physicians
laymen, and interviews are preferable to medical sources when
information is sought on symptoms or degree of disability or
impact on quality of life, or on mild short-term diseases that are
unlikely to bring the patient to a doctor or to be present at the time
of an examination conducted in the course of a survey. As far as
'general health' is concerned, it has been said that 'the bulk of the
research evidence can be interpreted as indicating that a clinical
assessment of general health and the responses to survey questions
about health are only slightly correlated phenomena'.[2]

A health appraisal by a clinician is not necessarily more useful
than a self-appraisal. Numerous studies have shown that unfavourable responses to a question like 'In general, would you say your
health at present is excellent, very good, good, fair, or poor?' are
predictive of subsequent mortality.[3] Mortality has been found to be
higher for elderly people who rate their health as unfavourable
than for those who rate their health as favourable, independently
of the physician's rating of their health. In at least one study,

mortality was more closely related to the subjective rating than to an objective rating.

Different medical sources may also yield differing information. Death certificates or autopsies will not reveal cases who have survived; official notifications of disease may not cover all cases; clinical records will tell us nothing about patients who have not attended for care or have attended and been misdiagnosed; and ordinary examinations will not reveal myocardial infarcts that have healed, leaving no symptoms or electrocardiographic traces, although ample evidence of the disease may be found in previous clinical records. In fact, any morbidity survey using information from only one source is likely to be incomplete.

The choice of methods of data collection is largely based on the accuracy and relevance of the information they will yield—will the method provide sufficiently precise measures of the variables the investigator wishes to study, taking account of the purposes and objectives of the study? Two aspects of accuracy, reliability and validity, will be discussed in Chapters 16 and 17.

The selection of a method is also based on practical considerations, such as:

1. The need for personnel, skills, equipment, etc. in relation to what is available, and the urgency with which results are needed.
2. The subjects' preparedness and capacity to participate, as influenced by, for example, the 'friendliness' of the procedures (absence of undue inconvenience or unpleasantness or untoward consequences) and requirements for literacy or numeracy skills or special motivation.
3. The probability that the method will provide a good coverage, i.e. will supply the required information about all or almost all members of the population or sample. If many people will not know the answer to a question, the question is not an appropriate one. If many of the clinical records of a factory health service do not show blood pressure, the use of these records is not a very practicable way of studying blood pressure. If laboratory tests require prolonged fasting or the collection of all urine passed during a 24-hour period, they may be difficult to perform in a survey of apparently healthy people living at home, although the test may be a practicable one in a hospital situation.
4. The investigator's familiarity with a study procedure may be a valid consideration, but keep the 'Law of the Hammer' in mind: 'Give a small boy a hammer, and he will find that everything he

encounters needs pounding. It comes as no particular surprise to discover that a scientist formulates problems in a way which requires for their solution just those techniques in which he himself is especially skilled'.[4]

These practical aspects should be considered not only in relation to the measurement of each separate variable, but also in relation to the methods of data collection as a whole. Each of a long series of questions or clinical tests may itself be a 'practicable' one, but put together, they may make up a 3-hour interview or examination, which may be impracticable in terms of the time available to the study personnel, or unacceptable to the subjects.

Accuracy and 'practicability' are often inversely correlated. A method providing more satisfactory information will often be more elaborate, expensive or inconvenient. Clinical examinations provide more accurate information on chronic diseases than do interviews, but they are more expensive, require medical or paramedical personnel, and are less acceptable to the subjects and hence associated with a higher refusal rate. Accuracy must be balanced against practical considerations by choosing a method that will provide the required accuracy within the bounds of the investigator's resources and other practical limitations. In making this choice, account must be taken of the importance of the data, in the light of the purposes and objectives of the study. If the information is not very important, a simple although less accurate method may suffice; if more accurate information is essential, an elaborate or inconvenient method may be unavoidable. The aim is not 100% accuracy, but the maximal accuracy required for the purposes of the study and consistent with practical possibilities. Rapid epidemiological methods that sacrifice some accuracy in the interests of practicability will be discussed in Chapter 31.

Information on the accuracy and practicability of the proposed methods can often be obtained from previous methodological studies or from experiences in other investigations. In reading the literature on his study topic, the investigator should pay especial attention to methodological aspects.

Usually, however, it is found that there is a need to test at least some of the projected methods. It may be necessary to determine, for example, how long an interview or examination will take, how acceptable it is, whether questions are clearly intelligible and unambiguous, or whether the requisite data are available in clinical records. (Such 'pretests' are discussed in Ch. 24.) There may be a need for specific tests of reliability and validity (Ch. 16 and 17). Even if use is made of 'ready-made' questionnaires or other procedures developed elsewhere, it may be necessary to test them in the context of the planned study.

BLIND METHODS

Use is often made of 'blind' methods—i.e. the concealment of facts from observers, interviewers, the study subjects, people extracting information from documents, or anyone else who may influence the results—where such concealment may increase accuracy by avoiding bias. This applies to nonexperimental studies as well as to trials.

A *single-blind* experiment (or a *single-masked* one, to use a term preferred by researchers on eye diseases),[5] may be one in which the researcher makes his observations without knowing whether the subject is in the treatment or control group, or one where this information is kept from the subjects. A *double-blind*[6] experiment is one where neither observers nor subjects know to which group the subjects belong. In a double-blind experiment to test the efficacy of prayer, some patients were prayed for and others not; the patients were not told of the prayers, and the physicians appraising their clinical progress did not know for which cases divine intercession had been requested.[7] If the processing and analysis or monitoring of data are also done 'blind', an experiment may be called *triple-blind*.

Blinding is not always possible, and it often fails. Keeping subjects blind to their treatment generally requires a placebo or alternative treatment that cannot be identified by its appearance, taste, smell or effects. Elaborate stratagems may be needed to maintain the secret, such as the production of special pharmaceutical preparations and the use of containers identified only by symbols or numbers. Even then, the truth will often out. To test for breakdowns of secrecy it is helpful to ask subjects or physicians to guess the treatments, so as to see whether correct guesses outnumber what might be expected by chance. In a double-blind trial of the prevention and treatment of colds by vitamin C, half the subjects said they knew whether they were getting vitamin C or placebo— and were generally right (many admitted opening and tasting the capsules); colds were reported to be milder and of shorter duration in the vitamin C treatment group, but only among subjects who thought they knew what capsules they were having—there was no apparent effect among other subjects.[8]

If it is essential for the doctors who treat the subjects of a clinical trial to know what their patients are receiving, or if there is no way of hiding this information, it may be decided to base the evaluation on appraisals made by independent 'blinded' investigators. This reduces the chance of biased assessments, but does not control any effects the physician may have on the patient's progress as a result of his awareness of the treatment.

In nonexperimental studies, 'blind' methods may prevent bias caused by the observer's or interviewer's knowledge that the subject is a case or a control (*exposure suspicion bias*, p. 301), or that there has or has not been exposure to the causal factor under study (*diagnostic suspicion bias*), or in other situations where the findings may be influenced by a 'halo effect' due to the observer's prior impression of the individual he is studying. In a methodological study of the validity of wives' reports of their husbands' circumcision status, foreskins should be sought without knowledge of the wives' tales. The effect of prior knowledge may be especially troublesome in a longitudinal study in which subjects are examined repeatedly. In such a study it may be advisable to plan a record system that ensures that the examiner will not see the previous findings when he makes his observations.[9]

A double-blind method may be used in nonexperimental studies. This was done in a case-control study of the relationship of childhood leukaemia to parents' exposure to diagnostic X-rays (the mother before or during pregnancy, the father before conception).[10] The interviewer was not told whether a leukaemic patient's or control's household was being visited, and the questions that might reveal this were left to the the the end of the schedule. The person interviewed was told that this was a health survey, but did not know it had to do with leukaemia. Efforts are often made to conceal the specific hypotheses from both interviewers and subjects, in so far as this is feasible and ethical.

QUALITATIVE RESEARCH[11]

Some study methods are 'qualitative' rather than quantitative, i.e. they are not based on measures of quantity or frequency— their findings are described in words rather than numbers. Many investigators pooh-pooh qualitative studies, and research is often considered real and serious only if it is quantitative. But what has been called 'our love affair with numbers'[12] should not blind us to the fact that in some situations qualitative methods are more appropriate than quantitative methods, and in others a combination of qualitative and quantitative methods offers advantages.

Qualitative methods are widely used in studies of concepts of health and disease and other cultural factors affecting health and health care. They are especially useful in investigations of beliefs, perceptions and practices regarding health, the prevention and treatment of illness, and the utilization of traditional and other health care. A study of patients who had a heart attack, for example, pinpointed the misconceptions (about heart attack symptoms) that contributed to delay in calling for medical help.[13] Qualitative research provides 'culture specific maps [that] can help to improve the 'fit' of programmes to people'—maps that show the presence of beliefs and behaviours, but not their numerical prevalence in the population.[14] Proponents of the use of qualitative methods in evaluations of health care point out that they involve the researcher in new and close relationships with informants, open up dialogues on basic questions of health and health care, and 'can help to extend public health beyond an exclusively biomedical model'.[15]

Qualitative and quantitative approaches may often be regarded as complementary.[16] In a study of the reasons for incomplete immunization in Haiti, for example, qualitative methods were used to identify barriers to the use of preventive services, and these were then measured in a quantitative survey.[17] Qualitative methods can also be used as a follow-up to a quantitative study, to explain and expand the findings, and they may be a fruitful source of hypotheses for quantitative testing. Qualitative inquiries can also uncover and explain deficiencies in the manner of collection of quantitative data.[12]

Qualitative methods[11] encompass 'field studies' (observations of 'ongoing social life in its natural setting'),[18] including observations in health care facilities and the community at large; *participant observation*[19] (where the researcher is personally involved in the action being observed); interviews and conversations with key informants and other members of the community, in which people can express their attitudes, perceptions, motivations, feelings and behaviour; *focus group interviews*,[20] in which a small group of informants talk freely and spontaneously about themes considered important to the investigator; the study of case histories; and other methods.

If done properly, qualitative research is as rigorous as quantitative research, and the need for accuracy and for reaching conclusions that a repeated study (were it feasible) would replicate is as important as for quantitative research. Methods available for these purposes include 'triangulation' (use of more than one qualitative method, to ascertain their common conclusions) and independent analyses of data by more than one investigator. Three suggested questions for use in appraising the conclusions of a qualitative study of beliefs and practices are:

1. How well do the conclusions explain why people behave in the way they do?
2. How comprehensible would this explanation be to a thoughtful participant in the setting?
3. How well does it cohere with what we already know?[21]

Full-blown qualitative research requires professional training, and this book discusses only a few simpler applications, such as 'rapid ethnographic assessment' procedures (see p. 348), the Nominal Group technique (Ch. 20), and the use of qualitative methods in exploratory studies (see p. 30) and as part of the process by which a practitioner of community medicine 'gets to know' a community (Ch. 34).

NOTES AND REFERENCES

1. Nafstad P, Botten G, Hagen J A, Zahlsen K, Nilsen O G, Silsand T, Kongerud J 1995 Comparison of three methods for estimating environmental tobacco smoke exposure among children aged between 12 and 36 months. International Journal of Epidemiology 24: 88.
2. Feldman J 1960 The household interview survey as a technique for the collection of morbidity data. Journal of Chronic Diseases 11: 535.
3. Idler E L, Benyamini Y 1997 Self-rated health and mortality: a review of twenty-seven community studies. Journal of Health and Social Behavior 38: 21.
4. Kaplan A 1964 The conduct of inquiry. Harper & Row, New York.
5. The term 'double-masked' is recommended by Ederer F 1975 (Practical problems in collaborative trials. American Journal of Epidemiology 102: 111), who goes on to say 'Carrying out masking successfully is usually more easily said than done ... One ophthalmologist measured patients' visual acuity with their bodies draped with a cloth and their heads covered with a hood'. Ingelfinger F J 1973 (Blind as a clinical investigator. New England Journal of Medicine 288: 1299) criticizes the term 'blind' ('The sections were read blindly under high-powered magnification'), especially if it supersedes a detailed account of the precautions taken to prevent bias (in such instances, he suggests that 'double-purblind' might be a good term!).
6. 'A fascinating instance of the blind leading the blind. With this, neither the physician nor the patient knows whether a drug or a placebo is being given—

until, that is, the patient either recovers or expires. Some think this technique was borrowed from Russian roulette' (Armous R 1971 It all started with Hippocrates. Bantam Books, New York, p. 132).

7. Joyce C R B, Welldon R M C 1965 The objective efficacy of prayer. Journal of Chronic Diseases 18: 367.
8. Lewis T L, Karlowski T R, Kapikian A Z, Lynch J M, Shaffer G W, George D A 1975 A controlled clinical trial of ascorbic acid for the common cold. Annals of the New York Academy of Sciences 258: 505.
9. Ignorance of the previous findings may also have disadvantages (Feinstein A R 1987 Clinimetrics. Yale University Press, New Haven, p. 98; Guyatt G H, Berman L B, Townsend M, Taylor D W 1985 Should study subjects see their previous response? Journal of Chronic Diseases 38: 1003).
10. Bross I D J, Natajaran N 1977 Genetic damage from diagnostic radiation. Journal of the American Medical Association 237: 2399.
11. Mays N, Pope C 1996 Qualitative research in health care. BMJ Publishing Group, London; Greenhaigh T, Taylor R 1997 How to read a paper: Papers that go beyond numbers (qualitative research). British Medical Journal 315: 740; Heggenhaugen H K, Pedersen D 1997 Beyond quantitative measures: the relevance of anthropology for public health. In: Detels R, Holland W W, McEwen J, Omenn G S (eds) 1997 Oxford Textbook of public health, 3rd edn, vol 2. The methods of public health. Oxford University Press, New York, pp 815–828; Morse J M, Field P A 1995 Qualitative research methods for health professionals, 2nd edn. Sage Publications, Beverly Hills; Bloor M, Taraborelli P (eds) 1994 Qualitative studies in health and medicine (Cardiff papers in qualitative research), Avebury; Smith R B, Manning P K (eds) 1982 A handbook of social science methods, vol 2. Qualitative methods. Ballinger, Cambridge, Mass.
    Guidelists for the collection of qualitative data on topics related to health and health care are provided by Scrimshaw S C M, Hurtado E 1987 (Rapid assessment procedures for nutrition and primary health care: anthropological approaches to improving programme effectiveness. UCLA Latin American Center Publications, Los Angeles, Cal.).
12. Black N 1994 Editorial: why we need qualitative research. Journal of Epidemiology and Community Health 48: 425.
13. Ruston A, Clayton J, Calnan M 1998. Patients' action during their cardiac event: qualitative study exploring differences and modifiable factors. British Medical Journal 316: 1060.
14. Scrimshaw S C M, Hurtado E 1987 (see note 11).
15. See Beattie A 1995 (Evaluation in community development for health: an opportunity for dialogue. Health Education Journal 54: 465. Reprinted in Sidell M, Jones L, Katz J, Peberdy A 1997 Debates and dilemmas in promoting health: a reader. MacMillan Press, Houndmills), who lists the evaluation methods used in community development for health projects in the United Kingdom and describes some of the features of *pluralistic evaluation*, which combines different approaches.
16. Kroeger A 1983 Anthropological and socio-medical health care research in developing countries. Social Science and Medicine 17: 147; and Health interview surveys in developing countries: a review of the methods and results. International Journal of Epidemiology 12: 465.
17. Coreil J, Augustin A, Holt E, Halsey N A 1989 Use of ethnographic research for instrument development in a case-control study of immunization use in Haiti. International Journal of Epidemiology 18: S33.
18. Arnold D O 1982 In: Smith R B, Manning P K (see note 11).
19. *Participant observation* is a technique widely used in anthropology but little used in health research. An example would be a study of doctor-patient relationships, carried out by the physician or patient participating in the

relationships. The hazards of this method are that the observer may influence the action, and may have a biased viewpoint.

20. *Focus groups.* See: Powell R A, Single H M 1996 (Focus groups. International Journal of Quality in Health Care 8: 499); Khan M E, Anker M, Patel B C, Barge S, Sadhwani H, Kohle R 1991 (The use of focus groups in social and behavioural research: some methodological issues. World Health Statistics Quarterly 44: 145); Bowling A 1997 (Research methods in health: investigating health and health services. Open University Press, Buckingham, pp 352–355).

21. Mays N, Pope C 1996 (see note 11).

16 Reliability

'Reliability' (also termed 'reproducibility' or 'repeatability') refers to the stability or consistency of information, i.e. the extent to which similar information is obtained when a measurement is performed more than once. The reliability of a procedure of measurement is equivalent to a marksman's capacity to hit the same spot each time he shoots, irrespective of whether this spot is the bull's-eye.

The concept is best explained by case illustrations:

1. In a study in rural India, in which the incidence of accidental injuries was studied by paying periodic home visits and asking about injuries occurring since the last home visit, the incidence was doubled when inquiries were made at intervals of 2 weeks instead of a month.[1]
2. In the USA, a comparison of death certificates with census records completed shortly before death showed that only 72% of white persons recorded as divorced on their census records were also recorded as divorced on their death certificates; 17% were recorded as widowed, 5% as single, and 6% as married.[2]
3. A film was prepared, portraying the measuring of the blood pressures of seven subjects; it showed the mercury column in the sphygmomanometer, while the sound track played the accompanying sounds. When nurses were shown the film and asked to read the subjects' blood pressures, there was much variation between the pressures recorded by different nurses. The same film was later used to test physicians, with similar results ('some of the best results have been achieved by

statisticians who had never taken a blood pressure before but who had been trained in objective and accurate recording of data')[3]

4. In a study of the utilization of hospital beds, panels of four physicians made appraisals of whether randomly selected beds were being appropriately used, i.e. whether the patient required hospital care on the day of observation. All four agreed in only 75% of cases.[4]

5. In Taiwan, two highly skilled ophthalmologists examined the same population sample, seeking evidence of trachoma, an infective disease of the eye often leading to disfigurement and sometimes to blindness. They used the same criteria (physical signs) and the same examination procedure; both had exceptionally keen vision. One found 122 cases of active trachoma, and the other found 136; but these included only 75 who were diagnosed by both experts; the other 108 were diagnosed by only one or other of them.[5]

6. The same chest X-ray films were examined independently by five experts in order to determine the presence of tuberculosis. Of 131 films which were recorded as positive by at least one reader, there were only 27 where all five observers agreed; in 17 cases, four observers gave a 'positive' verdict; in another 17, three said 'positive' and two said 'negative'; in 23, two said 'positive'; and in 47, one said 'positive' and four said 'negative'. The films were later reread by the same observers, and there were many reversals of verdict. For instance, one radiologist, who had found 59 positive cases the first time, found 78 the second time, comprising 55 who had been positive the first time, and 23 new cases.[6]

7. Material with a known concentration of haemoglobin (9.8 g per 100 ml) was sent to a number of hospital laboratories, and a separate determination of haemoglobin was performed in each laboratory; the results ranged from 8 to 15.5 g per 100 ml.[7]

8. A standard suspension of red blood cells was examined in a number of laboratories; when visual counting was performed the red blood cell counts ranged from 2.2 to 4.5 million cells per mm^3; when electronic cell counters were used the range was from 0.7 to 4.7 million.[8]

9. In a study of the medications taken by patients with congestive heart failure who were treated by a sample of general practitioners and internists in private practice in a city in the USA, information was obtained both from patients and from their

physicians. Medications that could be obtained without prescription were not included. Discrepancies were found in 73% of cases: 22% of the patients were not taking drugs their doctors thought they were, another 22% were taking drugs without their doctors' knowledge, and both these discrepancies occurred together in another 29%.[9]

10. A number of studies have shown that if children are measured during the morning they are on average taller, by half a centimetre or more, than if they are measured in the afternoon.[10]

High reliability does not necessarily mean that a procedure is a satisfactory one; measurements that are 'far from the bull's-eye' may not provide the investigator with helpful information (what is more reliable—or less useful—than a broken watch?). On the other hand it is obvious that the less reliable the procedure the less useful it will be. The problem of reliability is especially acute in longitudinal studies where an attempt is being made to assess change, since the findings may express variability in the measurements rather than a real change in the attribute that is being measured (see p. 85). In a study designed to measure the incidence rate of new cases of a chronic disease, performed by repeating a diagnostic procedure after a period of time, unreliability of the procedure will tend to produce an unduly high estimate of incidence. This is because persons who are falsely diagnosed as new cases on the second occasion, and ill persons falsely diagnosed as being healthy on the first occasion, will usually outnumber new cases that are missed, while well persons misdiagnosed as ill at the first examination will be excluded from the population at risk of developing the disease, thus further increasing the incidence rate.

If, when duplicate tests are performed by two laboratories, one laboratory consistently yields lower readings than another, a comparison of laboratory reports will show *systematic* or *one-sided variation*. This will pose a problem in a study using both laboratories, since (at best) only one of the laboratories can be providing correct results.

If the variation is random in direction, or if variations in the two directions cancel each other out, this is *non-systematic variation*. In a large study in England and Wales, for example, it was found that in only 65% of the cases where death was ascribed to arteriosclerotic heart disease by the treating physician, was the assignment to this cause confirmed by autopsy. However, there were other cases that were diagnosed on autopsy only, so that the total numbers of deaths ascribed to this disease by clinicians and pathologists were fairly similar.[11]

The fact that variation is nonsystematic offers no guarantee against erroneous conclusions. If our marksman's arrows are widely scattered, but centred on the bull's-eye, the average or overall measurement may indeed be accurate. But it is obvious that the individual measurements cannot all be correct. If we use an unreliable measure we are likely—whether the variation is systematic or nonsystematic—to obtain incorrect information and (if the scale is categorical) to *misclassify* individuals (as sick or well, smokers or non-smokers, etc.) and hence to obtain deceptive information about relationships between characteristics (see p. 188). Moreover, even if variation is on the whole nonsystematic, it is never easy to be sure that one-sided variation is not present in some part of the study population, since the balance between the opposing tendencies may differ in different strata. In the above study, for example, the findings varied in different age groups. Among people aged 45–64 years, slightly *more* deaths were ascribed to arteriosclerotic heart disease by clinicians than by pathologists; whereas among people aged 75 and more, 22% *fewer* cases were ascribed to this cause by clinicians.

The term 'error' should preferably not be used to describe variation (although it often is), unless there is definite knowledge that a particular value is correct.

SOURCES OF VARIATION

Variation between measurements[12] may have its source in (1) changes in the *characteristics* being measured (a lack of 'constancy');[13] (2) the *measuring instrument*, i.e. variation between readings (a lack of 'precision',[13] or between instruments (a lack of 'congruency');[13] and (3) the *person* collecting the information (a lack of 'objectivity').[13] For example, if two clinicians measure the same subject's blood pressure and record different readings, the possible explanations are (1) that the blood pressure altered between the two measurements; (2) that the sphygmomanometer or the measuring procedure as a whole provides variable results or, if different sphygmomanometers or procedures were used, that these provide different results; and (3) that the clinicians differ in the way they read or record blood pressure measurements.

1. *Variation in the characteristic being measured* may be caused by variation in any of the whole complex of factors which determine the characteristic. These factors include the measuring procedure itself. For example, blood pressure may be affected by the conditions under which the measurement is performed— the subject's posture and emotional state, the clinician's sex and pulchritude, etc. The response to a question may be affected (and 'response instability' thus produced) by the respondent's motivations, his state of fatigue or boredom, the circumstances of the interview (at home or in hospital, the presence of other persons, etc.), the interviewer's sex, appearance and manner, etc. Behaviour may be changed by the subject's awareness that he is being studied; he may modify his diet if he is aware that what and how much he eats are being observed and measured. In a clinical trial the subject's condition may be influenced by his awareness of whether he is receiving the treatment under test or is a member of a control group.

2. *The measuring instruments* (a term that may be extended to include not only mechanical devices, but biochemical and other tests, questions, questionnaires, and the measuring procedure as an entity) may not yield consistent results, or different instruments may give different results.

3. *The persons collecting the information* (observers, interviewers, or persons extracting data from documentary sources) may vary in what they perceive, in their skill, integrity, propensity to make mistakes, etc. They may be influenced, consciously or unconsciously, by their preconceptions and motivations; in a clinical trial, an investigator's awareness of whether he is dealing with an experimental or control subject may bias his observations. Observers tend to find what they expect to find. This (the 'Rosenthal effect') has been demonstrated repeatedly; for example, experimenters who compared groups of rats that they had been told came from 'clever' and 'stupid' strains found that the 'clever' rats were much better at learning to negotiate mazes—although in fact the two groups were genetically identical.[14] In a reliability study in which auscultatory measurements of the fetal heart rate were compared with the electronically recorded rate, it was found that when the true rate was under 130 beats per minute the hospital staff tended to overestimate it, and when it was over 150 they tended to underestimate it.[15]

Observer variation

'Observer variation' is a term which, strictly speaking, refers to variation arising from the persons making the observations, and not from changes in the characteristic being measured or from the measuring instrument. In practice, it is often extremely difficult to separate these aspects completely, and the term is therefore used to indicate any differences between observations by different observers (interobserver variation) or by the same observer on different occasions (intraobserver variation). Interobserver variation in blood pressure measurements may be caused not only by the way in which the measurements are read and recorded, but by the effect of the clinicians' demeanour on the subjects' blood pressure or by differences in the procedure of measurement (the rate at which the cuff is deflated, the level at which the sphygmomanometer is placed, etc.). Inter-interviewer variation may be due not only to the way in which the interviewers perceive, interpret and record what the respondents say, but to the way they ask questions and their influence on the respondent.

In clinical examinations, observer variation is often due to the fact that different clinicians use different definitions of what they are measuring. This is one reason for the unreliability of diagnosis which besets studies in psychiatric epidemiology.[16] Clinicians may also be influenced by what they have come to regard as 'normal'. A physician working in a malnourished population may regard as well nourished a child who, if seen by a physician accustomed to a better nourished population, would be appraised as malnourished. There may also be a tendency for the examiner to find what he thinks he ought to find.

MEASURING RELIABILITY

Although efforts should obviously be made to collect reliable information, it must be stressed that complete reliability is not essential. The measurement of a phenomenon should not be given up simply because there is some degree of unreliability. 'There is a danger in studies of reliability of permitting the perfect to become the enemy of the good or committing the error of errorlessness.'[17] It is important, however, to know *how much* unreliability there is, particularly with regard to the variables that play an important part in the investigation—how much variation arises from the method of measurement, as compared with the variation between the individuals or groups being studied? Unless this is known it may be difficult to avoid reaching unwarranted conclusions. Sometimes previous methodological studies may provide a sufficient guide. However, it is often necessary to measure reliability, either before embarking on the study, i.e. by performing a pretest (see Ch. 24), or by building reliability tests into the study itself.

Reliability is measured by performing two or more independent measurements and comparing the findings, using an appropriate statistical index, such as *kappa*[18] for a measure of a categorical variable, or a suitable coefficient for an interval- or ratio-scale measure.[19] The comparison may be based on observations by different observers or interviews by different observers, on repeated measurements or interviews using the same instrument or questionnaire (the *test–retest* method), or on measurements with different instruments. Replicate tests may be made on the same blood specimens. A question may be repeated in the same questionnaire, or differently worded questions asking for the same information may be included.

The results of a test–retest comparison depend on the interval between the tests. A questionnaire-based measure of overall health, for example, was found to have a test–retest reliability of about 0.85 (this was the proportion of variance not attributable to random variation) over a 1-month period, but only about 0.56 over a 3-year interval.[20] The purpose of the measurement should be kept in mind when reliability is tested. Long-term reliability is appropriate if the aim is to measure a fairly stable attribute, such as a personality trait, but not if the aim is to measure transient or changeable characteristics. Tests of an 'anxiety inventory' demonstrated that test–retest reliability (for intervals of 1 hour to 104 days) was much higher for questions designed to measure 'anxiety-trait' ('how you feel in general') than for those designed to measure 'anxiety-state' ('how you feel right now').[21]

It is often advisable to appraise reliability in different subgroups of the sample. The test–retest reliability of the anxiety-state questionnaire, for example, was much higher for men than for women. The Minnesota Leisure Time Physical Activity Questionnaire has a high test–retest reliability (5-week interval), but reliability is somewhat lower among people who report more activity.[22] For investigators using a set of questions on the frequency of consumption of various foods, it was important to know that test–retest reliability (over a 9-month period) was unaffected by age or relative weight.[23]

Reliability may of course differ for different items in an examination or interview. Repeated questioning of a sample of postmenopausal women, for example, revealed a high degree of concordance for a history of hysterectomy and a family history of breast cancer, but many disagreements with respect to a history of hot flushes.[24]

Sometimes it is impracticable or inadvisable to make repeated measurements of the same persons. In a test of an interview schedule, for instance, the two sets of responses may not be independent. The first interview may lead the respondent to give more thought to the survey topic, and change his mind; or he may try to be consistent in his two sets of replies, be less careful to give accurate answers the second time of asking, etc. Under such conditions, reliability may be tested by randomly dividing the subjects among a number of observers or interviewers, in order to see whether the differences between the groups are greater than are likely to be produced by the random allocation itself. If repeated measurements are made on the same subjects although there is reason to believe that their sequence may affect the findings, the order in which subjects are examined by different observers or interviewers or with different instruments should be determined by random allocation (see p. 359) or a satisfactory equivalent method.

Intraobserver variation may be particularly difficult to study in instances where the measurements are made by direct observations on human subjects, since the observer may remember the subjects and attempt (consciously or unconsciously) to be consistent in his two sets of observations. This difficulty is possibly less acute when the observations are based on X-ray plates, electrocardiogram tracings, etc., which may be less distinctive than faces and personalities.

If reliability is low, the possible role of each possible source of variation should in principle be measured, by testing each source separately. For example, in studying the reliability of haemoglobin determinations, one factor at a time may be varied, while the rest of the procedure is kept constant. In this way, separate attention can be given to the effect of the time of day that blood is sampled, the effect of using capillary or venous blood, the effect of using a tourniquet, the effect of delay in examining the specimen, the differences between biochemical methods, instruments, or technicians, the variation of results from a single photometer or technician, etc. Such tests can provide a rational basis for solutions; that is, they may indicate methods of correcting or allowing for the variation produced by each source. It may be difficult and sometimes impossible, however, to separate the different sources of error; moreover, this kind of methodological study is a formidable undertaking. In small-scale investigations, what is usually done instead is to make assumptions concerning the probable major sources of variation, and to take arbitrary steps aimed at counteracting them.

The reliability of a combination score—one that combines the scores of component items in order to measure a composite variable (see p. 153)—can be measured not only by the test–retest and other methods described above, but also by appraising internal consistency. If the items in a scale are measures of the same attribute, the extent to which they give the same result is a function of their reliability. Cronbach's *alpha* (see p. 156) is often called a measure of consistency-reliability and is commonly used for this purpose (but if the items are heterogeneous, *alpha* usually underestimates the true reliability).[25] It is customary to use more than one index of reliability.[26] Internal consistency is sometimes measured by the *split-half* method, in which a questionnaire that was administered to measure a single attribute is divided, purposively or randomly, into two parts, and the findings they yield are compared; if there is little variation, this is taken as evidence of consistency.

ENHANCING RELIABILITY

Steps should be taken, not to attain complete reliability, but to reduce variation to reasonable limits.

To this end, clearly defined standardized procedures are required. The variables should have clear operational definitions, a standard procedure of examination should be used, and standard questions should be asked in a standard way. There should be detailed step-by-step descriptions of the methods (but remember that 'a carefully detailed manual of methods, however massive, is not good for much, if ignored by the field workers').[27]

The instrument should be one that supplies relatively consistent measurements. In particular, the variation associated with the instrument should be small in relation to the total range of variation of the attribute being measured; a ruler with coarse calibrations is sufficient if a large expanse is to be measured, but one with finer calibrations is needed if a short length is to be measured (an instrument or test meeting this requirement may be called *precise* or of high *discrimination*). If more than one measuring device is used, they should be of the same model and/or standardized against each other. Equipment should be tested from time to time. Quality control procedures should be undertaken, e.g. chemical tests on a standard reference solution and comparisons of replicate tests of the same specimens.

The use of scores based on a number of related items generally increases reliability. In this context it may be noted that disease diagnoses based on a combination of manifestations are often of higher reliability than the data on the separate items. The use of repeated measures may also increase reliability: with quantitative measurements that show appreciable variation, the mean of two or more readings may be used.

If the procedure is one requiring special skill, the necessary training should be provided. If there is more than one observer, they should attune·their methods, possibly by working together for a while. Where necessary, they should have standard reference pictures, such as colour photographs of different stages of a skin disorder, or X-ray plates showing radiological abnormalities.

If it is not possible to use a single observer, and much inter-observer variation is expected, each individual should if possible be independently examined by more than one examiner. An advantage of this is that the disagreements can be exploited to produce a more discriminatory scale of measurement.[28] For example, if the severity of a disease is graded as 1 (mild), 2 (moderate) or 3 (severe), it may be assumed that subjects allocated to grade 1 by one clinician and to grade 2 by another lie close to the borderline between grades 1 and 2; such cases could be placed in an intermediate category, 1½, lying between grades 1 and 2 in the ordinal scale. Alternatively, when there is disagreement the cases may be re-examined and discussed until agreement is reached, or a referee may be called in for a casting vote; these latter procedures have been criticized, however, on the grounds that 'forced' agreement may not mean a correct decision, but submission to the more experienced or forceful of the observers. Parallel observations of this kind are facilitated if there are permanent records of the observations, such as electrocardiogram tracings or retinal photographs.

NOTES AND REFERENCES

1. Gordon J E, Gulati P V, Wyon J B 1962 Archives of Environmental Health 4: 575.
2. National Center for Health Statistics 1969 Comparability of marital status, race, nativity, and country of origin on the death certificate and matching

census record, United States, May–August, 1960. Vital and Health Statistics, series 2, no 34. Public Health Service, Washington D C.

3. Wilcox J 1962 Observer factors in the measurement of blood pressure. Journal of the American Medical Association 179: 53; Rose G A, Holland W W, Crowley E A 1964 A sphygmomanometer for epidemiologists. Lancet i: 296.

4. Zimmer J G 1967 An evaluation of observer variability in a hospital bed utilization study. Medical Care 5: 221.

5. Assaad F A, Maxwell-Lyons F 1967 Systematic observer variation in trachoma studies. Bulletin of the World Health Organization 36: 885.

6. Birkelo C C, Chamberlain W E, Phelps P S, Schools P E, Zacks D, Yerushalmy J 1947 Tuberculosis case finding: a comparison of the effectiveness of various roentgenographic and photofluorographic methods. Journal of the American Medical Association 133: 359.

7. Belk W P, Sunderman F W 1947 A survey of the accuracy of chemical analyses in clinical laboratories. American Journal of Clinical Pathology 17: 853.

8. Lewis S M, Burgess B J 1969 Quality control in haematology: report of interlaboratory trials in Britain. British Medical Journal iv: 253.

9. Hulka B S, Kupper L L, Cassel J C, Efird R L, Burdette J A 1975 Medication use and misuse: physician–patient discrepancies. Journal of Chronic Diseases 28: 7.

10. Baker I A, Hughes J, Jones M 1978 Temporal variation in the height of children during the day. Lancet 1: 1320.

11. Heasman L A, Lipworth L 1966 Accuracy of certification of causes of death. General Register Officer, Studies on Medical and Population Subjects no 20. HMSO, London, pp 84, 118.

12. A mathematical model of reliability expresses a measurement as the sum of its (unknown) true score, a random error, and a systematic error. Reliability theory is summarized by Guilford J P, Fruchter B 1986 (Fundamental statistics in psychology and education, 6th edn. McGraw-Hill, Auckland, Ch 7). See Healy M J K 1989 (Measuring measuring errors. Statistics in Medicine 8: 893). For a simple graphic explanation: trochim.human. cornell.edu/kb/reliable.htm (on the Internet).

13. Zetterberg H L 1963 On theory and verification in sociology. Bedminster Press, Totowa, N J, pp 50–51.

14. Rosenthal R 1976 Experimenter effects in behavioural research. Irvington, New York.

15. Day E, Maddern L, Wood C 1968 Auscultation of foetal heart rate: an assessment of its error and significance. British Medical Journal ii: 422.

16. See note 7, page 139.

17. Elison J 1972 In: Levine S, Reeder L G, Freeman H E (eds) Handbook of medical sociology, 2nd edn. Prentice Hall, Englewood Cliffs, N J, p. 493.

18. The simple 'reliability coefficient' or 'per cent agreement' (the proportion of cases placed in identical categories by two independent determinations) may be misleading, since agreement may occur by chance. *Kappa* is a better index for categorical measures, since it makes allowance for the contribution of chance agreement; kappa can also be used for ordered categories; see Fleiss J L 1981 (Statistical methods for rates and proportions, 2nd edn. Wiley, New York, pp 212–236).

    A kappa of 75% or more may be taken to represent excellent agreement, and values of 40–74% indicate fair to good agreement; most comparisons of clinical examinations, as well as interpretations of X-rays, electrocardiograms and microscopic specimens yield values of 40–74%; see Sackett D L, Haynes R B, Tugwell P 1985 (Clinical epidemiology: a basic science for clinical medicine. Little, Brown, Boston, Ch 2). In a study in which the commonly used Rose chest pain questionnaire for angina pectoris was administered repeatedly to various groups, *kappa* (after one year) was only 20 to 41% in men and 19 to 33% in women, reflecting the combined effects of the reliability of the instrument, differences in how it was administered (different interviewers, face-to-face or by phone) and possible changes in health status (Sorlie P D, Cooper L, Schreiner P J, Rosamond W, Szklo M 1995 Repeatability and validity of the Rose questionnaire for angina pectoris in the Atherosclerosis Risk in Communities study. Journal of Clinical Epidemiology 49: 719). In a study with a shorter interval (usually same day, several months at most) *kappa* for this questionnaire was 77% in men and 48% in women (Harris R B, Weissfeld L A 1991 Gender differences in the reliability of reporting symptoms of angina pectoris. Journal of Clinical Epidemiology 44: 1071).

Kappa may be affected by disparity in the prevalences of the categories and by systematic variation between the ratings (Byrt T, Bishop J, Carlin J B 1993 Bias, prevalence and kappa. Journal of Clinical Epidemiology 46: 423). KAPPA, in the PEPI package (see note 7, p. 292), which computes *kappa* and its confidence intervals, can make adjustments for these effects.

19. Reliability indices for use with interval-scale and ratio-scale variables include the correlation coefficient, an intraclass correlation coefficient (and the components of variation derived from analysis of variance), the concordance correlation coefficient, the mean, frequency distribution and quantiles of the differences, and the *limits of agreement* (the confidence interval of the crude or log-transformed difference). The term 'reliability coefficient' generally refers to an intraclass correlation coefficient. PAIRS, in the PEPI package (see note 7, p. 292) can compute the indices.

Different indices of reliability may be appropriate, depending on the purpose of the measurement. If the purpose is 'discrimination' (i.e. to compare individuals or groups), the correlation between replicate measures may be an appropriate index; for a predictive measure, the intraclass correlation coefficient or *kappa* is appropriate; and if the purpose is to measure change there should be little variation between replicate measures in stable subjects and large variation when the intensity of the attribute alters (Kirshner B, Guyatt G 1985 A methodologic framework for assessing health indices. Journal of Chronic Diseases 38: 27).

See Streiner D L, Norman G R 1995 (Health measurement scales: a practical guide to their development and use, 2nd edn. Oxford University Press, Oxford, Ch 8); Bartko J J 1994 (General methodology II: measures of agreement: a single procedure. Statistics in Medicine 13: 737); Chinn S 1990 (The assessment of methods of measurement. Statistics in Medicine 9: 351); Bland J M, Altmann D G 1986 (Statistical methods for assessing agreement between two methods of clinical measurement. Lancet i: 307) and 1995 (Comparing methods of measurement: why plotting differences against standard method is misleading. Lancet 346: 1085). For examples, see Sarmandal P, Bailey S M, Grant J M 1989 (A comparison of three methods of assessing inter-observer variation applied to ultrasonic fetal measurement in the third trimester. British Journal of Obstetrics and Gynaecology 96: 1261); and Bhushan V, Paneth N 1991 (The reliability of neonatal head circumference measurement. Journal of Clinical Epidemiology 44: 1027).

20. Ware J E Jr 1984 Methodological considerations in the selection of health status assessment procedures. In: Wenger N K, Mattson M E, Furberg C D, Elinson J (eds) Assessment of quality of life in clinical trials of cardiovascular therapies. LeJacq Publishing, pp 87–111.

21. Spielberger C D, Gorsuch R I, Lushene R E 1970 Manual for the state–trait anxiety inventory. Consulting Psychologists Press, Palo Alto, Cal. Cited by Siegel J M, Feinstein L G, Stone A J 1985 Personality and cardiovascular

disease: measurement of personality variables. In: Ostfeld A M, Eaker E D (eds) Measuring psychosocial variables in epidemiologic studies of cardiovascular disease. NIH publication no 85–2270. National Institutes of Health, US Department of Health and Human Services, pp 367–401.

22. Folsom A R, Jacobs D R Jr, Caspersen C J, Gomez-Martin O, Knudsen J 1986 Test–retest reliability of the Minnesota Leisure Time Physical Activity Questionnaire. Journal of Chronic Diseases 39: 505.

23. Colditz G A, Willett W C, Stampfer M J et al 1987 The influence of age, relative weight, smoking and alcohol intake on the reproducibility of a dietary questionnaire. International Journal of Epidemiology 16: 392.

24. Horwitz R I, Yu E C 1985 Problems and proposals for interview data in epidemiological research. International Journal of Epidemiology 14: 463.

25. Lord F M, Novick R 1968 Statistical theories of mental test scores. McGraw Hill, New York.

26. As an example, the findings of an appraisal in Sheffield of the reliability of 8 combination scores provided by the SF-36 health survey questionnaire (re-administered after two weeks) were: reliability coefficients, 0.74 to 0.93; correlation coefficients, 0.60 to 0.81; mean difference (on 100-point scale) 0.1 to 0.7 (regarded as 'of no practical significance'); Cronbach's *alpha*, 0.73 to 0.96. The authors concluded that the findings supported the internal consistency of the questionnaire and that 'since an instrument with a high discriminatory power may be unreliable it was reassuring to find that test–retest reliability was excellent' (Brazier J E, Harper R, Jones N M B, O'Cathain A, Thomas K J, Usherwood T, Westlake L 1992 Validating the SF-36 health survey questionnaire: new outcome measure for primary care. British Medical Journal 305: 160).

27. Anderson D W, Mantel N 1983 On epidemiologic surveys. American Journal of Epidemiology 118: 613.

28. Fletcher C K, Oldham P D 1964 Diagnosis in group research. In: Witts L J (ed) Medical surveys and clinical trials, 2nd edn. Oxford University Press, London, pp 25–49.

17 Validity

This chapter deals with the validity of *measures*; the validity of *studies*—i.e. their capacity to produce sound conclusions—will be covered in later chapters. We will consider the ways in which validity can be appraised, and the evaluation of screening and diagnostic tests and risk markers.

The *validity of a measure* refers to the adequacy with which the method of measurement does its job—how well does it measure the characteristic that the investigator actually wants to measure? It is equivalent to a marksman's capacity to hit the bull's-eye—if all arrows hit the bull's-eye (Robin Hood style) the measure is both valid and reliable.

If we wish to know how much sugar a person consumes, we may obtain more valid information by asking how many spoons of sugar he puts in his tea or coffee and how many cups he drinks a day, than by merely asking him whether he has a 'sweet tooth'. The data will be still more valid if we obtain information about everything he eats or drinks, and calculate his sugar intake by using tables showing the average sugar content of various foodstuffs; and they will be even more valid if, instead of using these tables, we perform laboratory analyses of samples of the foods and drinks he actually consumes.

Clearly, if a measure is not reliable (see Ch. 16) this must reduce its validity; if the shots are scattered they cannot all hit the bull's-eye. If reliability is high the measure is not necessarily valid—the shots may all hit an innocent bystander. ('Just because it's reliable doesn't mean that you can use it').[1] But if reliability is low the measure cannot have a high validity.

There is little point in considering whether a measurement is valid in relation to the operational definition of the variable being measured. If the operational definition is a good one, it will be phrased in terms of observable facts. These facts are hence automatically ('by definition') valid as a measure of the variable, as operationally defined. If prematurity is defined in terms of birth weight, as recorded in hospital records, then information on birth weight must constitute a valid measure of prematurity, so defined. If intelligence is defined as 'what is measured by an intelligence test', then an intelligence test must obviously be a valid measure of intelligence. To appraise validity meaningfully, it must be considered in relation to the conceptual definition of the variable.

In planning a study we should satisfy ourselves that every variable is measured as validly as its importance in the study requires, taking account of available resources and other practical constraints. If validity is low, the measure will be a poor proxy for the characteristic that we want to measure. Serum triglyceride estimations based on blood samples taken from people who have recently had a meal may be a reflection of what they ate rather

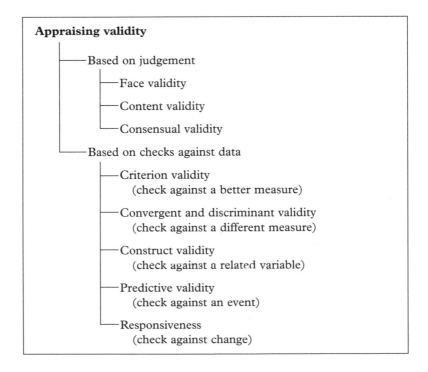

Appraising validity

- Based on judgement
  - Face validity
  - Content validity
  - Consensual validity
- Based on checks against data
  - Criterion validity
    (check against a better measure)
  - Convergent and discriminant validity
    (check against a different measure)
  - Construct validity
    (check against a related variable)
  - Predictive validity
    (check against an event)
  - Responsiveness
    (check against change)

than of the metabolic pattern that interests us. If the presence of a hernia is reported by only 54% of men who turn out to have obvious bulging inguinal hernias, and if hernias are reported by men who have none,[2] the *misclassification* of study subjects by interview data is likely to produce a biased picture of prevalence, the direction of the bias depending on the balance between false nonreports and false reports. This is an example of *information bias* (bias attributable to shortcomings in the way information is obtained or handled).

There are various ways of appraising validity. Some are essentially based on judgement alone (face, content and consensual validity), the issue being whether the operational definition of the variable being measured appears to be an appropriate rendering of its conceptual definition. Others are based on checks against data, permitting a judgement to be made about how well the measure does its job in the particular context represented by a specific sample or samples. The data may be available at the time the measure is used (sometimes called 'concurrent validity'), or may pertain to the future (predictive validity). The 'types of validity' listed on the previous page and discussed below express different approaches to the question 'How valid is the measure?'.

Common sense is the first requisite. Feinstein speaks of a measure's *sensibility* (not to be confused with sensitivity)—i.e. how sensible is the measure? does it make good sense? This requires consideration not only of face and content validity, but also of the measure's purpose (what is it supposed to do, and is it needed?), its comprehensibility (is it simple and transparent?), its replicability (are the instructions for its use clear enough?), the suitability of the scale (is it logical, comprehensive and sufficiently discriminatory?), and ease of use.[3]

No measure should be used unless its validity has been appraised—a reasonable degree of face validity is a *sine qua non*. If validity is uncertain and the variable is of more than peripheral interest in the study, a check against data should be considered. This may be done in a pretest, or during the study proper (in a sample of the study population), or even (if doubts arise only later) by collecting new data during the analysis phase. In some instances a simple tryout may be enough to raise or dispel doubts about the capacity of the measure to yield 'reasonable' and full responses. Appraisals of validity may influence the choice of study methods and, at a later stage, the interpretation of the findings.

Sometimes the results of previous tests of validity are available.

These may be very helpful, but it is important to realize that the validity of a measure may differ in different groups or populations or in different circumstances. The significance of the WHO definition of low birth weight (less than 2500 g), for example, will differ in populations whose neonates, like their adults, are large or small for genetic reasons. A measure of chronic bronchitis based on the prevalence of cough and phlegm may be of high validity in one population, but less so in another where there is a low prevalence of chronic bronchitis and a high prevalence of other diseases (such as pulmonary tuberculosis) that may cause cough and phlegm. Indirect sphygmomanometer readings are a better index of intra-arterial blood pressure in leaner than in fatter people. The validity of simple questionnaires and tests for identifying people with presenile or senile dementia is seriously impaired by the effect of educational level on the responses.[4] In surveys in the United States, under-reporting of hospitalization varied in different ethnic groups.[5] In Boston, mothers tended to under-report their children's attendances at outpatient clinics if there had been many such attendances, and to over-report them if there had been few.[6]

This possibility of *differential validity* should always be kept in mind—it is often advisable to test validity in different subgroups of the study population. If the validity of measures is not uniform this can easily produce deceptive information about associations between variables. Suppose we want to compare the prevalence of a disease in two groups, using a measure that makes errors when classifying people as well or ill. Patients will be 'diluted' with healthy people, and/or healthy people will be 'contaminated' by patients. It has been shown that if the measure has the same validity in the two groups we are comparing ('nondifferential validity'), the misclassification will tend to reduce any true difference between the prevalence in the two groups, or may even make it dwindle to vanishing point.[7] If the measure is of different validity in the two groups the difference may be lessened, obscured or increased, or its direction may change; also, a difference may be seen when really there is none. The possibility of a spurious association exists whenever differential validity is suspected; if women who have borne deformed babies are for this reason especially prone to recall and report minor injuries that occurred during early pregnancy,[8] a retrospective comparison with mothers of normal babies may produce deceptive evidence of an association between deformities and these injuries. The direction of information bias (are relationships spuriously strengthened or attenuated?) is especially difficult to predict if both the variables involved in an association (e.g. disease and personality type) are subject to misclassification—any kind of distortion may then occur. This is not an uncommon situation.

Possible differential validity should also be considered if we plan to use a study method that others have developed and tested—we should satisfy ourselves of its validity in our own study, performing a test if necessary. The earlier validation suffices only if we are reasonably sure that the study populations and circumstances are so similar that the method will be valid here too. Problems are especially likely if a questionnaire has to be translated from another language[9] or into terms that will be understood by a specific study population.

A number of statistical indices may be used to express the results of validity checks.[10] Those commonly used for criterion validity will be explained below.

Face validity

The relevance of a measurement may appear obvious to the investigator. This is referred to as *face validity* (or *logical validity*). It may be obvious, for instance, that the dates of birth recorded on birth certificates provide a valid measure of age. In choosing between different measures, common sense may indicate that some are more valid than others. It may be self-evident that the records kept in an obstetrics ward will provide a more valid indication of birth weights than information obtained by questioning mothers, or that an appraisal of the neurological status of neonates will provide a more valid measure of prematurity (as the investigator conceives it) than information on birth weights.

In formulating the questions to be included in a questionnaire, a prime consideration is whether they have face validity—do they seem likely to yield information of real relevance to what the investigator wants to measure? It must be remembered, however, that face validity may be deceptive. The question 'Do you have frequent headaches?', for example, may not necessarily provide a valid measure of the occurrence of frequent headaches. A positive response may reflect a general propensity to complain, or a state of emotional ill health, and have little relevance to headaches per se.

Sometimes the findings (of a pretest or the study itself) point to poor face validity. If there are many 'don't know' answers to a question, this is *ipso facto* evidence that the question does not supply the information the investigator needs. 'Unreasonable' findings—their non-conformity with expectations—may be evidence of poor validity: if the prevalence of acne in adolescents turns out to be only 1%, the measure is probably invalid. *Digit preference* points to impaired validity. For instance, if the question 'How old are you?' yields an undue number of replies of '20', '30', '40', etc., compared with the number of replies ending in digits other than zero, this may be taken as evidence of low face validity; in this instance it would probably be decided to use grouped ages, rather than single years, as the scale of measurement, and not to use ages ending in zero in defining the categories (i.e. to use '25–34', '35–44', etc., rather than '20–29', '30–39', etc.). Similarly, a question on the date of the first day of the last menstrual period, put to pregnant women, has been found to yield unduly high numbers of certain dates—the 1st, 10th, 15th, 20th and 25th days of the month.[11] In Canada 90% of newborn babies have weights (in grams) that end with '0', and 16% have weights ending with '00',[12] and in a questionnaire survey in Yemen 55% of reported birth weights were multiples of 500, and 23% were clustered at 2500 g[13] (low birth weight is defined by WHO as < 2500 g). A question concerning the number of days since the onset of symptoms, put to patients seeking care for infectious diseases, may yield high numbers of replies of 1, 2, 3, 4, 7, 10 and 14 days. In the measurement of blood pressures, digit preference—usually a high proportion of readings ending in zero—is a well known phenomenon, and one that makes it more difficult to assess associations between blood pressure and other variables.[14]

Content validity

If the variable to be measured is a composite one, one way of appraising validity is to see whether all the component elements of the variable (as conceived) are measured. This is *content validity*. Like face validity, this is a judgement of whether the conceptual definition has been appropriately translated into operational terms.

A composite scale for measuring satisfaction with medical care, for example, should specifically include attitudes to all important features of medical care, such as the way doctors and nurses relate with patients, the technical quality of care, convenience, cost, the efficacy of care, continuity of care, the physical environment, and the availability of facilities and care providers;[15] questions about specific aspects are more likely to tap dissatisfaction than general questions.[16] Thyrotoxicosis will be measured more validly if metabolic and biochemical tests are used as well as symptoms and clinical signs.

Consensual validity

When a number of experts agree that a measure is valid, this is *consensual validity*. Many experts agree, for example, that the British Registrar-General's classification (p. 124) is a valid measure of social class, or that a specific index based on the presence, frequency and duration of cough and phlegm is a valid indicator of chronic bronchitis. It must be remembered, however, that different groups of experts may differ in their consensus of opinion, and that a consensus may change—expert committees frequently recommend changes in diagnostic criteria (see p. 137).

Criterion validity

The best and most obvious way of appraising validity is to find a *criterion* (a reference standard or, in epidemiological jargon, a 'gold standard') that is known or believed to be close to the truth, and to compare the results of the measure with this criterion (*criterion validity*).

The ideal criterion is the 'true value' of the attribute that is being measured. A perfectly valid measure is one that correlates completely with 'God's opinion' concerning the attribute.[17] As 'God's opinion' is difficult to determine, the best criterion is a measure that has higher face validity than the measure being tested, or that has been tested previously and found to be of high criterion validity. As examples, questionnaire data on birth weights may be checked against the weights recorded in obstetric records, self-reports of overweight against weight and height measurements, and self-reported use of health care services with medical records. Blood pressure measured by indirect sphygmomanometry can be checked against direct intra-arterial pressure measurements; the causes of death recorded on death certificates may be compared with those inferred from post-mortem examinations, and readings of electrocardiogram tracings with the appraisals made by a panel of experts; biochemical results may be checked by using standard solutions whose composition has been measured by tests of established accuracy. The responses to a 'yes–no' question on stiffness in the joints or muscles on waking in the morning (one of the diagnostic criteria of rheumatoid arthritis) may be validated by comparing them with the responses elicited by a skilled interviewer who asks additional questions to ensure that the sensation is really one of stiffness, and not of 'pins and needles', general lassitude, etc. Similarly, the validity of a simple dietary questionnaire may be tested by a comparison with the findings obtained by a Burke research dietary history, a method involving very detailed questioning, with built-in cross-checks, by an experienced interviewer.[18] The validity of a new blood test for the diagnosis of a disease may be tested by examining its correlation with diagnoses established by clinicians after comprehensive examinations, using their own individual diagnostic criteria (which have face validity), generally accepted diagnostic criteria (which have consensual validity), or diagnostic criteria that have themselves been tested against some criterion.

If an unquestionably 'more valid' measure of the characteristic is available for use as a criterion, the comparison can provide convincing evidence of validity. It must be kept in mind, however, that validity measured in this way may not be quite as well founded as it appears, since (like face validity) it is in the last resort based on judgement—if only the judgement that the criterion is of higher validity than the measure that is being tested.

It is often—in fact, usually—impossible to use the above approach. For one thing, there may be no measure which can be unequivocally regarded as a more valid one. If we wish to test the validity of a composite measure of social class, based on occupation, education and income, what unquestionably 'more valid' measure can we find? If we wish to test the validity of information on an attitude—a man's attitude to his work or his wife or whether he approves of contraceptive practices—how can we come close to the 'true value' of the attitude, to obtain a criterion of validity? Furthermore, even when a 'more valid' measure is theoretically available, the information required may not be available in practice, e.g. if it requires a biopsy or autopsy.

The criterion validity of a 'yes–no' measure of a 'yes–no' attribute (e.g. the presence of a disease) is usually expressed in terms of *sensitivity* and *specificity*. The findings may be shown in a simple table (Table 17.1) representing the observations in two samples, 'Attribute present' and 'Attribute absent'. *TP* represents the 'true positives', *FP* the 'false positives', *FN* the 'false negatives, and *TN* the 'true negatives'. The measure's *sensitivity* is the proportion with a positive result, among people who truly have the attribute

Table 17.1 Results of a 'yes–no' measure of a 'yes–no' attribute

	Attribute present	Attribute absent
Positive finding	TP	FP
Negative finding	FN	TN

(e.g. the disease), i.e. $TP/(TP + FN)$. The *specificity* of the measure is the proportion with a negative result, among people who truly do not have the attribute, i.e. $TN/(FP + TN)$. The *false positive rate* is $FP/(FP + TN)$.

If both sensitivity and specificity are high, the measure is of high validity. Sensitivity and specificity must be considered together; separately, neither is very meaningful; the presence of a nose is a highly sensitive measure of kwashiorkor (100% of cases have noses) but its specificity is 0% (no individuals free of kwashiorkor are noseless); conversely, a bright green coloration of the ears (with purple stripes) is a highly specific index of kwashiorkor (100%), but its sensitivity is 0%.

If the measure (of, say, a disease) is not dichotomous, but has responses expressed on an ordinal, interval or ratio scale, its sensitivity etc. can be computed for different cut-points; i.e. at each of a number of selected points the scale is converted to a dichotomy (e.g. 120 or more = positive test, below 120 = negative test) and true and false positives and negatives are counted. Sensitivity can then be plotted against the false positive rate to produce a *ROC (receiver operating characteristics) curve*,[19] and the *area under the ROC curve* can be computed and used as an overall index that expresses the probability that the measure will correctly rank two randomly chosen persons, one with and one without the disease.

It must again be stressed that the validity of a measure may vary in different situations. A combination of signs and symptoms used as an index of a disease, for example, may have a higher sensitivity in a population where the disease tends to take a severe form than in one where the disease is generally mild (and therefore not detected by the test). For example, sensitivity may be higher in hospital patients than in diseased persons found in a household survey. On the other hand, specificity may be lower in a hospital population, where patients free of this disease are more likely to have other diseases producing the same manifestations.

Convergent and discriminant validity

Convergent validity is based on a comparison with other measures—not necessarily better ones—of the same variable or a closely related one. A new measure of social class, for example, could be checked against other measures of social class. If it is uncertain whether the other measure is superior to the one under test, convergent validity is being tested, rather than criterion validity. Validation studies of the SF-36 health survey questionnaire, for example, included comparisons with quality-of-life scales and the Nottingham Health Profile.[20]

This approach is generally used for measures of composite variables. A new measure of mental health would be expected to show a strong correlation with other mental health measures (but if the correlation is *too* high the need for the new measure may be questioned, unless there are practical advantages unrelated to validity). If it is a valid measure of mental health it would not be expected to show such a strong correlation with a measure of physical health. This latter aspect—i.e. *not* showing a strong correlation with measures of variables that are not closely related—is called *discriminant validity*. Convergent and discriminant validity can be examined simultaneously by the *multitrait-multimethod matrix* technique.[21]

Qualitative research methods are commonly validated by *triangulation*, i.e. by seeing whether the results are confirmed when other methods are used or investigations are repeated.

Construct validity

Another way of appraising validity is to see whether there are associations with other variables that there is reason to believe should be linked with the characteristic under study. This is *construct validity*[22]—'the extent to which a particular measure relates to other measures consistent with theoretically derived hypotheses concerning the concepts (or constructs) that are being measured'.[23] The usual question here is whether the measure discriminates between groups who are thought to differ with respect to the attribute that (it is hoped) it measures.

Examples abound. A measure of job satisfaction might be compared with information on what the subjects actually do (absenteeism, frequency of disputes at work, etc.), since it is reasonable to predicate some degree of association—although certainly not a one-to-one relationship—between these activities and the 'true' attitude to work. A scale measuring reported satisfaction with medical care might be validated in a similar way, using such criteria as the changing of doctors, the abandonment of health insurance, or the submission of formal complaints about the care received. If there are theoretical reasons for believing that satisfaction with medical care is correlated with income or ethnic group or emotional health, evidence of such correlations might be taken as indirect evidence of validity. Tests of physical fitness might be used to validate a questionnaire on habitual physical activity, and habitual physical activity has been used to validate an index of physical health.[24] A study of the Rose questionnaire for angina pectoris validated it against the thickness of carotid artery walls (measured by ultrasound imaging), on the assumption that atherosclerosis of the coronary and carotid arteries are correlated.[25] Age is often used; twenty operational definitions of benign prostatic hyperplasia, for example, were rejected because they did not show an increased prevalence with age.[26]

One way of checking construct validity is to see how well the measure discriminates between groups that there is reason to believe should differ in the characteristic under study. In a validation study of the SF-36 health survey questionnaire, for example, these groups were selected on the assumptions that poorer perceived health was to be expected in women than in men, in older people than in younger, in people in social classes IV and V than in higher social classes, and in users of health services than in nonusers.[27]

Construct validity is obviously less convincing than criterion validity. The value of this approach depends not only on how well the measure does its job, but on the validity of the underlying hypotheses leading to the selection of variables or groups.

Predictive validity

If the measure under consideration is to be used as a predictor of a future event, the occurrence of this event is an appropriate gauge of validity: the prophetic value of the measure is examined. This is *predictive validity*, a particularly convincing way of testing validity.

As an example, the validity of a 9-item mortality risk indicator was tested in a nested case-control study that compared elderly men who were and were not alive five years after the start of a cohort study. The risk of dying was found to be five-fold in men whom this measure identified as being at high risk.[28] The indicator's validity was subsequently confirmed by testing it in women, although the relative risk was not as high.

This approach may also be used in other instances, when prediction is not the measure's primary aim. For example, the validity of measures of prematurity (birth weight, gestation period, neurological maturity, etc.) may be tested by examining their association with death or survival during the first month of life, on the assumption that since prematurity is associated with neonatal mortality, the more strongly the measure is associated with neonatal mortality, the more valid it is. The validity of various minor ECG abnormalities as measures of coronary heart disease may be tested by examining their relationship to the subsequent occurrence of myocardial infarction. The validity of measures of social support may be appraised by examining their capacity to predict mortality, psychiatric symptoms, and other adverse health outcomes,[29] and the validity of clinical appraisals of disease severity by their capacity to predict a fatal outcome.[30]

Responsiveness

Some measures are used to gauge within-person change with time, and are required to be sufficiently *responsive* (sensitive to change) to serve this purpose. A measure of the effect of a treatment, for example, should ideally detect and measure any clinically meaningful change, however small. A measure may be a valid indicator of the presence and intensity of an attribute, and be useful for comparing individuals or groups, without being very responsive.

One way of appraising responsiveness is to compare findings before and after treatment. For example, administration of the SF-36 questionnaire to patients with migraine before treatment and a month later revealed differences in the responsiveness of the various scores derived from the questionnaire. The pain score decreased more than the other scores, one of which (the score for the impact of emotional problems on role performance) showed no significant change. The pain score also showed a change six months after treatment for back pain, whereas the general health score did not. The SF-36 health scores were more responsive to changes after treatment for asthma if the questions were asked about a single week rather than the previous four weeks.[31]

Another method is to compare the changes observed in groups of patients who differ in their progress (according to an external criterion). This was done in tests of two measures of functional status, the Barthel Index and the Rehabilitation Activities Profile, which were administered to hospitalized patients two weeks after a stroke and repeated after various periods. The criterion of improvement was that the patient was living at home 26 weeks after the stroke. The change in scores (2-week scores were compared with 12-week and 26-week scores) in the two groups of patients showed that responsiveness was high for both measures, but more so for the Rehabilitation Activities Profile.[32]

EVALUATION OF SCREENING AND DIAGNOSTIC TESTS

The testing of validity plays a central role in the evaluation of tests used to detect diseases. This applies both to *screening tests*, which are simple tests to identify people who are particularly likely to have the disease and therefore merit fuller examination, and to *diagnostic tests*, which establish the presence or absence of diseases more definitively.

Numerous indices of validity are available,[33] but the key ones are sensitivity (the test's capacity to correctly identify people who have the disease) and specificity (its capacity to correctly identify people free of the disease). If both sensitivity and specificity are high, the test is unquestionably a valid indicator of the disease (it has a high *discriminatory capacity*). Frequently, however, they are inversely related. A positive sputum culture, for example, is a very specific test for pulmonary tuberculosis, but one of low sensitivity; whereas radiological examination is more sensitive but less specific.

The sensitivity and specificity of a test may vary in different circumstances, e.g. when it is used in apparently healthy people or in hospital patients. Validity should therefore be measured whenever possible in the kind of group or population in which the test will be used—is it to be used in a mass programme for the examination of apparently healthy people, or as a component of periodic health examinations, or as a routine test for all patients who seek medical care, or for patients in a defined high-risk group, or is it for use only in the presence of symptoms or other evidence suggestive of the disease? For the measurement of sensitivity, there may unfortunately be little choice—to find a large enough sample of people with the disease it is sometimes necessary to use any means available. Specificity, however, should always be measured in an appropriate sample of people free of the disease—selected from the general population, or from people who seek medical care, or from a defined high-risk group, in accordance with the way the test will be used.

It is often helpful to estimate the *predictive value*[33] of a positive or negative result and (in clinical contexts) the *gain in certainty*,[33] which expresses the change that the test can be expected to make in the estimated likelihood that the disease is present or absent. These indices vary with the prevalence of the disease in the population or group of patients in whom the test is done, and this prevalence (known or assumed) is required for their computation.

Consideration should be given to the purpose[34] of the test: discovery of a disease, confirmation of its suspected presence, or exclusion of its presence. Some tests are used for only one of these purposes, some for two, and some for all three. A *discovery test*, used when there is no special reason to suspect the presence of the disease, may be a screening test or a diagnostic one. The aim is usually to find as many of the cases as possible, and high sensitivity is therefore of special importance. But specificity cannot be ignored; a screening test with a low specificity will yield an unduly large number of 'false positive' cases requiring further examination.

A *confirmation test* is one used when the presence of disease is suspected. Its purpose is to verify this suspicion. The presence of tubercle bacilli in the sputum, for example, will confirm a diagnosis of tuberculosis (but their absence does not exclude the diagnosis). For this purpose, specificity must be high; sensitivity is less important. The specificity of the test should be measured in patients in whom the disease is suspected, but who turn out to be free of the disease.

An *exclusion test* has the purpose of 'ruling out' the presence of a suspected disease. Some exclusion tests are elaborate procedures, such as computerized tomography or magnetic resonance imaging. Their essential feature for this purpose is an extremely high sensitivity; there must be very few false negative results.

Validity is not the only consideration when evaluating a screening procedure. It is also important to know what benefit or harm is to be expected from the screening procedure and the action that it sets in motion. Simple questions about eyesight, for example, are valid tests for visual impairment; but a meta-analysis of randomized control trials of these tests in people aged 65 or more yielded no evidence that they led to an improvement in vision.[35] A second illustration is the controversy about the value of the prostate specific antigen screening test, which can detect most cases of early prostate cancer but may lead to unnecessary prostatectomies and complications, and has an as yet uncertain effect on mortality.[36] Another example is the consensus that possible benefits are enough to warrant repeated measurements of blood pressure during pregnancy as a screening test for pre-eclampsia, despite low sensitivity and specificity.[37]

Applying the basic evaluation scheme shown on page 56, the following are the kinds of question that are usually asked:

1. *Requisiteness.* Is the test needed? Are other satisfactory tests not available? How important is it to detect the disease? What is the impact of the disease on the individual (shortening of life, disability, pain and discomfort, cost of care), on the individual's family, and on the community (mortality, morbidity rate, reduced productivity, cost of care)? Is effective intervention possible, and how good is the evidence for this? Does early detection make treatment easier? Does it make it more effective?

2. *Quality.* How well does the test achieve its desired effects, i.e. how valid is it (sensitivity, specificity, etc.)? Are there potential adverse effects? May the 'labelling' of symptom-free people as 'diseased' have undesirable effects? What is the impact of false positive results (false 'labelling')?

3. *Efficiency.* What is the cost per test and per case found, in comparison with other tests? What is the cost compared with the cost of *not* detecting the disease? What resources are needed—are highly-trained personnel required? What is the cost-effectiveness of the test, using, say, the detection of one case or the prevention of one death as a measure of effectiveness?

4. *Satisfaction.* How acceptable is the test? What is the level of compliance? Is there a demand—is there dissatisfaction if the test is *not* done?

5. *Differential value.* How do the size of the problem, the need for the test, and the acceptability of the test vary in different groups or populations? Is the validity of the test consistent in different groups?

EVALUATION OF RISK MARKERS

The same questions should be asked in the evaluation of a risk marker, which aims to identify individuals or groups who are especially likely to develop a given disorder in the future (see p. 45). A high level of predictive validity is not enough. There must also be good reason to think that the detection of vulnerability is likely to be beneficial, i.e. that techniques and resources are available for reducing the risk, and that the expected benefit outweighs any harm that may be done by 'labelling' and intervention. The use of the marker must also be practical in terms of cost, resources, acceptability and convenience. The most useful risk markers are probably those whose presence can be determined by questions, or simple procedures that can be built into ordinary clinical care.

With respect to validity, the primary requirement is a high sensitivity, since the usual aim is to find as many of the vulnerable individuals as possible. Account must also be taken of false positives; if these are numerous the predictive value of a positive test will be low, and the more intensive care recommended for vulnerable people will often be given unnecessarily.

An important consideration is the prevalence of the risk marker. This may be high either because the disorder it predicts is a very common one, or (if the disorder is less common) because the risk marker has a low specificity. If over half the children under care fall into a high-risk group needing special attention, it may be decided that the risk marker is of little value, since modification of the care programme so as to give extra care to *all* children may be a more efficient and effective solution.

NOTES AND REFERENCES

1. Baer D M 1977 Reviewer's comment: 'Just because it's reliable doesn't mean that you can use it'. Journal of Applied Behavior Analysis 10: 117.
2. Abramson J H, Gofin J, Hopp C, Makler A, Epstein L M 1978 Epidemiology of inguinal hernia: a survey in western Jerusalem. Journal of Epidemiology and Community Health 32: 59.
3. Feinstein A R 1987 Clinimetrics. Yale University Press, New Haven, Chapter 10.
4. The results of tests for dementia can be adjusted so as to remove the effect of education, but the role of education or education-related factors in the aetiology of dementia is then difficult to study.
   See Kittner S J, White L R, Farmer M E et al 1986 (Methodological issues in screening for dementia: the problem of education adjustment. Journal of Chronic Diseases 39: 163) and Berkman L F 1986 (The association between educational attainment and mental status examinations: of etiological significance for senile dementias or not? Journal of Chronic Diseases 39: 171).
5. National Center for Health Statistics 1965 Reporting of hospitalization in the Health Interview Survey, and comparison of hospitalization reporting in three survey procedures. Vital and Health Statistics, series 2, nos 6, 8. Public Health Service, Washington, D C.
6. Kosa J, Alpert J J, Haggerty R J 1967 On the reliability of family health information: a comparative study of mothers' reports on illness and related behavior. Social Science and Medicine 1: 165.
7. If a measure is wrong more often than it is right (false positive rate plus false

negative rate exceeds 100%) spurious associations may be produced even if misclassification is nondifferential. Validity as low as this is unusual. The effects of *misclassification* are described by Fleiss J L 1981 (Statistical methods for rates and proportions, 2nd edn. Wiley, New York, pp 188–200) and Kleinbaum D G, Kupper L L, Morgenstern H 1982 (Epidemiologic research: principles and quantitative methods. Lifetime Learning Publications, Belmont, Cal., Ch 12); see also Abramson J H 1994 Making sense of data: a self-instruction manual on the interpretation of epidemiological data, 2nd edn. Oxford University Press, New York, Units C3–C6.

MISCLASS, in the PEPI package (see note 7, p. 292), uses estimates of sensitivity and specificity to correct for misclassification in a 2 × 2 table.

8. A study in Boston of the reporting of events during pregnancy, in comparison with antenatal records, showed that the mothers of malformed infants reported urinary tract and yeast infections, and the use of birth control after conception, much more fully than the mothers of normal children. There were slight or no differences in the completeness of reports of other events (Werler M M, Pober B R, Nelson K, Holmes L B 1989 Reporting accuracy among mothers of malformed and nonmalformed infants. American Journal of Epidemiology 129: 415).

9. *Translation of questionnaires*. After a questionnaire has been translated to another language (preferably by several independent translators) it should be translated back for comparison with the original version. Alterations of some questions may be unavoidable, and response categories such as 'excellent/very good/good/fair/poor' may not have exact equivalents. However good the translation, cultural differences can affect validity.

Typical adaptations (from original physical health questions in American English): 'Bowling or playing golf' became 'walks in the forest or gardening' (in Swedish); 'walking one block' became 'walking 100 yards' (in British English) or 'going for a walk in the vicinity of your house' (in Hebrew); and 'scrubbing floors' became 'lifting and beating carpets or scraping and painting walls' (in Hebrew).

See: Ware J E Jr, Keller S D, Gandek B, Brazier J E, Sullivan M 1995 (Evaluating translations of health status questionnaires: methods from the IQOLA Project: International Quality of Life Assessment. International Journal of Technology Assessment in Health Care 11: 525); Bullinger M 1995 (German translation and psychometric testing of the SF-36 health survey: preliminary results from the IQOLA Project. Social Science and Medicine 41: 1359); Sullivan M, Karlsson J, Ware J E Jr 1995 (The Swedish SF-36 Health Survey: I. Evaluation of data quality, scaling assumptions, reliability and construct validity across general populations in Sweden. Social Science and Medicine 41: 1349); Bucquet D, Condon S, Ritchie K 1990 (The French version of the Nottingham Health Profile. Social Science and Medicine 30: 829); Ware J E Jr 1993 (Measuring patients' views: the optimum outcome measure. British Medical Journal 306: 1429); Abramson J H, Ritter M, Gofin J, Kark J D 1992 (A simplified index of physical health for use in epidemiological studies. Journal of Clinical Epidemiology 45: 651).

10. *Indices of validity*. Various indices (in addition to those mentioned in the text) may be used to express a measure's relationship with a criterion or other measure, e.g. correlation coefficients, *kappa*, and the size and direction of the differences. Reliability can be taken into account by computing what the correlation *would* be if reliability (of one or both measures) were perfect (Streiner D L, Norman G R 1995 Health measurement scales: a practical guide to their development and use, 2nd edn. Oxford University Press, Oxford, Ch 11).

Indices for measuring responsiveness: see Streiner and Norman 1995 (Ch 11) and Van Bennekom C A M, Jelles F, Lankhorst G J, Bouter L M

1996 (Responsiveness of the Rehabilitation Activities Profile and the Barthel Index. Journal of Clinical Epidemiology 49: 39).

11. Frazier T M 1959 Error in reported date of last menstrual period. American Journal of Obstetrics and Gynecology 77: 915.

12. Edouard L, Senthilselvan A 1997 Observer error and birthweight: digit preference in recording. Public Health 111: 77.

13. Boerma J T, Weinstein K I, Rutstein S O, Sommerfelt A E 1996 Data birth weight in developing countries: can surveys help? Bulletin of the World Health Organization 74: 209.

14. Hessel P A 1986 Terminal digit preference in blood pressure measurements: effects on epidemiological associations. International Journal of Epidemiology 15: 122.

15. This list of dimensions of *satisfaction with care* is by Ware J E, Snyder M K, Wright R, Davies A R 1983 (Defining and measuring patient satisfaction with medical care. Evaluation and Program Planning 6: 247). For a recent review, see Sitzia J, Wood N 1997 (Patient satisfaction: a review of issues and concepts. Social Science and Medicine 45: 1829).

16. Williams S J, Calnan M 1991 Convergence and divergence: assessing criteria of consumer satisfaction across general practice, dental, and hospital care settings. Social Science and Medicine 33: 707.

17. A concept attributed to A L Cochrane.

18. Burke B S 1947 The dietary history as a tool in research. Journal of the American Dietetic Association 23: 1041.

    Recent studies of the validity of dietary assessments will be found in Margetts B M, Pietinen P (eds) 1997 (EPIC European Prospective Investigation into Cancer and Nutrition: validity studies on dietary assessment methods. International Journal of Epidemiology 26 [suppl 1]: S1–S189).

19. *ROC curves*: see Zweig M H, Campbell G 1993 (Receiver-operating characteristics (ROC) plots: a fundamental evaluation tool in clinical medicine. Clinical Chemistry 39: 561). The area under the ROC curve is 50% if the measure does not discriminate.

    SCRN, in the PEPI package (see note 7, p. 292), draws a ROC curve and computes the area under it.

20. Bullinger M 1995 (see note 9); Brazier J E, Harper R, Jones N M B, O'Catham A, Thomas K J, Usherwood T, Westlake L 1992 Validating the SF-36 health survey questionnaire: new outcome measure for primary care. British Medical Journal 305: 160.

21. The *multitrait-multimethod matrix* (MTMM) requires measurement of two or more traits by two or more methods. A matrix of correlations provides a basis for assessments of convergent and discriminant validity (Campbell D T, Fiske D W 1959 Convergent and discriminant validation by the multitrait-multimethod matrix. Psychological Bulletin 56: 81).

    For examples, see Brazier J E et al 1992 (see note 20) and, with fuller explanations, Trochim W M K 1996 (The multitrait-multimethod matrix. Internet: trochim.human/cornell.edu/kb/mtmmmat.htm). A short explanation is given by Streiner and Norman 1995 (see note 10).

22. The *construct validity* of a measure can also be defined differently, as the extent to which the measure reflects the conceptual definition (or construct) of the variable. So defined, construct validity is an overriding term, and the various ways of appraising validity refer to specific aspects of construct validity. First, does the translation to an operational definition appear to be appropriate (face and content validity)? Secondly, how does the measure perform when checked against data, i.e. predictive validity, concurrent validity (a gold standard, or a variable believed to be linked with the variable under study), and convergent validity and discriminant validity? See Trochim

W M K 1996 (Measurement validity types. Internet: trochim.human.cornell. edu/kb/measval.htm).

23. Carmines E G, Zeller R A 1979 Reliability and validity assessment. Sage Publications, Beverly Hills, pp 22–26.
24. Abramson et al 1992 (see note 9).
25. Sorlie P D, Cooper L, Schreiner P J, Rosamond W, Szklo M 1995 Repeatability and validity of the Rose questionnaire for angina pectoris in the Atherosclerosis Risk in Communities study. Journal of Clinical Epidemiology 49: 719.
26. Bosch J L, Hop W C, Kirkels W J, Schroder F H 1995 Natural history of benign prostatic hyperplasia: appropriate case definition and estimation of its prevalence in the community. Urology 46(3 suppl A): 34.
27. Brazier J E et al 1992 (see note 20).
28. Abramson J H, Gofin R, Peritz E 1982 Risk markers for mortality among elderly men—a community study in Jerusalem. Journal of Chronic Diseases 35: 565.
29. Orth-Gomer K, Unden A-L 1987 The measurement of social support in population surveys. Social Science and Medicine 24: 83.
30. Charlson M, Sax F L, MacKenzie R, Fields S D, Braham R L, Douglas R G Jr 1987 Assessing illness severity: does clinical judgment work? Journal of Chronic Diseases 39: 439.
31. Bullinger M 1995 (see note 9); Keller S D, Bayliss M S, Ware J E Jr, Hsu M A, Damiano A M, Goss T F 1997 Comparison of responses to SF-36 Health Survey questions with one-week and four-week recall periods. Health Services Research 32: 367.
32. Van Bennekom et al 1996 (see note 10).
33. *Indices of validity for screening and diagnostic tests* include *sensitivity and specificity*, *chance-corrected sensitivity and specificity*, which make allowance for the occurrence of chance agreement between the test result and the true status (Brenner H, Gefeller O 1994 Chance-corrected measures of the validity of a binary test. Journal of Clinical Epidemiology 47: 627) and *likelihood ratios* for positive and negative tests (the ratio of the prevalence of a positive or negative finding in people with the disease to the prevalence of the same finding in people without the disease). Likelihood ratios are particularly useful aids in clinical practice (Sackett D L, Richardson W S, Rosenberg W, Haynes K B 1997 Evidence-based medicine: How to practice & teach EBM. Churchill Livingstone, New York, pp 118–128, 221–222).

If the prevalence of the disease in the group or population in which the test is to be used is known or assumed, other useful indices include the *predictive value of a positive test* (*positive predictive value, PPV*—if a test is positive what is the probability that the disease is present?), the *predictive value of a negative test* (*negative predictive value*—if the test is negative what is the probability that the disease is absent?) and *measures of gain in certainty*—i.e. of the change that the test can be expected to make in the clinical estimate of the patient's likelihood of having or not having the disease (Connell F A, Koepsell T D 1985 Measures of gain in certainty from a diagnostic test. American Journal of Epidemiology 121: 744)—as well as the *number of positive tests per case identified* and the *total number of tests per case identified*.

For a test that provides results on an ordinal, interval or ratio scale, useful indices include sensitivity, specificity and post-test probabilities for different cut-points, and the *area under the ROC curve* (see note 19). Optimal cut-points (yielding minimal errors) can be identified, conditional on the prevalence of the disease and the relative undesirability attached to false negatives and false positives (McNeil B J, Keeler E, Adelstein S J 1975. Primer on certain elements of medical decision making. New England Journal of Medicine 293: 211; Linnet K 1988 A review on the methodology for assessing diagnostic tests. Clinical Chemistry 34: 1379; Zweig and Campbell 1993 [see note 19]).

SCRN, in the PEPI package (see note 7, p. 292) computes these indices, with confidence intervals.

34. Feinstein A R 1977 Clinical biostatistics. C V Mosby, St Louis, Chapter 15.
35. Smeeth L, Iliffe S 1998 Effectiveness of screening older people for impaired vision in community setting: systematic review of evidence from randomized controlled trials. British Medical Journal 316: 660.
36. Woolf S H 1997 Editorial: Should we screen for prostate cancer? Men over 50 have a right to decide for themselves. British Medical Journal 314: 989; Brawley O W 1997 Prostate cancer incidence and patient mortality: the effects of screening and early detection. Cancer 80: 1857; Smart C R 1997 The results of prostate carcinoma screening in the U.S. as reflected in the Surveillance, Epidemiology, and End Results Program. Cancer 80: 1835.

In 1996 the US Preventive Services Task Force recommended that prostate cancer antigen screening should be excluded from consideration in a periodic health examination (US Preventive Services Task Force 1996 Guide to clinical preventive services, 2nd edn. US Department of Health and Human Services, Washington DC, pp 119–134).
37. US Preventive Services Task Force 1996 (see note 36), pp 419–424.

18 Interviews and self-administered questionnaires

Interviews may be less or more structured. A clinician uses a relatively unstructured interview—his approach is flexible, he follows leads as they arise, and the content, wording and order of the questions vary from interview to interview. In the same way, a public health worker conducting interviews as part of the investigation of a local outbreak of disease has an idea of what he wants to learn— the nature and time of onset of the symptoms, the patients' prior movements, their contacts with other ill persons, their recent meals, their milk and water supply, and so on—but does not decide in advance exactly what questions will be asked, or in what order.

In other situations a more standardized technique may be used, the wording and order of the questions being decided in advance. This may take the form of a *highly structured interview*, in which the questions are asked orally, or a *self-administered questionnaire*, in which case the respondent reads the questions and fills in the answers by himself (sometimes in the presence of an interviewer who 'stands by' to give assistance if necessary). For simplicity, we will use the term 'questionnaire' to indicate the list of questions prepared for either of these purposes. (In the behavioural sciences, a 'questionnaire' usually means a self-administered questionnaire, and the term is not applied to the interview schedule used by an interviewer.)

Standardized methods of asking questions are usually preferred in community medicine research, since they provide more assurance that the data will be reproducible. Less structured interviews may be useful in a preliminary survey, where the purpose is to obtain information to help in the subsequent planning of a study rather than facts for analysis, and in intensive studies of perceptions, attitudes, motivations and affective reactions. Unstructured ('free-style') interviews are characteristic of qualitative (non-quantitative) research (see p. 166).

MODE OF ADMINISTRATION

The choice between a self-administered questionnaire and a highly structured interview may not be an easy one. The use of self-administered questionnaires is simpler and cheaper; such questionnaires can be administered to many persons simultaneously (e.g. to a class of schoolchildren) and, unlike interviews, can be sent by post. On the other hand, they demand a certain level of education and skill on the part of the respondent; people of a low socioeconomic status are less likely to respond to a mailed questionnaire.

Face-to-face or phone interviews have many advantages. A good interviewer can stimulate and maintain the respondent's interest, and can create a rapport and atmosphere conductive to the answering of questions.[1] If anxiety is aroused (e.g. 'Why am *I* being asked these questions?—Have I an illness they haven't told me about?'), the interviewer can allay it. If a question is not understood an interviewer can repeat it and if necessary (and in accordance with guidelines decided in advance) provide an explanation or alternative wording. Optional follow-up or probing questions that are to be asked only if prior responses are inconclusive or inconsistent cannot easily be built into self-administered questionnaires. A self-administered questionnaire is perforce restricted to simple questions with simple instructions, designed to elicit simple data. In a face-to-face interview, observations can be made as well; the so-called 'coronary-prone behaviour pattern', for example, was originally detected in interviews during which note was taken not only of what the subject said but of how he said it, whether he clenched his fists and his teeth, etc.[2] Furthermore, the interviewer can use visual aids; cups and saucers of various sizes and models of food servings can be an invaluable aid in a quantitative dietary interview.

In general, apart from their expense, interviews are preferable to self-administered questionnaires, with the important proviso that they are conducted by skilled interviewers. Otherwise, there is much truth in the statement that 'to gain information by interview resembles the use of questionnaires, except that questionnaires only contain errors caused by the patient, but interviews include errors caused by the interviewer as well.[3] Self-administered questionnaires are widely and successfully used, and appear to be better for some purposes.[4] They have been found to yield appreciably more reports of disability, pain and emotional disturbance than interviewer-administered questionnaires, and in a study of women's health they significantly increased the reported number of sexual partners and reports of sexually transmitted diseases and condom use; in general, there is a reduced tendency to refrain from giving socially undesirable responses. A decision on the use of a self-administered questionnaire may require a pretest to obtain information on the response rate, rates of unanswered items, and the quality of responses.

The main problems with postal questionnaires are that response rates tend to be relatively low, and that there may be under-representation of less literate subjects. The questionnaires often find their way to wastepaper baskets, even if they are simple, attractively designed, accompanied by a persuasive covering letter and a stamped return envelope, preceded by a courteous 'pre-letter' and followed by one or more reminders. Response rates may be high, however, in surveys where subjects have a special motivation, as in the instance of questionnaires sent to patients or ex-patients by their own physicians or treating agencies, enquiring about their progress. If the questions are formulated suitably the replies are in general similar to those obtained in interviews,[5] but there may be more missing answers.

Phone interviews are sometimes preferred to mailed questionnaires and face-to-face interviews. Selection of a method depends on feasibility (e.g. the prevalence of telephones), costs and the nature and purpose of the study. Comparisons yield inconsistent findings;[6] phone interviews sometimes elicit fewer reports of ill health than mailed questionnaires. Some studies show little difference in cost or data quality between phone and personal interviews; some questions are easier to ask on the telephone, and others are easier to ask face-to-face, but the differences between these two interview modes are not consistent. One expert jubilates that 'it seems almost too good to be true that telephone interviewing produces results that are practically no different from face-to-face interviewing, and I continue to be surprised at our good fortune'.[7] Some comparisons have found phone surveys satisfactory in studies of mental health, but others have found that phone surveys yield fewer reports of smoking and drinking, that phone surveys on drug use incite more refusals than face-to-face interviews, and that more questions go unanswered.

There is sometimes less concealment of socially undesirable behaviour when a more impersonal mode is used. In a study of the use of seat restraints for children in cars, nonuse of a restraint on the last trip was reported by 30% of parents in phone interviews and 26% in postal questionnaires, but by only 18% in face-to-face interviews.[8] In another comparative study the proportion of respondents who admitted to 'nervousness, worry or depression or trouble sleeping' (symptoms that might be considered embarrassing) was somewhat higher for mailed questionnaires than for phone interviews.[9]

Mixed strategies are often used—for example, trying mail or telephone first, and using home interviews only for persistent non-respondents.[9]

COMPUTER-ASSISTED INTERVIEWS

Computer-aided interviewing has become increasingly popular. The questions are shown on a computer screen, and the keyboard or mouse is used for entering the answers. Skipping and branching patterns (i.e. 'if so-and-so, go to Question such-and-such') are built into the program, so that the screen automatically displays the appropriate question. Checks can be built in and an immediate warning given if a reply lies outside an acceptable range or is inconsistent with previous replies; revision of previous replies is permitted, with automatic return to the current question. The responses are entered directly on to the computer record, avoiding the need for subsequent coding and data entry. The technique may be especially helpful if question structure is complicated or there are many possible responses, as in a survey that required information about asthma medication, in terms of 486 possible combinations of drug, dose and delivery system.[10] The program can make an automatic selection of subjects who require additional procedures, such as special tests, supplementary questionnaires, or follow-up visits.

The advantages of the procedure are obvious, but consideration should also be given to its drawbacks. Apart from the need to write and test a computer program, there is also a possibility of errors, mainly caused by typing slips when entering the answers. In one careful comparison it was found that 2.0% of recorded responses were erroneous, as compared with 1.1% when a paper-and-pencil technique was used.[11] This is counterbalanced by the avoidance of errors that may occur during the transfer and entry of ordinary interview data. The automatic skip patterns can, however, lead to other and irremediable errors. Suppose that subjects are asked if they smoke and, if they say 'yes', are then asked about the number and kind of cigarettes smoked. In an ordinary interview, if the response to the first question is 'yes' but is erroneously entered as 'no', and the subsequent questions are (correctly) asked and answered, the inconsistency can be detected when the data are checked, and the reply to the first question can be corrected. In a computer-aided interview, if 'no' is entered by mistake the other questions will not be asked at all. Also, if the interviewer has to code responses before keying them in, there is later no way of detecting coding errors, since there is no record of the actual responses. Other drawbacks are that the use of a computer lengthens the interview slightly, and that interviewers may find their work boring. Printed questionnaires must be available for emergency use; in one study using computer-aided personal interviews, printed forms were needed in 5% of instances.[11]

If the right software is available,[12] the preparations for computer-assisted interviewing present no technical problems.

The various methods of computer-assisted interviewing (*CAI*) have catchy nicknames. For example, *CAPI* is computer-assisted personal interviewing (face-to-face); *CATI* is computer-assisted telephone interviewing (the interviewer uses both a phone and a computer); and *CASI* is computer-assisted self-interviewing, alias *CSAQ* (computerized self-administered questionnaire).[13] All these are contrasted with *PAPI*, or paper-and-pen interviewing.

The use of self-administered computer questionnaires is sure to increase. Like self-administered paper questionnaires, they apparently boost willingness to report socially undesirable behaviours.[14] In a randomized trial in a study of drinking habits in Edinburgh, men who entered their own responses reported the consumption of 30% more alcohol than men asked the same questions in face-to-face interviews.[15] In a controlled comparison, more responses suggesting the possibility of HIV infection were provided by self-administered computer questionnaires than by self-administered paper questionnaires and face-to-face interviews.[16]

Audio-CASI,[17] with audio playback of the questions shown on the screen, is a promising enhancement, and a multimedia approach, embracing pictures as well, has been warmly advocated: 'Computers can conduct personalized, in-depth interviews without interviewers;

provide standardized data collection with appropriate levels of probing; automate data entry; encourage subjects to review and correct inconsistent data; and ensure that responses are complete. Interactive multimedia tools can motivate subjects and improve participation. Visual and aural cues may stimulate recall and improve data quality. CASI is appropriate for use in populations in which literacy is low and in multiple ethnic groups'.[18] The Internet is a natural home for multimedia CASI questionnaires.

VALIDITY

Information obtained by interviewing and questioning is often referred to as 'soft' data, as opposed to the presumably 'hard' data[19] derived from observations. A man who says he has heart disease may have a non-cardiac disease, or none at all. In a study of questionnaire responses by registered nurses in the United States, only 74% of cases of cancer of the uterus reported in questionnaires were confirmed by medical records.[20] In a Californian study, the proportions of various chronic diseases (recorded in medical records) that were not reported in interviews ranged from 15 to 79%, and the over-reporting rate from 1 to 83%.[21] A person who says he does not have a disease may be unaware that he has it, or may have forgotten, or may be unwilling (on a conscious or unconscious level) to admit its presence—particularly if the disease carries a stigma (this has been called 'unacceptable disease bias'). In a survey in which comparisons were made with cancer registry data, it was found that only 51% of men with a previous diagnosis of cancer of the lip reported this condition when asked about previous illnesses, and only another 13% reported it when they were specifically asked about cancer.[22] When a survey shows that more reports of severe sexual abuse in childhood are provided by depressed women than by non-depressed women,[23] it is legitimate to ask whether this reflects differential validity rather than an aftermath of sexual abuse.

People may be reluctant to admit to induced abortions, drug abuse, overindulgence in alcohol or tobacco, or other socially undesirable behaviour—a study in Holland showed that a question-based survey of alcoholism would miss over half the known problem drinkers.[24] Self-reported weight may tend to be an underestimate, and self-reported height an overestimate; in one study the prevalence of obesity (using a definition based on weight and height) was 50% higher when based on actual measurements than when based on reported weights and heights.[25] A mother reporting that her children have an abundance of milk, fruit, vegetables and meat may be saying this only to put herself into a favourable light, whereas a mother reporting that her children have none of these foodstuffs may be trying to elicit sympathy or welfare assistance.

Interviews conducted at home and in a clinic may elicit different information, and the responses may depend on who else is present. Suspicions about the interviewers' motives may influence responses. Different answers may be given to an interviewer who is older than, younger than, or the same age as the respondent, or who is of the same, a higher or lower social class, or of the same or a different ethnic group. Doctors and lay interviewers may obtain different responses to the same questions—the easiest way to ensure a high degree of satisfaction with medical care is to base the appraisal on interviews conducted by the treating physicians themselves.

A tactic sometimes used is to have the interviewer make an appraisal of the respondent's 'reliability' (trustworthiness), based on impressions gained during the interview; this appraisal may be aided by asking additional informal questions (preferably after the structured part of the interview) that plumb consistency and accuracy. These appraisals can be taken into account when the data are analyzed, e.g. by comparing the results for 'reliable' and 'unreliable' informants.

The interviewer, as well as the respondent, may be a source of bias—his or her expectations or preferences may influence the answers or the way they are interpreted and recorded. An interviewer who knows what hypothesis the study is testing may tend to get responses that fit in with his or her view of the validity of the hypothesis. Bias of this sort is least likely to occur in cohort studies in which the interviewer is unaware of the subject's prior exposure to the causal factors under study, and is most likely to occur in a case-control study in which the interviewer knows whether the subject is a case or a control.

Answers may also be influenced by the wording of the questions (see Ch. 19). A greater number of surgical procedures may be reported in reply to a question about 'stitches' or 'sutures' than to one about 'operations'. In one study 'How old were you when you had our first child?' was found to be a much more reliable question (*kappa* = 88%) than 'How old is your eldest child?' (*kappa* = 66%).[26] The sequence of the questions may also affect the responses.

Memory is fallible, and *recall bias* often occurs. Mild injuries and illnesses, brief stays in hospital, and other past episodes and experiences that made little impact on the respondent may be forgotten and not reported, especially if the time lapse is long. On the other hand, if the question refers to the recent past (say the last month), episodes that occurred longer ago may also be reported (*telescoping bias*). As a compromise, questions about acute illnesses and injuries are usually confined to the previous 2 weeks. Test-retest reliability of interview data on 'simple' events (such as hysterectomy) is high, but it is lower for more complicated data, such as age at occurrence of menopause or other events, or the reasons for starting or stopping drug treatment.[27] When there is an option it is preferable to ask for current rather than historical information. Population studies of age at menarche or menopause and duration of breast-feeding, for example, are more accurate if they use current status than if they rely on 'When did you ...' questions.[28]

Cues may be needed to tickle the memory. When mothers were asked about the taking of prescription drugs during pregnancy, for example, specific mention of headache, nausea, and various other symptoms increased the number of reports of having taken drugs by 32–58%, and mentioning the drugs by name increased the reports by an extra 6–40%.[29] The number of chronic diseases reported can be doubled if a check-list (phrased in lay terms) is shown or read to the respondents,[30] and can be further increased by using an extensive questionnaire that provides multiple cues and includes probing questions.[31] Reporting of symptoms may be doubled if a check-list is shown to the respondents.[32] Responses become more accurate in studies in which respondents can use memory aids, such as health diaries or wall calendars maintained for this purpose (see p. 251); in a randomized controlled study, 50% more symptom episodes were reported by subjects who had been given wall calendars for the recording of symptoms.[33]

'Simple memory failure' of this sort can produce biased estimates of prevalence or incidence and (if groups are being compared) can make it more difficult to detect differences that actually exist. Other effects may occur if there is 'differential memory failure', i.e. where the validity of what is recalled varies in the groups that are compared (see *differential validity*, p. 188). True differences between the groups may then be diminished, magnified or masked, and spurious differences may be produced. Precautions can be taken to detect and deal with this form of recall bias.[34] For example, in a case-control study where an association with a specific drug is postulated and it is believed that taking of the drug may be over-reported by cases and/or under-reported by controls, questions may be asked about other drugs (or other factors) known to be unrelated to the disease, to see whether they are reported more frequently by cases than by controls; these results will provide an indication of the degree of recall bias, and can be taken into account when analyzing or interpreting the study findings. Also, at the end of the interview the subjects may be asked about their beliefs concerning the cause of the disorder; recall bias is especially likely if the respondents suspect the drug under study to be a cause.

The replies to questions also depend on who is asked. Husbands and wives tend to report more illness for themselves than for their spouses ('the health of the nation improves markedly when proxy respondents are used; differences are even more noticeable when the respondent for a family is Uncle Joe').[35] Respondents may be unaware of most of the diseases suffered by their brothers and sisters, may not correctly report the causes of their relatives' deaths, and may be more likely to report that family members have a given disease if they themselves have the disease.[36] Details of a man's drinking and smoking habits may be reported differently by himself and his wife,[37] and agreement between parents and children with respect to information about the children varies from excellent (e.g. for eye and hair colour) to very poor (e.g. for a history of peeling sunburn).[38]

Whatever the variable we are trying to measure, we are dealing with statements, and not with direct measurements. This applies as much to attitudes, for which there are no more direct methods of measurement, as to any other variable. If a respondent says he feels well, we have not necessarily learnt his self-perception of his health, but only his reported self-perception of his health—which, however useful it may be as a datum in its own right, is not quite the same thing.

The validity of responses may be appraised by the methods described in Chapter 17. Many studies have compared interview responses with presumably accurate medical records. These found that only 30–53% of documented diagnoses were reported; most hospital admissions and operations were reported, but diagnostic X-ray examinations and many medications were poorly reported.[39] Comparisons with old records may permit tests of the validity of interview data about long past events or experiences; the validity of such data is sometimes surprisingly high.[40] Observational data that can be used as criteria are sometimes available. A comparison with angiographic findings, for example, showed that the sensitivity of the WHO questionnaire on intermittent claudication, as an indicator of severe grades of peripheral arterial disease, was 50%, and its specificity was over 98%.[41] Where suitable criteria are not available, construct validity (see p. 194) may be examined. A questionnaire on habitual physical activity, for example, was validated by finding the expected associations with age, sex, kind of job, self-appraisals of physical activity, caloric intake, maximal oxygen intake, body fatness, and exposure to health promotion programmes.[42] When possible, differential validity in different subgroups of the study population should be examined.

INTERVIEW TECHNIQUE

The accuracy of interview data can be boosted not only by the choice of an appropriate mode of administration, the use of memory aids, and careful attention to the construction of the questionnaire and the selection and wording of questions, but by proper interview technique.[1] It is important, but not sufficient, to follow the 'golden rule of survey research':[43] 'Do unto your respondents as you would have them do unto you' (thank them at the start and end of the interview, be sensitive to their needs, and watch for signs of discomfort). In the interests of accuracy, the main requirement is that the interviewer should beware of influencing the responses. Questions should be asked precisely as they were written, and re-worded or supplemented by explanations only when this is absolutely necessary. The questions should be asked in a neutral manner, without showing (by words, inflection or expression) a preference for any particular response. Agreement, disagreement or surprise should not be shown, and the precise answers should be recorded, without sifting or interpreting them. This, like the ability to encourage the respondents' participation and other necessary skills, demands training and practical experience. Good interviewers are made, not born (although some people are congenitally incapable of becoming good interviewers).

It may be noted that physicians, nurses and social workers often make poor interviewers in a research setting. They have been trained to see their role as the provision of help to patients or clients, and often have difficulty in accepting or fulfilling the different role of collecting standardized data. They may be incapable of merely reading out questions, but insist on rephrasing them or altering their order. They are often skilled interviewers, but have been trained to conduct interviews of a different type, in which selective information is sought to clarify a specific case problem, and efforts are made to exert influence by providing advice, directions, information or reassurance; these habits are not easily unlearned.

NOTES AND REFERENCES

1. For useful practical advice on the art of interviewing, see: Bowling A 1997 (Research methods in health: investigating health and health services. Open University Press, Buckingham, Ch. 13); Kornhauser A, Sheatsley P B 1976 (Questionnaire construction and interview procedure. In: Selltiz C, Wrightsman L S, Cook S W, eds. Research methods in social relations, 3rd edn. Holt, Rinehart & Winston, New York); or Trochim W M K 1997 (Interviews [on the Internet: trochim.human/cornell.edu/kb/interview.htm]).
2. Rosenman R H, Friedman M, Straus R et al 1964 A predictive study of coronary heart disease: the Western Collaborative Group Study. Journal of the American Medical Association 189: 15 (appendix; included in reprints only).
3. Glaser E M 1964 Volunteers, controls, placebos and questionaires in clinical trials. In: Witts L J (ed) Medical surveys and clinical trials. Oxford University Press, Oxford, pp 115–129.
4. Self-administered compared with interviewer-administered questionnaires: Picavet H S J, Van den Bos G A M 1996 (Comparing survey data on functional disability: the impact of some methodological differences. Journal of Epidemiology and Community Health 50: 86); Grootendorst P V, Feeny D H, Furlong W 1997 (Does it matter whom and how you ask? Inter- and intra-rater agreement in the Ontario Health Survey. Journal of Clinical Epidemiology 50: 127); Tourangeau R, Jobe J B, Pratt W F, Rasinski K 1997 (Design and results of the Women's Health Study. NIDA Research Monographs 167: 344 [on the Internet: www.nida.nih.gov/pdt/monographs/ monograph167/344–365_Tourangeau.pdf]); De Leeuw E D 1993 (Data quality in mail, telephone and face-to-face surveys. TT-Publikaties, Amsterdam).
   In the Rand Health Insurance Study, 70% of participants opted for self-administered questionnaires and 12% for interviews; 18% stated no preference (Ware J E Jr 1984 In: Wenger N K, Mattson M E, Furberg C D, Elinson J, eds. Assessment of quality of life in clinical trials of cardiovascular therapies. LeJacq Publishing [Haymarket-Doyma], New York, pp 87–111).
5. In a survey of women's experiences with childbearing, a randomized comparison showed a lower response for *postal interviews* (75%) than for home interviews (92%). Replies on painful and delicate subjects were similar for the two methods; there were differences in reports of attitudes and of doing the 'right' or 'wrong' thing, but some were in one direction and some in the other (Cartwright A 1988 Interviews or postal questionnaires? Comparisons of data about women's experiences with maternity services. Milbank Quarterly 66: 172).
6. Comparisons of *modes of interview*: Donovan R J, Holman C D, Corti B, Jalleh G 1997 (Face-to-face houschold interviews versus telephone interviews for health surveys. Australian and New Zealand Journal of Public Health 21: 134); McHorney C A, Kosinski M, Ware J E Jr 1994 (Comparisons of the costs and quality of norms for the SF-36 Health Survey collected by mail

versus telephone interview: results from a national survey. Medical Care
32: 551); Mickey R M, Worden J K, Vacek P M, Skelly J M, Costanza M C
1994 (Comparability of telephone and household breast cancer screening
surveys with differing response rates. Epidemiology 5: 462); Fox T A,
Heimendinger J, Block G 1992 (Telephone surveys as a method for obtaining
dietary information: a review. Journal of the American Dietetic Association
92: 729); American Journal of Public Health 83: 896; Brambilla D J,
McKinlay S M 1987 (A comparison of responses to mailed questionnaires
and telephone interviews in a mixed mode health survey. American Journal
of Epidemiology 126: 962); O'Toole B I, Battistutta D, Long A, Crouch K
1986 (A comparison of costs and data quality of three health survey methods:
mail, telephone and personal home interview. American Journal of
Epidemiology 124: 317); Siemiatycki J 1979 (A comparison of mail,
telephone and home interview strategies for household health surveys.
American Journal of Public Health 69: 238).

In mental health and drug use surveys: Revicki D A, Tohen M, Gyulai L,
Thompson C, Pike S, Davis-Vogel A, Zarate C 1997 (Telephone versus
in-person interviews in patients with bipolar disorder. Harvard Review of
Psychiatry 5: 75); Simon G E, Revicki D, VonKorff M 1993 (Telephone
assessment of depression severity. Journal of Psychiatric Research 27: 247);
Fenig S, Levav I, Kohn R, Yelin N 1993 (Telephone vs face-to-face
interviewing in a community psychiatric survey); Aquilino W S 1992
(Telephone versus face-to-face interviewing for household drug use surveys.
International Journal of the Addictions 27: 71).

7. Bradburn N M 1984 Discussion: telephone service methodology. In: Cannell
   C F, Groves R M (eds) Health survey research methods DHHS publication
   no (PHS) 84–3346. National Center for Health Services Research,
   Washington, DC, pp 146–148.
8. Pless I B, Miller J R 1979 Apparent validity of alternative survey methods.
   Journal of Community Health 5: 22.
9. Siematycki 1979 (see note 6).
10. Anie K A, Jones P W, Hilton S R, Anderson H R 1996 A computer-assisted
    telephone interview technique for assessment of asthma morbidity and drug
    use in adult asthma. Journal of Clinical Epidemiology 49: 653.
11. Birkett N J 1988 Computer-aided personal interviewing: a new technique for
    data collection in epidemiologic surveys. American Journal of Epidemiology
    127: 684.
12. *Epi Info* is a public domain program that can prepare questionnaires for
    computer-assisted interviews (see note 3, p. 292).
13. For a detailed review of computer-assisted methods, see De Leeuw E,
    Nicholls W II 1996 (Technological innovations in data collection:
    acceptance, data quality and costs. Sociological Research Online 1[4] [on
    the Internet: www.socresonline.org.uk/socresonline/1/4/leeuw.html]).
14. De Leeuw and Nicholls 1996 (see note 13) cite a meta-analysis showing that
    CASI reduces social desirability bias, but suggesting that although this effect
    remains significant, it may be weaker than it was in earlier years.
15. Waterton J, Duffy J C 1984 A comparison of computer interviewing
    techniques and traditional methods in the collection of self-report alcohol
    consumption data in a field survey. International Statistical Review 52: 173.
16. Locke S E, Kowaloff H B, Hoff R G et al 1994 Computer interview for
    screening blood donors for risk of HIV transmission. MD Computing 11: 26.
17. Lessler J T, O'Reilly J M 1997 Mode of interview and reporting of sensitive
    issues: design and implementation of audio computer-assisted self-
    interviewing. NIDA Research Monographs 167: 366 (on the Internet:
    www.nida.nih.gov/pdt/monographs/monograph167/366–382_Lessler.pdf).
18. Kohlmeier L, Mendez M, McDuffie J, Miller M 1997 Computer-assisted

self-interviewing: a multimedia approach to dietary assessment. American Journal of Clinical Nutrition 65(4 suppl): 1275S.

19. In a review of what *hard data* means, Feinstein (1983) considers five attributes—preservability, objectivity, dimensionality, accuracy (criterion validity) and consistency—and, after citing examples of data that are not regarded as 'soft' although they are ephemeral, subjective, non-dimensional, or inaccurate—concludes that the fundamental quality of 'hard' data is their consistency—they are 'repeatable by the same observer and reproducible by another' (Feinstein A R 1983 An additional basic science for clinical medicine: IV. The development of clinimetrics. Annals of Internal Medicine 99: 843).

20. Colditz G A, Martin P, Stampfer M J et al 1986 Validation of questionnaire information on risk factors and disease outcomes in a prospective cohort study of women. American Journal of Epidemiology 123: 894.

21. Madow W G 1973 Net differences in interview data on chronic conditions and information derived from medical records. Vital and Health Statistics series 2: 57.

22. Chambers L W, Spitzer W O, Hill G B, Helliwell B E 1976 Underreporting of cancer in medical surveys: a source of systematic error in cancer research. American Journal of Epidemiology 104: 41.

23. Cheasty M, Clare A W, Collins C 1998 Relation between sexual abuse in childhood and adult depression: case-control study. British Medical Journal 316: 198.

24. Mulder P G H, Garretsen H F L 1983 Are epidemiological and sociological surveys a proper instrument for detecting true problem drinkers? International Journal of Epidemiology 12: 442.

25. Stewart A W, Jackson R T, Ford M A, Beaglehole R 1987 Underestimation of relative weight by use of self-reported height and weight. American Journal of Epidemiology 125: 122.

26. Yorkshire Breast Cancer Group 1977 Observer variation in recording clinical data from women presenting with breast lesions. British Medical Journal 2: 1196.

27. When interviews of postmenopausal women were repeated after 2–22 months, kappa values were 89–93% for data on hysterectomy, a family history of breast cancer, hot flushes, and other 'simple' variables; in 22% there were discrepancies of over 2 years in reported age at menopause (Horwitz R I, Yu E C 1985 Problems and proposals for interview data in epidemiological research. International Journal of Epidemiology 14: 463).

28. This requires *probit analysis*. As an example, data on current breast-feeding status were converted to an estimate of the average duration of breast-feeding by Ferreira M U, Cardoso M A, Santos A L, Ferreira C S, Szarfarc S C 1996 (Rapid epidemiologic assessment of breastfeeding practices: probit analysis of current status data. Journal of Tropical Pediatrics 42: 50).

29. Mitchell A A, Cottler L B, Shapiro S 1986 Effect of questionnaire design on recall of drug exposure in pregnancy. American Journal of Epidemiology 123: 670.

30. Linder F E 1965 National health interview surveys. In: Trends in the study of morbidity and mortality. Public Health Papers 27. WHO, Geneva, p. 78.

31. National Center for Health Statistics 1972 Reporting health events in household interviews: effects of an extensive questionnaire and a diary procedure. Vital and Health Statistics, series 2, no 49. Public Health Service, Washington, DC.

32. Spilker A, Kessler J 1987 Comparison of symptoms elicited by checklist and fill-in-the-blank questionnaires. Pharmaco-Epidemiology Newsletter 3: 8.

33. Marcus A C 1982 Memory aids in longitudinal health surveys: results from a field experiment. American Journal of Public Health 72: 567.

34. Raphael K 1987 Recall bias: a proposal for assessment and control. International Journal of Epidemiology 16: 167. Also, see Coughlin S S 1990 (Recall bias in epidemiologic studies. Journal of Clinical Epidemiology 43: 87).
35. Kirscht J P 1971 Social and psychological problems of surveys in health and illness. Social Science and Medicine 5: 519.
36. *Family histories of disease* should be used with caution. Diseases of relatives tend to be under-reported (Grootendorst P V, Feeny D H, Furlong W 1997 Does it matter whom and how you ask? Inter- and intra-rater agreement in the Ontario Health Survey. Journal of Clinical Epidemiology 50: 127), and reported causes of death often differ from the certified causes (Napier J A, Metzner H, Johnson B C 1972 Limitations of morbidity and mortality data obtained from family histories—a report from the Tecumseh Community Health Study. American Journal of Public Health 62: 30).

    When people with rheumatoid arthritis were questioned, 27% reported that their parents were free of arthritis; but when their unaffected siblings were questioned, 50% reported that the same parents were free of arthritis (Schull W J, Cobb S 1969 The intrafamilial transmission of rheumatoid arthritis. Journal of Chronic Diseases 22: 217).

    Children aged 10 or more can accurately report their parents' smoking status (Barnett T, O'Loughlin J, Paradis G, Renaud L 1997 Reliability of proxy reports of parental smoking by elementary schoolchildren. Annals of Epidemiology 7: 396), and women's current use of contraceptives can be accurately reported by their husbands, less so by their mothers and sisters (Poulter N R Chang C I, Farley T M M, Marmot M G 1996 Reliability of data from proxy respondents in an international case-control study of cardiovascular disease and oral contraceptives. Journal of Epidemiology and Community Health 50: 674).
37. Passaro K T, Noss J, Savitz D A, Little R E, ALSPAC Study Team 1997 Agreement between self and partner reports of paternal drinking and smoking. International Journal of Epidemiology 26: 315.
38. Whiteman D, Green A 1997 Wherein lies the truth? Assessment of agreement between parent proxy and child respondents. International Journal of Epidemiology 26: 855.
39. Harlow S D, Linet M S 1989 Agreement between questionnaire data and medical records: the evidence for accuracy of recall. American Journal of Epidemiology 129: 233.
40. Interview data about the remote past can sometimes be compared with old records. A study in Iowa found that the reported birth weights of adolescents were accurate enough to permit inferences about relationships with other factors (Burns T L, Moll P P, Rost C A, Lauer R M 1987 Mothers remember birth weights of adolescent children: the Muscatine Ponderosity Family Study. International Journal of Epidemiology 16: 550). In Jerusalem, mothers were found to provide valid information (*kappa* = 80%) about the breast-feeding of army recruits (in their infancy) (Kark J D, Troya G, Friedlander Y, Slater P E, Stein Y 1984 Validity of maternal reporting of breast feeding history and the association with blood lipids in 17 year olds. Journal of Epidemiology and Community Health 38: 218). Records of a cohort study showed that 8% of 36-year-old men who said they had never smoked regularly had reported regular smoking when questioned at younger ages (Britten N 1988 Validity of claims to lifelong nonsmoking at age 38 in a longitudinal study. International Journal of Epidemiology 17: 525).

    Improved interview methods have been recommended for obtaining past information. Careful interviews gave 'usefully accurate' information about social circumstances 50 years earlier (father's occupation, number of rooms, etc.), but not about illnesses and diet in childhood (Berney I R, Blane D B

1997 Collecting retrospective data: accuracy of recall after 50 years judged against historical records. Social Science and Medicine 45: 1519). The current diet exerts a strong influence on the recall of past diet, and probes and memory aids may be needed to obtain more accurate information about the past (Friedenreich C M, Slimani N, Riboli E 1992 Measurement of past diet: review of previous and proposed methods. Epidemiologic Reviews 14: 177).

41. Fowkes F G R 1988 The measurement of atherosclerotic peripheral arterial disease in epidemiological surveys. International Journal of Epidemiology 17: 248.
42. Blair S N, Haskell W L, Ho P et al 1985 Assessment of habitual physical activity by a 7-day recall in a community survey and controlled experiments. American Journal of Epidemiology 122: 794.
43. The golden rule according to Trochim M K 1997 (Question placement and sequence. On the Internet: trochim.human/cornell.edu/kb/quesplac.htm). See also: Matthew 7: 12.

19 Constructing a questionnaire

Before a questionnaire is constructed the variables it is designed to measure should be listed (see Ch. 10). This done, suitable questions should be formulated, i.e. questions that have (at least) face validity (see p. 189) as measures of these variables, and that also meet the other requirements listed below. To enhance validity, it may be decided to ask multiple questions on some topics, permitting the use of composite scales of measurement (see Ch. 14), both because it may not be possible to cover all facets of the variable in a single question, and because reliance on a single question may increase the chances of inaccuracy due to misunderstanding or other factors. In some cases, to enhance comparability with other studies, questions are borrowed from other sources rather than creating them anew.

'Something old, something new, something borrowed, something blue'—apart maybe from the last ingredient, this is the recipe for most questionnaires. The use of borrowed questions or 'standard' questionnaires has the advantage that they have already been tested and found to be serviceable. But comparability is sometimes an illusion, since the same questions may differ in their validity in different kinds of population or different circumstances. The investigator should always consider the possible need to revalidate the questions or questionnaire. A decision on what to borrow is not always easy. A researcher wanting to measure social support, for example, can choose between many different questionnaires, varying in their conceptual framework, content, convenience, applicability, and validity.[1]

This chapter will deal with the types of question (open or

closed), the requirements that a question should meet, ways of dealing with sensitive topics, and the structure of the questionnaire as a whole.

OPEN OR CLOSED?

Questions may take two general forms: they may be 'open-ended' (or 'free response') questions, which the subject answers in his own words, or 'closed' (or 'fixed-alternative') questions, which are answered by choosing from a number of fixed alternative responses.

Open-ended questions often produce difficulties when it comes to interpreting the responses. Suppose, for example, we were interested in knowing how many people had given up smoking for reasons connected with health. The question 'Why did you stop smoking? State your main reason' might excite such responses as: 'I thought it was better not to smoke'; 'I'd been smoking for 30 years, and decided it was time to give it up'; 'Because my wife said I should'. There is obvious difficulty in categorizing these answers; in all three instances, it is impossible to tell whether the main reason was connected with health. In a self-administered questionnaire, even a question like 'What is your marital status?' may be answered 'Unsatisfactory' or 'Ask my wife'; a closed question ('Are you at present single, married, widowed or divorced?') is preferable. There is, of course, no difficulty in the use of open-ended questions in instances where the responses can be easily handled, e.g. 'How old were you at your last birthday?' or 'In what country were you born?'. Open-ended questions have an important role in exploratory surveys, where they indicate the range of likely replies and provide a guide to the formulation of alternative responses to closed questions. They may also be used to provide colourful case illustrations to brighten up an otherwise dull report. If followed by 'probe' questions, open-ended questions have certain advantages in the study of complicated or ill formed opinions or attitudes. Qualitative research (see p. 166) uses open-ended rather than closed questions.

Closed questions make for greater uniformity and simplify the analysis, and are therefore preferred for most purposes, although they limit the variety and detail of responses. They may provide two responses (such as 'yes–no', 'agree–disagree') or more (such as 'never', 'seldom', 'occasionally', 'fairly frequently', and 'very often'). The range of responses is equivalent to the scale of measurement we have previously spoken of (Ch. 13); it should be comprehensive, and the categories should be mutually exclusive. An 'other (specify) …' category is sometimes included, as insurance against oversights in the choice of categories; but respondents who mark 'other' very commonly fail to supply the specific information requested.[2]

When there is a range of responses extending from one extreme to the opposite extreme (e.g. from 'strongly disagree' to 'strongly agree'), an equal number of alternatives (generally two or three) should be presented on each side of the scale. Offering a central 'neutral', 'undecided' or 'no opinion' option reduces the nonresponse rate. This option is sometimes omitted, to try to force the respondent to make a stand; but some respondents may then be compelled to say 'I don't know' or skip the question (and be indistinguishable from those who fail to answer for other reasons). Labelling the middle category 'neutral' or 'undecided' may elicit different replies.

Sometimes more than one response is permitted, e.g. to the question 'Which of the following cereals do you eat?'; in this instance each item represents a separate 'yes–no' variable.

Except in simple instances such as 'yes–no' choices, the alternative responses should be read to the subject, or may be shown (e.g. on a card) or, in a self-administered questionnaire, specified after the question.

To avoid the need to express all the alternative responses in words, use may be made of graphic rating (visual analogue) scales. The subject is shown a line or ladder, and asked to answer the question by indicating an appropriate point on the scale. Points along the scale may be shown by numbers (often 0 to 10 or 1 to 10), or a score can be obtained by measuring the position of the point marked by the respondent. The scale can be labelled at its ends with the two extreme responses (e.g. 'very satisfied' and 'completely dissatisfied'), and intermediate labels may also be printed.

The formulation of response categories for a question like 'What was your main reason for giving up smoking?' often needs careful thought. A misguided selection of alternatives may, like a Procrustean bed, achieve conformity at a considerable price. It is sometimes advisable to use an open-ended question first (in a pretest), so that free responses can be collected and used as a basis for the design of 'closed' categories. Another approach is to follow the closed question with a suitable open-ended one on the same topic; in a pretest, this may demonstrate flaws in the closed question; in the study itself, the combination provides the advantages of both types of question.

REQUIREMENTS OF QUESTIONS

Questions are very easy to write. Good questions are hard to write. They require skill and experience (or expert advice),[3] careful thought, and practical testing. The answers they elicit may vary widely, depending on precisely how the questions are constructed and worded. The proportion of elderly people who say they are 'unable to walk', for example, can range from 4 to 16%, depending on how the question is phrased: walking 'a block' or '400 metres'—walking 'without help' or 'without standing still'—and with or without the specification 'using a cane if necessary'.[4] The propensity of competing public opinion polls with differently worded questions to supply conflicting results is notorious.

Requirements of questions

1. Must have (at least) face validity
2. Respondents can be expected to know the answer
3. Must be clear and unambiguous
4. Must be 'user-friendly' (not demanding undue effort)
5. Must not be offensive or embarrassing
6. Must be fair

The minimal requirement is, of course, that the question should have *face validity* as a measure of the variable it is wished to study. Implicit in this requirement is the obvious but sometimes neglected principle that questions should be asked only if they are necessary. Ensuring that a question accurately reflects what the investigator wishes to know may demand rethinking of the conceptual definition. Is information on 'ability to walk', for example, being requested as a measure of physical capacity or of independence in daily living?

The questions should be ones to which the respondents can be *expected to know the answers*. There is little point in asking 'Did your grandmother have piles?' or (from an Internet questionnaire) 'As a baby, did you have milk scurf (itching and scratched weeping lesions)?', or in inviting opinions on a matter the respondent has never thought about, or asking the respondent to state attitudes or motivations of which he may not be aware. People who have not been told they have diabetes cannot report that they have the disease. There is little value in questions concerning events or experiences that had little impact and that many subjects will not recall, such as minor injuries or food eaten 3 days previously. Many mild illnesses not requiring medical care and not restricting activity fail to be reported after the lapse of 1 week, and many hospitalizations are not recalled after 1 year. Illnesses requiring a single consultation with a physician are reported more poorly than those requiring many consultations, and conditions requiring a long stay in hospital or involving surgery are reported more fully than other conditions.

It is often decided that since the respondents cannot be expected to supply the required information in a direct way, indirect questions will be asked, the desired information being inferred from the responses to questions on other matters. Instead of asking the subject if he is emotionally healthy, he may be asked about a series of symptoms from which his emotional health can be inferred. Instead of asking a mother to state her attitudes concerning permissiveness towards children, she may be asked whether she carries or carried out specific actions, or what she would do in a specific situation, or how she thinks other mothers would feel or act, or how she thinks mothers *should* act. Instead of (or as well as) asking the respondent whether he is satisfied with his own medical care, he may be asked what he thinks of the medical care in his neighbourhood, or whether he agrees or disagrees with such statements as 'Most doctors take a real interest in their patients'.

The way in which questions are worded can 'make or break' a questionnaire. Questions must be *clear* and *unambiguous*. They must be phrased in language that it is believed the respondents will understand, and that all respondents will understand in the same way. This is more easily said than done—when a questionnaire is tested, unexpected double meanings are often found concealed in apparently crystal-clear questions. 'Single' may mean 'never married' to some people, and 'not married at present' to others; 'abortion' may mean different things to different people. 'Family' may be understood to mean the immediate family, or relatives in the same household, or the far-flung extended family, or forebears. To some people, 'family planning' means 'saving money for vacations'. The most everyday words may evoke different interpretations. In one methodological study it was found that when answering questions about 'usual' behaviour—where the intended meaning was 'in the ordinary course of events'—20% of respondents gave it other interpretations (e.g. 'more often than not' or 'at regular (even if infrequent) intervals') or 'sometimes', and 19% disregarded the term completely, and gave answers that were not constrained by it at all.[5]

Medical terms, even those commonly used in everyday speech, may occasion much difficulty. 'Anaemia' and 'heart disease' may have different connotations for the layman and the physician; to many laymen, 'palpitation' means a feeling of breathlessness or of fright, and 'flatulence' means an acid taste in the mouth.[6]

Questions should be as 'user-friendly' as possible—that is, as easy and convenient as their purpose and content will permit. Intricate or demanding questions, and questions requiring complicated responses or a choice between complicated alternatives, should if at all possible be avoided. 'Double-barrelled' questions like 'Do you take your child to a doctor when he has a cold or diarrhoea' may be difficult to answer (and the answers may be difficult to interpret), and should be split into separate questions. Questions requiring a 'yes' answer to indicate agreement with a negative statement may confuse respondents (e.g. 'Should a woman aged 50 not have regular breast X-rays?'). If closed questions are used, the possible responses should be clearly expressed, and stated at the end, not the beginning; i.e. not 'Do you very often, often, occasionally, hardly ever or never do the Highland fling?', but 'How often do you do the Highland fling—very often, often, occasionally, hardly ever or never?'. Also, the need for responses should be reduced where possible; for example, to find out to which of a list of sources of stress the respondent feels exposed, it may be better to ask for a mark against those that apply (with an added 'None of the above' category), rather than to request a 'yes–no' response to each; the former approach, which assumes a 'no' for unchecked items, was found to reduce the nonresponse rates for items from 12–50% to 2%.[2]

As examples of questions that some respondents would find burdensome, here are two from Internet surveys.

1. What is your weight? (in kilograms—multiply pounds by .45 to get kilograms).
2. Suppose, in the future, a woman finds out that she carries a gene which greatly increases her chances of developing endometriosis. Her own brothers, sisters and children would have a

50% chance of carrying this gene. The doctor tells the woman that she should inform her female relatives about her situation to let them decide if they want to learn if they are also at increased risk of developing endometriosis. Women known to be at an increased risk for endometriosis may choose to have children earlier in life or take some kind of drug as a possible form of prevention. The woman refuses to tell them, because she says they will only worry. What do you think the doctor should do?

- Go along with the woman's wishes and not tell the relatives.
- Tell the relatives whether or not they ask about endometriosis.
- Without talking specifically about the woman, recommend testing to relatives if they ask about endometriosis.
- Without talking specifically about the woman, recommend testing to relatives even if they do not ask about endometriosis.

Short questions are generally regarded as preferable to long ones. But experiments have shown that length may sometimes be a virtue—longer questions may elicit fuller responses.[7] More symptoms or chronic disorders, for example, tend to be reported if longer questions are used. This may partly be because the additional material helps the respondent's recall. But a longer question may evoke a fuller response even if the added verbiage seems redundant. In one study, the question 'The next question is about medicines during the past 4 weeks. We want to ask you about this. What medicines, if any, did you take or use during the past 4 weeks?' yielded more information than the same question with the first two sentences removed. The reasons for this are not clear—maybe asking a longer question inclines the respondent to answer at equal length, or maybe the extra material simply gives the respondent more time to think. Short, terse questions appear to be preferable for the study of attitudes,[8] but longer questions may have advantages for symptoms, disorders, and practices. One recommendation that has ensued from these findings is that questions should be short when possible, but interviews should be conducted at a slow pace, so that respondents have time to think. Longer questions should be used with discrimination—'if we larded all questions with "filler" phrases, a questionnaire would soon be bloated with too few, too fat questions'.[9]

It is wise to try to avoid questions that may *offend or embarrass* the respondent. If 'sensitive' questions of this sort must be asked, special care should be taken (see below).

The questions should be *fair*. They should not be phrased (or voiced) in a way that suggests a specific answer, and should not be loaded or one-sided. The question 'What are the main things that are wrong with the care you get from your doctor?' is an obviously unfair one. A format that 'begs the question' in this way (by assuming the truth of something not yet known) should be used, if at all, only in studies of attitudes in which it is felt that the best way to get a respondent to give voice to prejudices is to indicate that the questioner shares them.

'SENSITIVE' QUESTIONS

It may not be possible to avoid asking 'sensitive' questions that might offend or embarrass some respondents, e.g. requests for intimate or confidential information, questions that may seem to expose the respondent's ignorance, and questions that may elicit socially undesirable answers, such as admitting to a sexually transmitted disease or a shameful habit.

Simple solutions are sometimes feasible. For example, reluctance to disclose age or income may be countered by using broad categories of response (if these satisfy the needs of the study), such as '45–64 years', '65 or more', instead of an open-ended question like 'How old are you?', and questions to measure level of knowledge can be presented as requests for an opinion ('Do you think that...?').

Possible offence or embarrassment can often be mitigated by including a statement designed to show that the questioner's interest is non-judgemental: 'We know that all married couples sometimes quarrel with each other; how often does it happen that *you* quarrel with your husband?'. Possible tactics, as amusingly described by Barton,[10] are:

1. *The everybody approach*: 'As you know, many people have been killing their wives these days. Do you happen to have killed yours?'.
2. *The other people approach*: (a) 'Do you know any people who have murdered their wives?' (b) 'How about yourself?'.
3. *The Kinsey technique*: Stare firmly into the respondent's eyes and ask in simple, clear-cut language such as that to which the respondent is accustomed, and with an air of assuming that everybody has done everything, 'Did you ever kill your wife?'.

Self-administered questionnaires usually elicit a greater number of socially undesirable responses. But a study of reactions to questions concerning behaviour about which many people are reluctant to talk fully and honestly, in three large samples in the United States, showed that the effects of mode of administration (face-to-face, phone, or self-administered) were small, whereas the construction of the question made a great deal of difference.[11] In particular, there were two ploys that produced a two- to threefold increase in the amount of reporting of behaviour. The first was the use of a long introduction to the question, and the second was the use of an open-ended question. In this study the open-ended format was used only for questions about the amount or frequency of behaviour (how much liquor do you drink? how many times a week do you drink?), where the answers could be fairly easily coded. The findings suggested that long questions and an open-ended format should routinely be used when asking about the frequency of sensitive behaviour. The open-ended questions gave significantly higher frequencies for beer, wine and liquor drinking, petting, intercourse, and masturbation. A suggested reason is that the presence of low-frequency categories ('never, once a year or less, every few months, once a month, every few weeks ...') made people less willing to admit to higher frequencies.

Another recommended approach, which increased the reported frequencies of socially undesirable behaviour by about 15%, is the use of words familiar to the respondent. A suggested method is to let the respondent decide what term should be used, and then to use this in subsequent questions. For example, 'Different people use different words for sexual intercourse [or marijuana, masturbation, etc.]. What word do you think we should use?' It may also be helpful to ask whether the respondent has engaged in the socially undesirable behaviour in the past ('Did you ever, even once ...'), before asking about current behaviour.[8]

Another simple technique is putting the possible responses on cards, so that the respondent need only point to the answer, without letting the offending words sully his lips.

PUTTING IT ALL TOGETHER

A questionnaire should always have an introductory explanation, stating the purposes and sponsorship of the study. A statement about confidentiality should be included, but anonymity should not be guaranteed unless there is really no way of tracing which questionnaire belongs to whom. If the questionnaire is self-administered, the introduction should include clear instructions and examples. If the questionnaire is to be used by an interviewer, it may be preferred to put the explanation and instructions in an accompanying guide or manual. The instructions to the interviewer should be full and explicit.

The introductory explanation must be drafted with care, since it may markedly affect the responses to the questions. In surveys of the elderly in Holland, the reported prevalence of disability was much lower if the introduction emphasized that the questions referred to longstanding rather than temporary limitations. This reduced the prevalence of disability in mobility by 13.7 percentage points.[4] In a questionnaire covering different topics, each new topic should have an introductory phrase (e.g. 'Now, about ...') or explanation.

The first questions should be easy to answer, of obvious relevance to the topic of the study and (if possible) interesting. 'Sensitive' questions, which may engender embarrassment or resentment, should be left until later—even questions about age, education, ethnic group, etc., are sometimes left to the end for this reason. It may be inadvisable to start a postal questionnaire with an open-ended question.

The sequence of the questions needs careful attention. They should follow an order that the respondent will see as natural, with smooth movement from item to item. On the other hand, if the questionnaire is long it may be wise to have breaks in the continuity by switching topics or altering the format of questions, since 'changes of scenery' may prevent boredom. Long successions of questions that can elicit repeated identical responses (e.g. 'yes') should be avoided, as the respondent may fall into a rut (a 'response set') and continue to give the same response unthinkingly.

With proper sequencing, irrelevant questions can be bypassed. A 'sieve' or 'filter' question about drinking, for example, might screen out people who take no alcohol, so that subsequent detailed questions about the consumption of alcoholic beverages are skipped, or might direct the respondent to an appropriate 'branch' (if, say, there are different questions for ex-drinkers and current drinkers). Skipping and branching patterns (indicated by 'go to' instructions or arrows) are usually acceptable in a self-administered questionnaire, provided that they are simple; but multistep branching and skipping schemes may be confusing, and should be avoided.

When arranged in order the questions should be gone through carefully ('put yourself in the respondent's boots') to examine the implications of the sequence. In particular, the answer to a prior question may influence the response to a later question (in which case the order should probably be reversed). If the questionnaire includes both specific and general questions about attitudes, the general question should come first, since specific questions tend to be answered in the same way wherever they are placed, whereas the response to a general question may be affected by prior specific questions. One study showed that the answer to a question about marital happiness was not influenced by a previous question about happiness in general, whereas the question on general happiness tended to be answered differently, depending on whether the marriage question was asked first.[12] Similarly, questions about general health and functional capacity should be put near the beginning of the questionnaire, unless the investigator wants the appraisal to be influenced by questions about specific illnesses, symptoms and disabilities. A run-through of the questionnaire may also reveal awkward sequences; for example, some women may resent being asked 'Are you married' after giving a positive answer to 'Do you have children?'

When the questionnaire is reconsidered and discussed with colleagues, it is invariably found to need modification. Usually, more than one redraft is needed. The questionnaire should then be tested in practice—'if you do not have the resources to pilot-test your questionnaire, don't do the study'.[8] It may be decided to try alternative versions of the same questions, in the same questionnaire or in questionnaires tested on different respondents. Pretests (see Ch. 24) are indispensable; they usually reveal a need for changes in the questions or their sequence or, very frequently, for shortening the questionnaire.

NOTES AND REFERENCES

1. Perrin K M, McDermott R J 1997 Instruments to measure social support and related constructs in pregnant adolescents: a review. Adolescence 32: 533.
2. Dengler R, Roberts H, Rushton L 1997 Lifestyle surveys—the complete answer? Journal of Epidemiology and Community Health 51: 46.
3. Fink A 1995 How to ask survey questions. Sage Publications, Beverly Hills; Fowler F J Jr 1995 Improving survey questions: design and evaluation. Sage Publications, Beverly Hills; Kornhauser A, Sheatsley P B 1976 Questionnaire construction and interview procedure. In: Selltiz C, Wrightsman L S, Cook S W (eds) Research methods in social relations, 3rd edn. Holt, Rinehart & Winston, New York; Payne S L 1965 The art of asking questions. Princeton

University Press, Princeton, N J; Converse J M, Presser S 1986 Survey questions: handcrafting the standardized questionnaire. Sage Publications, Beverly Hills; Sudman S, Bradburn N M 1983 Asking questions. Jossey-Bass, San Francisco.

Useful practical advice on questions and questionnaires (particularly mail questionnaires) is provided on the Internet (hammock.ifas.ufl.edu/txt/fairs/ 19814) by the Institute of Food and Agricultural Services, University of Florida: Taylor C L 1992 (Formatting a mail questionnaire); Summerhill W R, Taylor C L 1992 (Obtaining response to a mail questionnaire); Taylor C L, Summerhill W R 1992 (Writing options for mail questionnaires); Summerhill W R, Taylor C L 1992 (Writing questions for mail questionnaires). Also, see: Trochim W M K 1997 (Constructing the survey. Internet: trochim.human.cornell.edu/kb/survwrit.htm).

4. Picavet H S J, Van den Bos G A M 1996 Comparing survey data on functional disability: the impact of some methodological differences. Journal of Epidemiology and Community Health 50: 86.
5. Belson W A 1981 The design and understanding of survey questions. Gower, Aldershot, Hants.
6. Boyle C M 1970 Difference between patients' and doctors' interpretation of some common medical terms. British Medical Journal ii: 286.
7. Henson R, Cannell C F, Lawson S A 1979 In: Cannell C F, Oksenberg L, Converse J M (eds) Experiments in interviewing techniques. Institute for Social Research, Ann Arbor, Michigan; Laurent A 1972 Effects of question length on reporting behavior in the survey interview. Journal of the American Statistical Association 67: 298; Belson W A 1981 (see note 5).
8. Sudman S, Bradburn N M 1983 (see note 3).
9. Converse J M, Presser N M 1986 (see note 3).
10. Barton A J 1958 Asking the embarrassing question. Public Opinion Quarterly 22: 67.
11. Bradburn N M, Sudman S et al 1981 Improving interview method and questionnaire design. Jossey-Bass, San Francisco.
12. Turner C F 1984 Why do surveys disagree? Some preliminary hypotheses and some disagreeable examples. In: Turner C F, Martin E (eds) Surveying subjective phenomena, vol 2. Russell Sage, New York.

20 Surveying the opinions of a panel: consensus methods

There is sometimes interest in learning the opinions of a group of people with special knowledge or interests, in order to ascertain their consensus (majority opinion) or, if there is no consensus, to map their main disagreements. The group may be a panel of experts who have skills and knowledge relevant to some field of health care, or of professionals or laymen who have a special interest in some situation or topic, such as a specific community and its problems.

There may be two kinds of study objective:

1. To determine attitudes, concerns, appraisals of the relative importance of various factors or the desirability of various options, and the reasons for these judgements. When planning a health programme, for example, it may be helpful to know what knowledgeable people think are the chief problems and how they appraise the relative importance of these problems, or their opinions about the desirability, feasibility or pros and cons of various solutions. When a programme is to be evaluated, experts may be asked to choose criteria for the evaluation and to decide on the relative importance of these criteria, so that an appropriate weight can be allocated to each of them.
2. If objective facts about a situation are difficult or impossible to obtain, experts may be asked what they judge the facts to be. These 'guesstimates' may in some circumstances provide a basis for programme planning, on the assumption that an informed guess is better than no information at all. This use of experts' opinions may be especially appropriate in developing countries

in instances where 'hard' data cannot be gathered. In studies of cost-effectiveness, experts' estimates of the effectiveness of intervention procedures may be used as a substitute for objective measurements. In long-term planning, decisions may be based on experts' forecasts of the future situation.

Such surveys call for special methods. The main limitation of ordinary interview and questionnaire methods is that they permit no communication among the members of the group, who have no opportunity to reach a modified judgement after appraising the opinions of others. On the other hand, group techniques that permit free communication—focus groups and other group discussions, committee meetings and conference telephone calls—permit too much interaction. The group's decisions may be heavily influenced by this interaction, and may be unduly affected by a chairperson's bossiness or ineffectiveness, dominance by verbose or forceful speakers, deference to authority, power, prestige or age, or friendships or antagonisms between participants.

These problems can be minimized by methods that avoid or restrict interaction between participants, but provide interim feedback of the opinions of the group as a whole, which each participant can take into account before stating his final judgement. This is then pooled with other contributions to yield a group decision.

The *nominal group technique* is a simple method that may be used if the participants can be brought together at a meeting. The *Delphi technique* needs more elaborate preparation and organization but does not require the members of the panel to come together. With both techniques the findings depend, of course, on the selection of the participant experts. If these are not well chosen 'there is the danger of defining collective ignorance rather than wisdom'.[1] Both these consensus techniques are *qualitative methods* (see p. 166), although the results may be expressed in quantitative terms.

NOMINAL GROUP TECHNIQUE

The nominal group technique (NGT), which was developed by Van de Ven and Delbecq,[2] is so called because although the participants sit together, discussion is permitted only during specified phases of the process. Hence during most phases they are a group 'in name only'.

The technique may be used in a variety of situations requiring group decision-making. The participants may be any knowledge-

able or concerned individuals, professional or lay. The technique
was originally developed as a method of involving disadvantaged
citizens in community action agencies, and it has been recommended for use in exploratory studies of citizens' or professionals'
perceptions of health care problems (see p. 391).[2] It has been used
to learn why teenagers do or do not seek preventive health care[3]
and to study beliefs about susceptibility to AIDS,[4] and applied in
practice development and the selection of outcome measures for
use in clinical trials.[2]

The procedure[5] is simple. Five to nine participants (preferably
not more than seven) sit round a table, together with a leader (facil-
itator). If there are more participants they are divided into small
groups. A single session, which deals with a single question, usually
takes at least 60–90 minutes (longer if the judgements of different
groups are to be pooled).

For a typical meeting of a single small group, the following are
the successive steps.

1. Silent generation of ideas in writing
2. 'Round-robin' feedback of ideas
3. Serial discussion of ideas
4. Preliminary vote
5. Discussion of preliminary vote
6. Final vote

1. *Silent generation of ideas in writing.* After making a welcoming
   statement, which stresses the importance of the task and of each
   member's contribution, the leader reads out the question that
   the participants are required to answer. This is usually an open-
   ended question that calls for a list of items, e.g. the elements of
   a specified problem or of a proposed programme for dealing
   with a problem. Each member is given a worksheet (at the top
   of which the question appears) and is asked to take 5 minutes to
   write his ideas in response to the question. The leader also does
   this. Discussion is not permitted.
2. *'Round-robin' feedback of ideas.* The leader goes round the table
   and asks each member in turn to contribute one of the ideas he
   has written, summarized in a few words. The leader also takes a
   turn in each round. Each idea is numbered and written on a
   large blackboard or on a flip pad, completed sheets of which are
   taped or pinned where they are visible to all members. Members
   are asked not to contribute ideas that they regard as complete
   duplicates. Members are encouraged to add ideas to their work-

sheets at any time; they may 'pass' in one round and contribute in a later one. The process goes on until no further ideas are forthcoming. Discussion is not permitted during this stage.

3. *Serial discussion of ideas.* Each of the ideas listed on the board or flip pad is discussed in turn. For each one, the group is asked whether there are questions, or whether anyone wishes to clarify the item, explain the logic behind it, or express a view about its relative importance. The object of the discussion is to obtain clarity and to air points of view, but not to resolve differences of opinion. If there is much overlap between items it may be desirable to modify the list, after the serial discussion. One way of doing this is to rearrange the items so that variants of a single factor appear consecutively (retaining their original serial numbers) under a broad heading. Modest rewording may be undertaken if the group wishes to refine the list.

4. *Preliminary vote.* Each participant is asked to select a specified number (5–9) of 'most important' items from the total list, and copy them on to cards. If six are to be chosen, each participant is asked to write '6' (underlined or circled) on the 'most important' card, then '1' on the least important, then '5' on the most important of the remaining four, then '2', and so on. The leader also ranks the items. The cards are then collected and shuffled to maintain anonymity, and the votes are read out and recorded on a tally-chart that shows all the items and the rank numbers allocated to each.

5. *Discussion of preliminary vote.* Brief discussion of the voting pattern is now permitted. Members are told that the purpose of this discussion is additional clarification, and not to pressure them to change their votes.

6. *Final vote.* Step 4 is then repeated. The most important items may again be ranked, or they may be given ratings on a scale from 0 (unimportant) to 10 or 100 (very important). The rank numbers or ratings allotted to each item may be averaged by summing them and dividing by the total number of participants. Other rating methods may be used. For example, members may be asked to assign 100 points to the most important item and to give points to the other items in proportion to their relative importance, e.g. 50 points for an item half as important.[6]

If there are 10 or more participants they should be divided into small groups, and steps 1 to 4 are performed separately in each group. There is then a break, during which the group leaders meet to prepare a master list of items, including the top five to nine priorities identified by each group. Where necessary, items are reworded or combined. The master list shows the aggregated votes relating to each of the items included. All the participants then gather in a single large group, and discuss each item in the master list in turn, for clarification. The preliminary vote is then discussed. At any member's request, items not included in the master list can be added. A final vote is then conducted.

Modifications of this procedure may be used.[1] For example, the first step can be conducted by post, followed by the face-to-face meeting; a detailed literature review can be provided as background material; or there can also be a nonparticipant observer collecting qualitative data about the group.

DELPHI TECHNIQUE

The Delphi technique (named after the oracle) is more elaborate. It was first used to forecast what atom bomb targets might be selected by a potential enemy of the United States and how many bombs would be needed. Since then its applications have broadened considerably. It has been defined as a 'method for structuring a group communication process so that the process is effective in allowing a group of individuals, as a whole, to deal with a complex problem'.[7] The method has been applied extensively in the health field.[8]

Face-to-face contact between the participants is not required, although the 'Delphi' label is sometimes attached to procedures that include group discussion.[1] A series of mailed questionnaires is usually used, each one sent out after the results of the previous one have been analyzed. The time taken by this process may be cut down considerably by the use of modern communications.

The elements that are usually included are an opportunity for individuals to contribute ideas or information, an assessment of the group judgement, clarification of reasons for differences, a chance for individuals to revise their views, and some degree of anonymity for the individual responses. Votes may be cast and results fed back repeatedly, until stability or consensus is reached.

The Delphi procedure is protean in its manifestations, and no simple prescription can be given.[9] A learned compendium on the technique states that 'if anything is true about Delphi today, it is that in its design and use Delphi is more of an art than a science'.[7]

NOTES AND REFERENCES

1. Jones J, Hunter D 1995 Consensus methods for medical and health services research. British Medical Journal 311: 376. Also in: Mays N, Pope C (eds) 1996 Qualitative research in health care. BMJ Publishing Group, London.
2. Van de Ven A H, Delbecq A L 1972 American Journal of Public Health 62: 337.
3. Ginsburg K R, Menapace A S, Slap G B 1997 Factors affecting the decision to seek health care: the voice of adolescents. Pediatrics 100: 1997.
4. Manning D, Balson P M, Barenberg N, Moore T M 1989 Susceptibility to AIDS: what college students do and don't believe. Journal of the American College Health Association 38: 67.
5. The *nominal group technique* is fully described by Delbecq A L, Van de Ven A H, Gustafson D H 1975 (Techniques for program planning: a guide to nominal group and Delphi processes. Scott, Foreman, Glenview, Ill.) The procedure described in the text is based on detailed instructions given in Chapter 3 of that book.

    The authors point out the importance of asking the right questions and the right people, likening the nominal group technique to a microscope and a vacuum cleaner: 'NGT is like a microscope. Properly focused by a good question, NGT can provide a great deal of conceptual detail about the matter of concern to you. Improperly focused by a poor or misleading question, it tells you a great deal about something in which you are not interested' (p. 75). 'NGT is like a vacuum. It is a powerful means to draw out the insight and information possessed by group members. However, if there is nothing to "draw out" even a powerful vacuum is useless' (p. 79).
6. If the total points are assigned to the referent item, it may be desirable to standardize the scores by expressing each one as a proportion or percentage of the sum of all the points allocated by the person. See Edwards W, Guttentag M, Snapper K 1975 (A decision-theoretic approach to evaluation research. In: Struening E L, Guttentag M, eds. Handbook of evaluation research. Sage, Beverly Hills, Cal., p. 155).
7. Linstone H A, Turoff M (eds) 1975 The Delphi method: techniques and applications. Addison-Wesley, Reading, Mass., p. 3.
8. *Delphi method* (examples): Hunter D J W, McKee C M, Sanderson C F B, Black N A 1994 (Appropriate indications for prostatectomy in the UK: results of a consensus panel. Journal of Epidemiology and Community Health 48: 58); Attala J M, Gresley R S, McSweeney N, Jobe M A 1993 (Health needs of school-age children in two midwestern counties. Issues in Comprehensive Paediatric Nursing 16: 51); Clark A, Friedman M J 1982 (The relative importance of treatment outcomes: a Delphi group weighting in mental health. Evaluation Review 6: 79). Linstone H A, Turoff M (eds) 1975 The Delphi method: techniques and applications. Addison-Wesley, Reading, Mass., pp 79, 80, 124; Hallan J B, Harris B S H 1970 (Estimation of a potential hemodialysis population. Medical Care 8: 209); Milholland A V, Wheeler M S, Heieck J J 1973 (Medical assessment by a Delphi group technic. New England Journal of Medicine 288: 1272).
9. Interested readers may refer to Linstone & Turoff 1975 (see note 7) who give a number of detailed examples. Simple guidelines are provided by Jones and Hunter 1995 (see note 1) and Delbecq et al 1975 (see note 5).

21 The use of documentary sources

The use of documentary sources is attractive because it is a relatively easy way of obtaining data; documents can provide ready-made information both about the study population as a whole, and about its individual members. Documents may also constitute the best or only means of studying past events. ('There are two ways of telling the age of a rhinoceros. The first is to examine its teeth. The second is to collect the evidence of those who remember the beast when it was young, and may even have kept some newspaper cutting recording its birth.')[1]

The documents may be written, printed, or recorded electronically (computer tapes or disks, audio recordings). They include clinical records, 'vital records' (certificates of birth, death, marriage, etc.), other personal records (such as health diaries specially maintained for the purpose of a study), and registers, databases and archives containing aggregations of data on individuals. Use may also be made of documents that provide ready-made statistics and other information on populations (demography, mortality, morbidity, hospitalization rates, use of ambulatory medical services, etc.), sometimes derived from censuses or other surveys planned to collect this information, and sometimes based on data recorded in an ongoing way for administrative or other specific purposes.

Documents are frequently the only or the most convenient source of information at the investigator's disposal. But it must be remembered that if they were produced for clinical, administrative or fiscal ends rather than for research purposes, questions of their validity for study purposes are very likely to arise. There may be no uniform definitions (of diseases and demographic or other variables), methods of investigation may be unstandardized or used differentially, and the records may not have been maintained with the obsessive care that would be expected in a planned investigation. A study of cases of abortion in a national hospital register, for example, revealed that in over a third of cases the diagnostic code did not reflect the diagnosis in the discharge record.[2] In a hospital discharge data set in Kentucky, which contained 16 apparent cases of serious uncommon communicable diseases, six of these were coding errors and four were cases that had been suspected but not confirmed by subsequent workup.[3] Variables important to the investigator may be lacking, and even if uniform definitions and careful procedures were used, they may not be consistent with the investigator's concepts of the variables; for his purposes the data may hence be of low validity. Secondary data should always be used with circumspection.

The use of these records is of course also subject to practical constraints;[2] confidentially may present a problem, or they may be hard to access for other reasons, or the identifying information may be incomplete or inaccurate, or the records may be kept in a way that makes them inconvenient to use.

CLINICAL RECORDS

Medical records may be very disappointing as a source of data, unless they have been planned and maintained as a basis for research. To quote Mainland:

> Most of the people responsible for hospital and clinic records are not trained investigators, and moreover the pressure of routine work is commonly heavy. From experience gained in the making of clinical records myself, from watching others making them, and in trying to use them, I have come to believe that the only records trustworthy for anything more than superficial impressions, or as hints for further research, are: (a) The records made meticulously by a physician regarding his own patients because he wishes to learn from them; (b) Records kept regarding a particular group of patients by a suitable and adequately instructed person, specially assigned to the task.[4]

There are generally problems of reliability and validity. The information may have been collected by more than one person, using different definitions. Since the data are second-hand, it is possible that even if uniform definitions and procedures were used, these may not be consistent with the investigator's requirements.

Moreover, recording may be patchy; occupations, body weights and blood pressures may be recorded in some instances, not in others. If the presence of a symptom, sign or specific disease is not recorded, this may mean that it was found to be absent, or that no attempt was made to establish its presence, or that its presence was established but not recorded, whether by oversight or because it was regarded as unimportant or irrelevant.[5] In one study, mention of the presence or absence of urinary tract symptoms was found in the medical records of only 18% of a sample of older men, but 30% reported moderate to severe symptoms when questioned.[6] As an extreme example, only 2% of outpatients attending an African hospital were recorded as having avitaminoses or other deficiency states, although field surveys showed that most people in their neighbourhoods of residence had clinical evidence of malnutrition.

Nevertheless, routine records that include reasonably well-recorded information of reasonable quality can be reasonably useful as a basis for investigations. Special care must be taken not to make errors when the information is extracted from the records. These are especially likely to occur if handwritings are difficult to read or if the required information has to be hunted for, e.g. if it is not recorded in a standard place or is buried in long works of prose. A study of reliability, based on replicate extractions by carefully trained personnel from a set of hospital records, showed a good deal of interextractor and intraextractor variation; for example, in 23% of instances there was disagreement between extractors on the presence of a history of hypertension, and in 21% there were discrepancies between two extractions (6 or more months apart) by the same person. In about half these cases the disagreement concerned the presence or absence of the history, and in half the conflict was between 'negative' and 'uncertain'. The main reasons for disagreements were failure to find information recorded in un-expected places, and errors (despite careful training) in the coding of data.[7]

However good the records and however carefully the data are extracted, it is important to remember that the information in rou-tine clinical records is unlikely to be complete. Use is being made of selected facts—those that clinicians determined and recorded—concerning selected people—those who came for care.

The potential research benefits of high quality clinical databases are well recognized. The General Practice Research Database in the United Kingdom, for example, provides a basis for studies of drug safety, disease incidence, resource utilization and disease treatment and prevention.[8] The requirements for a good database are, however, too demanding to be easily met—'such databases must include individual data on all consecutive cases, use standard definitions of conditions and outcomes, ensure data are complete and accurate, and include data on all patient characteristics that affect outcome,'—but there is generally 'a lack of interest on the part of clinicians, managers, and researchers.'[9] The success of the *population-adjusted clinical epidemiology* (PACE) strategy in developing a comprehensive registry for patients with haematological cancers in northern England as a basis for observational studies and trials can be attributed to the co-operation of the haematological consultants in the region. The PACE approach stresses the importance of a defined population base and detailed demographic, treatment and outcome data on the cases; its advocates contrast their database with the usual disease register, which they say resembles 'the capital letter at the start of a sentence and the full stop at the end.'[10]

Routine clinical records from services other than hospitals and some clinics and health centres are generally of little value as a basis for research. This applies especially to general practice records, which usually give only a very rough guide to morbidity patterns and the utilization of services. Not only may the quality of the diagnostic information be unsatisfactory, for lack of suitable diagnostic facilities and other reasons, but the records are seldom full or maintained in a manner that lends itself to analysis. Records of home visits are usually especially incomplete; a study of the clinical records maintained in a medical care plan in New York indicated that half the home visits (as opposed to one sixth of the office visits) were not recorded, and that respiratory diseases were consequently under-represented in the diagnostic data.[11]

This is not to say that routine records from general practices or other primary-care services can never provide useful data. On the contrary, if pains are taken to collect and record information accurately, the records may be of immense value.[12] Not only do people who attend for primary medical care constitute a very much larger and more representative population group than patients treated in hospitals or specialty clinics, but the records of a primary-care service directed at a defined eligible population can sometimes provide data about all members of that population, including those who do not seek care. Moreover, primary-care records can yield data about mild illnesses as well as those that need specialized care, and in many instances can also provide information about incipient and potential illnesses and about factors that may endanger or promote health. They can provide a basis for research on the aetiology, natural history, prevention and care of common diseases and disabilities, processes of growth and development, and the effects of familial factors and social supports and pressures on health and health care. Networks of primary-care practices that engage in collaborative research have been set up in a number of countries.

The use of clinical records for epidemiological purposes is an essential element in community-oriented primary care (see Ch. 34).

There are a number of tools and procedures that can help physicians to conduct epidemiological, operational and other research based on their own work.[13] These include age–sex registers of the practice population, 'minimum data sets' that include a wider range of variables, registers of patients with selected disorders or risk factors, and 'problem-oriented' and other improved records. There is an increasing tendency to computerize primary-care records, but this is usually done to facilitate accounting or information retrieval at an individual level, rather than with an eye to statistical processing and epidemiological analysis.

MEDICAL AUDIT

In recent years much attention has been paid to the development of techniques of evaluating the quality of clinical care by measuring the performance of diagnostic, therapeutic and other procedures. These 'medical audit' and related techniques[14] are usually based upon an examination of clinical records. In order to enhance objectivity, use is generally made of explicit criteria. These may be *normative* standards, which express experts' opinions as to what procedures should be carried out in specific types of cases, or *empirical* standards, based upon studies of what is actually done in clinical facilities that are of an acceptable level. The review may cover all cases cared for, a representative sample, or defined categories, such as patients with selected conditions. Attention may be concentrated on the performance of specific *marker* procedures chosen as indicators of the quality of care, as in a study in inner-city New York, which showed that 74% of children cared for by private physicians were not fully immunized, 80% were not screened for lead, and 83% were not screened for tuberculosis.[15] It is often especially helpful to review the history of patients with poor outcomes, such as those with preventable disorders or complications. This may identify deficiencies not only in the care that was given, but also in compliance and in the availability and use of services.

Audit techniques have their main application in evaluative reviews (as opposed to trials) of clinical services. The audit is based on the assumption that the performance of certain procedures is likely to benefit patients, and care is favourably evaluated if the audit shows that these activities have been satisfactorily performed. The assumptions themselves are not tested. This means, of course, that the evaluation is valid only in so far as the assumptions are valid. Sceptics point out that evidence of the efficacy of the procedures is usually lacking; that is, there is seldom convincing proof of a cause–effect relationship between the recommended procedures and the outcome.[16]

An important advantage of the audit method is said to be the ease with which the evaluation results can be translated into practical recommendations. If the audit shows that X is *not* being done, then the recommendation is made that X *should* be done. It may also be a useful educational tool—a new doctor or nurse in a clinic will rapidly learn that it is expected that X *will* be done. However, the actual effect of audit programmes on the quality of care remains controversial, despite many observational studies and a number of trials; ('we will never really know ... audit will always be an act of faith').[17]

In some audit systems, account is taken of outcomes. The outcomes that are measured include not only end-results, but also intermediate outcomes, such as the establishment of correct diagnoses, or changes in the patient's health behaviour. The assumption is made that satisfactory end-results indicate that care was satisfactory. This is of course not necessarily true, but if patients do well, there is at least no cause for concern.

A basic problem of medical audit is that the records may not provide the required information unless they are planned for this purpose, and unless pains are taken to keep full clinical notes (computer recording does not necessarily solve these problems). Fuller notes may of course not mean better care. A comparison of the charts of patients treated for acute appendicitis, for example, revealed considerable disparity among three hospitals in the frequency of documentation of commonly sought symptoms and signs, yet at each hospital the disease was diagnosed with the same accuracy. Similarly, in cases with acute myocardial infarction the documentation of elements of the history, physical examination and special tests bore no relationship to the outcome of care, such as the length of time lost from work, or the occurrence of new angina pectoris, a repeated infarction, or death. 'Outstanding clinicians may keep inadequate records, whereas others less competent may write profusely ... The mere act of writing cannot improve a patient's outcome.'[18]

Administrative data accumulated as a byproduct of health service administration, reimbursement for services, etc., are at present of little value as a basis for assessing the quality of care. At best, they point to *possible* problem areas that may merit proper investigation.[19]

HOSPITAL STATISTICS

Hospital records have come a long way since Florence Nightingale wrote, 'In attempting to arrive at the truth, I have applied everywhere for information, but in scarcely an instance have I been able to obtain hospital records fit for any purposes of comparison'.[20] In most hospitals today, most diagnoses regarded as important are recorded, and most recorded diagnoses are reasonably well substantiated. Despite their shortcomings, hospital statistics provide a useful source of data on the morbidity pattern of a population. The same applies to diagnostic statistics based on the utilization of some health maintenance organizations and other medical care agencies.

Problems in the use of hospital statistics include the bias caused by selective factors influencing hospitalization, including possible Berksonian bias affecting associations between diseases and between diseases and other factors (see p. 74). Another problem is that diagnostic statistics based on hospital records are usually based on the selection of a single one of the patient's diagnoses. WHO makes the following recommendation:[21]

> The condition to be used for single-condition morbidity analysis is the main condition treated or investigated during the relevant episode of health care. The main condition is defined as the condition, diagnosed at the end of the episode of health care, primarily responsible for the patient's need for treatment or investigation. If there is more than one such condition, the one held most responsible for the greatest use of resources should be selected. If no diagnosis was made, the main symptom, abnormal finding or problem should be selected as the main condition.

It may be a physician—often a junior one—who makes the choice, or a medical recorder, and there may be no certainty that the detailed guidelines provided by WHO are followed, or indeed that any consistent method of selection is used. Diagnostic statistics based on hospital statistics should be treated with reserve, especially in studies of time trends. In the United States there was a substantial increase in reported hospitalizations for acute myocardial infarction between 1981 and 1986, caused by a change in the way diagnoses were selected.[22]

In some countries diagnosis-related groups (DRGs) are used for determining rates of payment for hospital care. The classification is based not only on the patient's main diagnosis, but on other factors as well, such as age, the occurrence of complications and associated disorders, and the form of treatment. Since the inclusion of additional data may increase the hospital's income, more information is likely to be used than merely a diagnosis—there is a higher rate of remuneration for 'complicated peptic ulcer' (such as a bleeding ulcer), for example, than for an uncomplicated ulcer. But there may also be bias, since a choice is often available (depending on clinical judgement) between DRGs with very different rates of reimbursement; one author who warns of possible 'shift in a hospital's reported case mix in order to improve reimbursement' refers to this possibility as 'DRG creep—a new hospital acquired disease'.[23] A study of hospital diagnostic statistics in the United States before and after the introduction of payment by DRGs showed differences consistent with the hypothesis that 'within the range of accepted medical practice, diagnoses will be recorded which maximize hospital revenues'.[24] Nevertheless, say the authors of that study, 'while it is true that epidemiologists must operate in a world of imperfect information, they should not be paralyzed by this lack of knowledge; rather they must become as aware as possible of the nature and extent of these imperfections. As Major Greenwood said: 'The scientific purist, who will wait for medical statistics until they are nosologically perfect, is no wiser than Horace's rustic waiting for the river to flow away'.[25]

DEATH CERTIFICATES AND MORTALITY STATISTICS

Mortality statistics are based on the causes of death reported in death certificates. As shown in this exerpt (see Table 21.1) from

---

Table 21.1 Part of the international form of the medical certificate of cause of death

Cause of death

I

Disease or condition directly leading to death*	(a) ....
	due to (or as a consequence of)
Antecedent causes: Morbid conditions, if any,	(b) ....
giving rise to the above cause, stating the	due to (or as a consequence of)
underlying condition last	(c) ....

II

Other significant conditions	....
contributing to the death, but not related to	
the disease or condition causing it	....

---

*This does not mean the mode of dying, e.g. heart failure, respiratory failure. It means the disease, injury or complication that caused death.

---

the international form, several causes may be entered. One of these is selected as the *underlying cause* of death; this is defined by WHO as '(a) the disease or injury which initiated the train of events leading directly to death, or (b) the circumstances of the accident or violence which produced the fatal injury'. If the certificate has been filled in correctly this is the last condition entered in part I of the certificate. This cause is not automatically selected—if it seems highly improbable that it was in fact the underlying cause of death, a different condition may be chosen, using a series of rules recommended by WHO.[26] The wording chosen for the diagnosis (e.g 'chronic ischaemic heart disease' or 'arteriosclerotic cardiovascular disease', or 'cancer of the uterus' or 'cancer of the cervix') may determine the coding category to which the cause is allotted.[27]

There are a number of obvious sources of inaccuracy. As any physician who fills in death certificates knows, it is not always easy to complete the form accurately. The certifier may not be sure of the true cause or causes of death, either because he has insufficient clinical information, or because the clinical picture is a complicated one—and may yet feel bound to specify a cause of death, so as to avoid forensic complications or for other reasons. It may not be easy to distinguish between direct, antecedent and contributory causes, or to determine a simple sequence of causes, as required by the certificate. The physician may in any case regard the certificate as 'red tape' rather than a scientific document, and not attempt to complete it conscientiously; even when an autopsy is performed, the certificate is often made out before the autopsy, and not modified in the light of the post-mortem findings. Add to this the known unreliability of clinical diagnoses, and the possibility that coders may vary in their selection of an underlying cause (largely because of disagreements as to whether what the physician has written can be taken at its face value),[28] and it is clear that death certificate data and mortality statistics must be treated with some reserve.[29]

In a study in England and Wales, where 9500 certificates completed by hospital physicians before autopsies were compared with certificates subsequently made out by pathologists (based upon both the autopsy and clinical findings), it was found that the underlying causes differed in 55% of cases. In half of these, the difference was one of wording or opinion; in the other half, there was a difference of 'fact'—either the clinician named an underlying cause that the pathologist did not mention in his certificate or notes, or the pathologist named one that the clinician did not mention even as a contributory cause or in the differential diagnosis that he was asked to append to his certificate. The proportion with differences of 'fact' was 16% in cases where the clinician had indicated that he was reasonably certain of his diagnosis (about two thirds of all cases), 33% in cases where the clinician stated that his diagnosis was 'probable' (a quarter of all cases) and 50% where he stated that the diagnosis was 'uncertain' (one tenth of all cases). For some disorders, the discrepancies tended to 'cancel each other out'; in other instances there was a definite bias, with a tendency for the clinician to 'underdiagnose' (e.g. chronic bronchitis, peptic ulcer and malignant neoplasms of the lung) or 'overdiagnose' (e.g. bronchopneumonia and cerebral haemorrhage).[30]

Although death certificate data and statistics based upon them must be treated with reserve, this certainly does not nullify their usefulness, since they undoubtedly contain a sufficient core of hard fact. Their lack of complete accuracy and possible biases must, however, be taken into consideration. One precaution to be taken is that mortality from broad groups of diseases, rather than specific diseases, should be considered. In the autopsy study cited above, for example, it was found that while for specific neoplasms there were differences between the statistics based on clinicians' and pathologists' diagnoses, there was fair agreement on the total number of malignant neoplasms. Similarly, when all categories relating to pneumonia and bronchitis were combined, this eliminated the inconsistencies shown by specific conditions.

It must of course be remembered that whatever the validity of death certificate data as a reflection of *causes* of death, they have less validity as a measure of the *presence* of diseases at death,[31] and still less as a measure of prevalence among the living.

NOTIFICATIONS

In most countries physicians are required by law to notify the public health authority of cases of certain (mainly communicable) diseases; doctors, laboratories and others may also be requested to make voluntary reports of certain other diseases to public health or other agencies.

The main problem besetting the use of disease notifications and statistics based on them is that reporting is often far from complete, even where notification is mandatory. One study showed that only 35% of cases of notifiable diseases treated in hospitals in Washington, D C, were notified; the notification rates ranged from 11% for viral hepatitis to 63% for tuberculosis.[32] Reporting is likely to be fuller when the physician feels that notification will benefit the patient or the community and less complete when he feels that it will bring no benefit, or may embarrass the patient. Furthermore, reporting may be selective; cases of venereal disease treated in public clinics may be far more fully notified than those treated by private practitioners. Such selective factors may introduce biases, in social class or other characteristics, that must be taken into account when inferences are drawn from the data.

These shortcomings apply to all reporting systems, such as those set up for the surveillance of hospital infections, drug reactions, movements into or out of a neighbourhood, etc. The information collected tends to be far from complete, unless a great deal of trouble is taken to ensure full reporting. Despite these shortcomings, the number of notifications can be a useful rough guide to time trends, provided that notification practices have not altered greatly over the period studied.

REGISTERS

Health services and other agencies often maintain registers of people who have specific disorders or who require defined types of care. These registers[33] may list patients with cancer, tuberculosis, or other diseases, people who are blind, housebound, or otherwise handicapped, pregnant women, infants, the elderly, children or families who are at risk of disease, etc. The diagnostic index of a hospital may be used as a disease register. The registers may be simple lists, card indexes, or computerized. In many cases they fulfil important functions in the day-to-day provision of a service, e.g. by identifying patients who require care and by providing a check on the performance of procedures, apart from collecting data that can be analyzed for epidemiological or evaluative purposes.

Registers, and the statistics based upon them, may provide valuable data. An investigator not connected with the responsible agency must remember, however, that the information is second-hand or, very often, third-hand—obtained by the agency from other sources—and he should acquaint himself with the definitions and procedures used, in order to decide on the suitability of the data for his purpose.

Registers should not contain more data than necessary: 'their failure ... in many instances has been due to the collection of too much data ... Some cancer registries have drowned under a weight of data suitable not for a register, but for a data bank'.[34]

Registers of patients with chronic or other selected conditions can be especially valuable in primary-care settings, as a basis for the planning and conduct of organized programmes (see p. 393). The maintenance of such registers is, however, not easy, unless clinical records are computerized, which can avoid the need to record the diagnosis twice, both in the clinical record and in a separate register. A register is likely to be complete only if the physician is convinced that it is helpful in his work or research. A check of computerized chronic disease registers in seven teaching general practices in Oxford showed that the registers included only 49–72% of all patients having care for diabetes, thyroid disease, asthma or epilepsy; in one practice, 97% of patients with diabetes were recorded, but in another, only 18%. Computers had been used in these practices for 4 or more years, but as an adjunct to, rather than as a substitute for, manual records; they were hardly ever used during consultations.[35]

The *capture–recapture* technique can be used to compensate for under-registration, if two or more overlapping registers (or other databases) for the same condition are available. This is a method originally used for estimating the size of an animal population, by marking and releasing a batch of captured animals and then seeing how many are recaptured in the next batch caught, thus permitting estimation of the chance of being caught. Similarly, the total number of cases of a disease in the population can be estimated from the numbers (totals and shared) in separate registers, which provide estimates of the 'chance of being caught' (the completeness of case ascertainment) in each register. In a study of childhood diabetes in Madrid, for example, 451 cases were identified—432 by one procedure and 138 by another, with 119 common to both; the estimated total, computed from these figures, was 501.[36] In Glasgow, where 2006 injecting drug users were ascertained from three sources, the computed 'ascertainment-corrected' total was 13 050, a number that the authors reduced to 9424 to compensate for possible false positive reports.[37] The capture–recapture method can be used to correct for underascertainment in any case-finding survey, if an appropriate independent case register is available. The results may be helpful, but must be used with caution:[38] the case totals may be underestimates, because registers or case-finding procedures are usually not independent, and cases ascertained by one may be especially likely to be identified by another; conversely, they may be overestimates if cases ascertained by one method are likely to be missed by the other. Elaborate methods of computation can largely control these and other biases, but even they may not provide completely valid estimates. If, for example, cases of a certain kind are 'uncatchable'—i.e. systematically missed by *all* procedures—no manipulation can estimate their number; or if all cases have in fact been found, the computed total will be an overestimate.

HEALTH DIARIES AND CALENDARS

In some studies, people are asked to record symptoms, illnesses or other events, physician contacts, self-medication, food consumption, or other data in diaries or calendars. These documents can then be used as direct sources of data, or as memory aids in face-to-face or phone interviews. They generally lead to a considerable increase in the reporting of symptoms and illnesses, especially minor ones.

A drawback of these methods is that not everyone is able or willing to maintain such a record; nonresponse tends to be higher for poorly educated and elderly subjects. Even in uneducated populations, however, appropriate techniques may be devised; in a study in Bangladesh, for example, health calendars were prepared in which diarrhoea, scabies and conjunctivitis were indicated by appropriate drawings, and parents were asked to record episodes by putting the affected child's handprint in the appropriate space.[39]

Also, the value of the record tends to decline if it has to be maintained for more than a short period ('fatigue effect')—reported symptoms or illness rates tend to decline after a month, and sometimes during the first month. In a study in Detroit, subjects who were of a higher social status were more likely to persist with a diary for 6 weeks. There is also evidence of a 'sensitization effect'—maintaining a health diary may make respondents more aware of health problems and may spur them to take greater care of their health; in the Detroit study, the average number of days spent in bed because of illness increased during the 6-week period.[40]

CENSUS DATA

Census data may be invaluable, but their shortcomings should not be ignored.

Population censuses cannot be assumed to be completely accurate. There may be underenumeration, especially of illegal immigrants and their families, members of minority ethnic groups, young adults, infants, and the very old. The 1991 British census, for example, missed an estimated 10% of men in their twenties and 8% of those aged 85 or more.[41] Common inaccuracies in the information reported in censuses include a tendency of divorced men to describe themselves as single (never married), and a tendency for elderly people to overstate their age. 'Investigations into the causes of reported 'superlongevity' invariably show that age misstatement, rather than eating yoghurt, lies behind them.'[42]

Special problems in the use of national census data face an investigator doing a survey in a small locality. Not only may the area be difficult to define in terms of the census tracts or subtracts, zip code areas, or other geographical entities used in the census and its reports, but data for small areas may be difficult to access, or may not include the required variables, or (if the information was collected from a population sample) may be subject to marked random sampling variation. Census figures for a small area are particularly liable to be distorted by a failure to include or exclude people temporarily away from their homes, such as students and migrant workers. The data may also be out-of-date if population size or composition is changing rapidly, as in a fast-developing town or urban neighbourhood. In a longitudinal study, changes between censuses in the boundaries of census tracts may pose a problem.

Census figures should not be used as denominators for specific rates (by ethnic group, income level, etc.) without confirming that the definitions used are equivalent to those used for the numerator data.

OTHER DOCUMENTARY SOURCES

A large variety of other documents may be useful as sources of information on morbidity or other characteristics—medical certificates, sick-absence records, medical insurance records, certificates of birth and fetal death, social welfare records, police records, school records, etc. Parish records have successfully been used in a study of long-term trends in infant mortality.[43]

In each instance, the investigator should acquaint himself with the possible limitations of the information provided. It is important, however, not to expect too much. These documents were designed for someone else's purposes, and it is no more than a happy chance if they meet the investigator's needs (see Finagle's Third Law).[44]

RECORD LINKAGE

With the advent of computers there has been increased interest in the bringing together of records from different sources to obtain a fuller picture than is provided by any single source (creating 'new data from old').[45] Different records relating to the same person may be linked, such as records from various hospitals, or death certificates and hospital or census data. Alternatively, the linkage may be of records relating to different people, such as members of a family; this is a useful method in genetic research. Record linkage presents considerable practical problems, and may be beset by the ethical problem of possible breaches of confidentiality. When practicable, it has extensive applications in epidemiological and other health research.[46]

NOTES AND REFERENCES

1. Morton J B 1966 The best of Beachcomber. Penguin Books, Harmondsworth, p. 102. (' "Fancy that," said the man who handed a rhinoceros to the pigeon fancier.' ibid. p. 219.)
2. Sorenson H T, Sabroe S, Olsen J 1996 A framework for evaluation of

secondary data sources for epidemiological research. International Journal of Epidemiology 25: 435.

3. Finger R, Auslander M B 1997 Results of a search for missed cases of reportable communicable diseases using hospital discharge data. Journal of the Kentucky Medical Association 95: 237.

4. Mainland D 1963 Elementary medical statistics, 2nd edn. W B Saunders, Philadelphia, p. 147.

5. A study at the Yale–New Haven Hospital showed that among postmenopausal women whose medical records provided no information on the presence or absence of certain phenomena, the proportion who reported the phenomenon on interview ranged from 72% for hot flashes, through 39% for benign breast disease, to 1% for the taking of beta-blockers or reserpine (Horwitz R I 1986 Comparison of epidemiologic data from multiple sources. Journal of Chronic Diseases 39: 889).

6. Collins M F, Friedman R H, Ash A, Hall R, Moskowitz M A 1996 Underdetection of clinical benign prostatic hyperplasia in a general medical practice. Journal of General Internal Medicine 11: 513.

7. Horwitz R I, Yu E C 1984 Assessing the reliability of epidemiologic data obtained from medical records. Journal of Chronic Diseases 37: 825.

8. Jick H 1997 A database worth saving. Lancet 350: 1045.

9. Black N 1997 Editorial: Developing high quality clinical databases: the key to a new research paradigm. British Medical Journal 315: 381.

10. Charlton B G, Taylor P R A, Proctor S J 1997 The PACE (population-adjusted clinical epidemiology) strategy: a new approach to multi-centred clinical research. Quarterly Journal of Medicine 90: 147; Engels E A, Spitz M R 1997 PACE-setting research. Lancet 350: 677; Legge A 1997 Is this the end of research as we know it? British Medical Journal 315: 388.

11. Densen P M, Balamuth E, Deardorff N R 1960 Medical care plan as a source of morbidity data: the prevalence of illness and associated volume of service. Milbank Memorial Fund Quarterly 38: 48.

12. Wood M, Mayo F, Marsland D 1986 (Practice-based recording as an epidemiological tool. Annual Reviews of Public Health 7: 357) review the reasons for *using primary-care records in epidemiology*, discuss methods and instruments, problems with diagnoses and their classification and problems with numerators (what is an illness episode?) and denominators, and give examples of collaborative and other research in primary-care settings.

13. Eimerl T S, Laidlay A J 1969 A handbook for research in general practice. Livingstone, Edinburgh.

14. *Medical audit* and similar techniques for evaluating clinical care—'self-audit', 'peer review' (by others), 'internal audit' (by colleagues in the same institution), 'external audit', 'medical care evaluation studies', 'nursing audit', etc.—may be based upon routine records, upon specially modified or designed records, or upon special investigations, including direct observations of practitioners at work.

15. Fairbrother G, Friedman S, DuMont K, Lobach K S 1996 Markers for primary care: missed opportunities to immunize and screen for lead and tuberculosis by private physicians serving large numbers of inner-city Medicaid-eligible children. Pediatrics 87: 785.

16. Brook R H 1973 Quality of care assessment: a comparison of five methods of peer review. DHEW Publication No HRA-74-3100. US Department of Health, Education, and Welfare, Rockville.

17. Lord J, Littlejohns P 1997 Evaluating healthcare policies: the case of clinical audit. British Medical Journal 315: 668. See also Forster D P 1997 Leading article: Uncertainties in medical audit. Public Health 111: 67; Robinson M B 1994 Evaluation of medical audit. Journal of Epidemiology and Community Health 48: 435.

18. Fessel W J, van Brunt E E 1972 Assessing quality of care from the medical record. New England Journal of Medicine 286: 134.
19. Jezzoni L I 1997 Assessing quality using administrative data. Annals of Internal Medicine 127: 666.
20. Nightingale F 1873 Notes on a hospital.
21. World Health Organization 1993 International statistical classification of diseases and related health problems: 10th revision, vol 2: Instruction manual. World Health Organization, Geneva, pp 96–123.
22. Statistics on hospitalizations for acute myocardial infarction in the United States were based on the 'first-listed' diagnosis until 1982, when it was decided that if this diagnosis was not the first one recorded, but occurred with other circulatory diagnoses, it would be moved to first place. As a result, the proportion of acute myocardial diagnoses that were regarded as the principal reason for hospitalization rose from 60% in 1981 to 87% in 1986 (Vital and Health Statistics series 13, no 96).
23. Simborg D W 1981 DRG creep: a new hospital-acquired disease. New England Journal of Medicine 304: 1602.
24. Cohen B B, Pokras S, Meads M S, Krushat W M 1987 How will diagnosis-related groups affect epidemiologic research? American Journal of Public Health 126: 1.
25. Greenwood M 1948 Medical statistics from Graunt to Farr. Cambridge University Press, Cambridge.
26. World Health Organization 1993 (see note 21), pp 30–96.
27. Nelson M, Farebrother M 1978 (The effect of inaccuracies in death certification and coding practices in the European Economic Community [EEC] on international cancer mortality statistics. International Journal of Epidemiology 16: 411) show how differences in certification and coding practices may affect international comparisons of cancers of the cervix and body of the uterus. Sorlie P D, Gold E B 1987 (The effect of physician terminology preference on coronary heart disease mortality; an artifact uncovered by the 9th Revision ICD. American Journal of Public Health 77: 148) show how the change in the 9th revision of the ICD, whereby 'arteriosclerotic cardiovascular disease' was no longer classified as 'ischemic heart disease', might account for part of the apparent decline in coronary heart disease mortality.
28. World Health Organization 1966 Studies on the accuracy and comparability of statistics on causes of death. Unpublished WHO document EURO-215.1/16. WHO, Geneva.
29. Sirken M G, Rosenberg H M, Chevarley F M, Curtin L R 1987 (The quality of cause-of-death statistics. American Journal of Public Health 77: 137) stress the need for periodic assessment of the quality of *cause-of-death statistics* in the USA. Grubb G S, Fortney J A, Saleh S et al 1988 (A comparison of two cause-of-death classification systems for deaths among women of reproductive age in Menoufia, Egypt. International Journal of Epidemiology 17: 385) show how the findings of a detailed local survey can reveal biases in official cause-of-death statistics in a developing country.
30. Heasman L A, Lipworth L 1966 Accuracy of certification of cause of death. A report on a survey conducted in 1959 in hospitals of the National Health Service to obtain information on the extent of agreement between clinical and post-mortem diagnoses. General Register Office, Studies on Medical and Population Subjects no 20 HMSO, London.
    Other studies of the validity of mortality statistics are described by Ashley J S A, Cole S K, Kilbane M P J 1997 (Health information resources in the United Kingdom. In: Detels R, Holland W W, McEwen J, Omenn G S, eds. 1997 Oxford Textbook of public health, 3rd edn, vol 2. The methods of public health. Oxford University Press, New York, pp 451–475).

31. Beadenkopf W G, Abrams M, Daoud A, Marks R U 1963 An assessment of certain medical aspects of death certificate data for epidemiologic study of arteriosclerotic heart disease. Journal of Chronic Diseases 16: 249; Abramson J H, Sacks M I, Cahana B 1971 Death certificate data as an indication of the presence of certain common diseases at death. Journal of Chronic Diseases 24: 417.

32. Marier R 1977 The reporting of communicable diseases. American Journal of Epidemiology 105: 587.
    Other studies of the validity of disease notifications are described by Ashley J S A, Cole S K, Kilbane M P J 1997 (see note 30).
    In France, GPs who were motivated towards disease surveillance displayed more interest in reporting serious or preventible diseases (Chauvin P, Valleron A-J 1995 Attitude of French general practitioners to the public health surveillance of communicable diseases. International Journal of Epidemiology 24: 435).

33. Thompson J R 1989 The role of registers in epidemiology: discussion paper. Journal of the Royal Society of Medicine 82: 151.

34. Brooke E M 1976 Problems of data collection in long-term health care. Medical Care 14(suppl): 165.

35. Coulter A, Brown S, Daniels A 1989 Computer held chronic disease registers in general practice: a validation study. Journal of Epidemiology and Community Health 43: 25.

36. McCarty D J, Tull E S, Moy C S, Twoh C K, LaPorte R E 1993 Ascertainment corrected rates: applications of capture–recapture methods. International Journal of Epidemiology 22: 559.

37. Frischer M, Bloor M, Finlay A et al 1991 A new method of estimating prevalence of injecting drug use in an urban population: results from a Scottish city. International Journal of Epidemiology 20: 997.

38. Other illustrations of the *capture–recapture method*: McCarty D Y, Manzi S, Medsger T A Jr 1995 (Incidence of systemic lupus erythematosus: race and gender differences. Arthritis and Rheumatism 38: 1260); Bobo J K, Thapa P B, Anderson J R, Gale J L 1994 (Acute encephalopathy and seizure rates in children under age two years in Oregon and Washington state. American Journal of Epidemiology 140: 27).
    The use of the capture–recapture method is discussed by: Schouten L J, Straatman H, Kiemeney L A L M, Gimbrere C H F, Verbeek A L M 1994 (The capture–recapture method for estimation of cancer registry completeness: a useful tool? International Journal of Epidemiology 23: 1111); Hook E B, Regal R R 1995 (Capture–recapture methods in epidemiology: methods and limitations. Epidemiological Reviews 17: 243); Hook E B 1996 (Capture–recapture estimates of cancer incidence, adjusting for geographic effects: an alternative perspective. American Journal of Public Health 86: 746); International Working Group for Disease Monitoring and Forecasting 1995 (Capture–recapture and multiple-record systems estimation: II. Applications in human diseases. American Journal of Epidemiology 142: 1059); Brenner H 1996 (Effects of misdiagnoses on disease monitoring with capture–recapture methods. Journal of Clinical Epidemiology 49: 1303); Stephen C 1996 (Capture–recapture methods in epidemiologic studies. Infection Control and Hospital Epidemiology 17: 262); Hook E B, Regal R R 1997 (Validity of methods for model selection, weighting for model uncertainty, and small sample adjustment in capture–recapture estimation. American Journal of Epidemiology 145: 1138); and Nanan D J, White F 1997 (Capture–recapture: reconaissance of a demographic technique in epidemiology. Chronic Diseases in Canada 18: 144).

39. Stanton B, Clemens J, Aziz K M A, Khatun K, Ahmed S, Khatun J 1987 Comparability of results obtained by 2-week home maintained diarrhoeal

calendar with 2-week diarrhoeal recall. International Journal of Epidemiology
16: 595.

40. Verbrugge L M 1984 Health diaries—problems and solutions in study design.
In: Cannell C F, Groves R M (eds) Health survey research methods. DHHS
publication no. PHS 84–3346. National Center for Health Services Research,
Rockville, MD, pp 171–192.
    Uses of health diaries in nursing research are described by Burman M E
1995 (Health diaries in nursing research and practice. Image—The Journal of
Nursing Scholarship 27: 147).

41. Heady P, Smith S, Avery V 1994 (1991 census validation survey: coverage
report. HMSO, London).

42. Grundy E M D 1997 (Populations and population dynamics. In: Detels R,
Holland W W, McEwen J, Omenn G S, eds. 1997 Oxford Textbook of
public health, 3rd edn, vol 1. The scope of public health. Oxford University
Press, New York, pp 75–94), citing Thatcher A R 1992 (Trends in numbers
and mortality at high ages in England and Wales. Population Studies
46: 411).

43. Armenian H K, Zurayk H C, Kazandjian V A 1986 The epidemiology of
infant deaths in the Armenian parish records of Lebanon. International
Journal of Epidemiology 15: 373.

44. Finagle's three laws on information state: '(1) The information you have is
not what you want. (2) The information you want is not what you need. (3)
The information you need is not what you can obtain'. Cited by Murnaghan
J H 1974 (Health indicators and information systems for the year 2000.
New England Journal of Medicine 290: 603).

45. Neutel C I, Johansen H L, Walop W 1991 'New data from old':
epidemiology and record linkage. Progress in Food and Nutrition Science
15: 85.

46. See: Gill L, Goldacre M, Simmons H, Bettley G, Griffith M 1993
(Computerized linking of medical records: methodological guidelines. Journal
of Epidemiology and Community Health 47: 316); Baldwin J A, Acheson
E D, Graham W J 1987 (Textbook of medical record linkage. Oxford
University Press, New York).
    For an example, showing how death certificate data on causes of death
were linked with census data on socio-economic and demographic attributes
to permit an appraisal of differential mortality, see Eisenbach Z, Manor O,
Peritz E, Hite Y 1997 (The Israel longitudinal mortality study: differential
mortality in Israel 1983–1992: objectives, materials, methods and preliminary
results. Israel Journal of Medical Sciences 33: 794).

22 Planning the records

Records cannot be properly planned until the study plan is almost complete. The planning of records requires prior decisions as to what variables will be studied, what scales of measurement will be used, and how the information will be collected and processed.

Apart from the forms used for recording the primary data collected in the study (which will be the main topic of this chapter), a variety of other records may be required to ensure smooth working. These may include lists of people to be examined or interviewed, lists of potential controls from which some are to be chosen by matching or random selection, 'appointment book'-type records showing when examinations or re-examinations are scheduled, and so on. In a study in which various procedures are applied to the same subjects on different occasions or in different places (interview, physical examination, glucose tolerance test, chest X-ray, etc.), it is often helpful to maintain a 'record of procedures' for each individual, showing what has been performed (and if not, why not). In a large study the organization of an efficient filing system may not be simple. Use may be made of computer database programs[1] or card registers (in which the cards of people awaiting different procedures can be kept in separate sections or marked with variously coloured tags).

The most important forms are those used for recording the primary data of the study. These forms, or 'data sheets', may take the shape of questionnaires, examination schedules, forms for laboratory or other test results, extraction forms on to which data are copied from clinical or other records, etc., or they may be multipurpose forms with different sections to meet these various purposes.

The form may be printed on paper or cards, or may be designed for a computer screen. It is usually advisable to use different forms for data (concerning a single individual) collected in different places, from different sources, by different observers or interviewers, or at different times. It may also be necessary to use different forms for different categories of subjects, e.g. when there are substantial differences in the questionnaires put to men and women, or to living patients and the surviving relatives of dead ones. If several forms are used, it may be helpful to use differently coloured paper.

These record forms should, if possible, meet the following four main requirements.

1. Only one individual per form

It is advisable to use a separate form for each individual studied. (As usual, 'individual' here means the individual unit of the study, even if this is a collective unit, such as a family or school.) This usually greatly facilitates the subsequent handling of the data. Lists showing many individuals, with columns for different pieces of information (the 'ledger', 'register', or 'exercise book' method), have limited value; if hand tallying (p. 272) is used, errors are likely if more than two or three variables are recorded in the list. Swaroop tells of a director of public health who analyzed several thousand registers of cholera patients to determine how many had died, then repeated the process to obtain the same information for each sex, and when he found that he was unable to obtain the same total 'threw up his hands and exclaimed, "Now I *really* wish those people had not died" '.[2]

It is generally necessary to identify the individual to whom the form refers. The identifying data are not necessarily used in the analysis. In addition to the person's name, use may be made of his or her sex, age, address, hospital number, personal identity number, etc. In a long-term follow-up study, it is often helpful to add the name and address of a close friend or relative, to help in finding the person after a change of address; an e-mail address may also be helpful. Each record should also have space for a number that distinctively indicates the individual to whom it refers. This identifying number is usually a *serial number* or 'study number' arbitrarily allocated for the specific purpose of the study. The same identifying number should appear on all records pertaining to a single individual. In an investigation where anonymity is guaranteed, this number will be the only identification on the record.

In studies where computers are used, a 'check digit'[3] may be added to the serial number. This is a digit that is derived from the digits in the number, using a predetermined rule, and that is placed after it to make a new serial number that has a logical consistency. An error made in transcribing or computer entry is likely to produce an 'illogical' number, which the computer can detect. A simple method is to choose a digit that will provide zero or a multiple of 10 when alternate digits are added and subtracted. If the original number is 1568, the check digit is 6, since $(+ 1 - 5 + 6 - 8 + 6) = 0$, and the new serial number is 15686. If this is accidentally rendered as 16586, the error can be detected, since $(+ 1 - 6 + 5 - 8 + 6) = -2$.

2. All the required information should be specified

Physical examination schedules are frequently unsatisfactory, in that they do not specify all the variables about which the investigator wishes to obtain information. If we wish to know about swelling of the legs, for instance, there is little point in using a form which merely has a heading 'Lower extremities', with a blank space beneath it. If the space remains blank after the examination, or if some other abnormality is noted, we will not know whether the examiner looked for oedema; even if the researcher has carried out the examinations himself, he cannot be sure that he did not forget to carry out a specific test for oedema. At the least, then, the heading 'oedema of legs' should be printed.

Furthermore (and this applies to questionnaires as well as to examination schedules) all the alternative categories of measurement should appear on the form. If the heading 'oedema' has only a space beneath it, which the examiner leaves empty, we will still be uncertain that this sign was sought. The words 'present' and 'absent' should be printed, for the examiner to mark whichever is applicable; the findings are then clear and unequivocal. This item in the schedule might have the following format:

Oedema:	Right	Left
Absent		
Present		

As an extra precaution, the examiner may be asked to write 'not examined' (and state the reason) if any part of the examination is omitted, or to enter a prearranged number, say 9, in the appropriate box.

The same principle applies to questionnaires, in which (except in the case of open-ended questions) all the possible responses to each question should be printed, including (if necessary) a category of 'other'—or, more usefully, 'other (specify) ...' One exception to this rule is that some investigators prefer not to include a 'don't know' or 'unknown' category, in order to reduce the frequency of such answers, which (if given to an interviewer) can be written in. To avoid the possibility of ambiguous 'blank' responses when a question requests a numerical answer ('On how many days of a week do you eat meat?'), the instruction 'If not at all, write 0' should be stated.

3. The form should be easy to use

The easier the form is to use, the fewer errors there will be.

The items should follow the sequence in which the data are to be collected. This requirement may present especial difficulties in the planning of a schedule for a clinical examination, and flaws in the schedule may not be detected until the form is submitted to a pretest.

As far as possible, the need for writing or entering text should be avoided, both to simplify the task of the observer, interviewer or extractor, and to reduce the need to decipher unintelligible scrawls. Wherever possible, the relevant findings or responses should be marked with a tick or cross or by circling or underlining or by a mouse click.

The form should, as far as possible, be self-explanatory. The main instructions should be clearly stated in the form itself, even if a more detailed manual has been prepared for examiners or interviewers. Although written instructions cannot always replace oral explanations, they serve as a constant guide and reminder. Instructions are particularly important when, as often happens, certain items are applicable only to some individuals. The instructions should be spelled out in detail, e.g. by saying 'If male and 17 years or older, ask:' or 'If "no", proceed to question 17. If "yes", ask next question'. Such instructions are best printed in a different type or shown in parentheses. Arrows may be helpful, as in the examples on the next page. In a 'skip' instruction in a self-administered questionnaire, a page number ('go to page 3') may be better than a question number ('go to question 17').

Other self-explanatory conventions may be used (not in self-administered questionnaires). For example, it is useful to divide a questionnaire into sections by horizontal lines, and instruct the interviewers that whenever the response they receive is one that is marked by double underlining, they should go on to the next section (see the second example below).

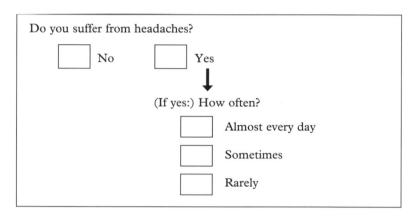

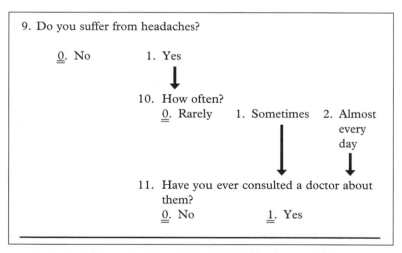

Clear and simple instructions are particularly important in self-administered questionnaires. The method of marking responses should be clearly explained. In a study to be carried out in Trinidad, for example, the introduction (after explaining who is performing the study and why, and inviting the respondent's co-operation) might state:

Most of the questions can be answered by putting an 'X' in the box next to the answer that fits you best. For example:

Do you live in Trinidad?   [X]   Yes   [   ]   No

The layout of the form should make for its easy use. The items should not be crowded, and the places for answers should be clearly shown.

4. The form should be geared to the needs of data processing

If responses to a paper questionnaire are to be coded manually, boxes should be printed for the codes; this will facilitate computer entry.

The use of a precoded form permits coding to be done at the time the data are collected. The code digits are printed on the form, and are either marked by circling or by checking an appropriately numbered box, or are written in a box provided for the purpose. Graphic rating scales (see p. 223) may also be used. A different approach is employed in each of the pot-pourri of items on the next page. (In practice, the use of such a medley of methods in a single form might be confusing.) The figures on the right are the numbers of the columns in which the data will be stored in the computer record,[4] and are not needed if a data-entry program is to be used.

An alternative approach, preferred by some investigators, is to provide an interviewer with only a single questionnaire, on which the coded alternatives to each question are stated, and to have a separate 'answer sheet' filled in for each respondent. This sheet need contain only the subject's name, etc., and the numbers of the questions, with either a box or a row of the alternative code numbers (for circling) next to each question number. This makes the form more compact, but there may be more errors when it is filled in.

A method that is likely to increase in popularity is the use of machine-readable forms, marks on which are read by an optical scanner and transferred to a computer record.

Precoding is best avoided in self-administered questionnaires, since it may confuse the respondent. It may, however, be used if

23. Acne vulgaris. (Check the appropriate box.)

0 ☐ Absent

1 ☐ Grade I

2 ☐ Grade II   41

3 ☐ Grade III

4 ☐ Grade IV

24. Pulse rate. (If under 100, put a zero in front of the number. If pulse rate is 72, write 072.)

☐ ☐ ☐   42–44

25. Systolic pulmonic murmur. (Circle the appropriate number.)
    1. Absent
    2. Present   45

26. Character of murmur. (Write the appropriate number in the box.)
    1. Blowing
    2. Musical   ☐   46
    3. Harsh

27. Diastolic murmurs. (Circle the appropriate numbers.)

	Absent	Present Grade of intensity						
Apical	0	1	2	3	4	5	6	47
Mid-precordial	0	1	2	3	4	5	6	48
Pulmonic	0	1	2	3	4	5	6	49
Aortic	0	1	2	3	4	5	6	50

28. Varicose veins. (Check the appropriate two boxes.)

	0. Absent	1. Present	
Right			51
Left			52

the code numbers are kept small and inconspicuous, as in the following example.

---

57. Is it time this chapter came to an end?

X	Definitely		Maybe		No
1		2		3	

NOTES AND REFERENCES

1. There are many easy-to-use PC programs that can be used for filing, updating, sorting, finding and printing individual records and for displaying or printing reports (lists and simple counts).
2. Swaroop S 1966 Statistical methods in malaria eradication. WHO, Geneva, p. 20.
3. Acheson E D 1968 Record linkage in medicine. Livingstone, Edinburgh, pp 181–183.
4. See note 2, page 291 .

23 Preparing for the analysis

During the planning phase of a study, decisions must be made about the coding, checking and processing of data. These decisions are interrelated.

DECISIONS ABOUT CODING

To facilitate computer processing and analysis, codes must be assigned to the categories of variables that have nominal, ordinal or dichotomous scales. Numbers (0, 1, 2, etc.) are generally used for this purpose. Coding is not needed for simple numerical data or for verbal data that will not be analyzed (e.g. subjects' names).

The codes should be decided in advance where possible, particularly if precoded records (see p. 264) are wanted. For questionnaires or other record forms to be displayed on a computer monitor, decisions on coding are an integral part of the programming process.

Coding requires the preparation of a *coding key* (or *dictionary file* for computer use) that shows the codes used for each variable, and their meanings. If coding is complicated, detailed *coding instructions* may be needed. These should be clear and unambiguous, in order to ensure coding reliability. Voluminous instructions may be needed if the responses to open-ended questions or statements made in relatively unstructured interviews have to be coded, particularly with respect to attitudes, motivation, etc. ('content analysis').

Standardized codes should be used wherever possible, so as to simplify both the coding process and the analysis. If there are 'yes–no' questions, for example, 1 might be allocated to all 'yes' answers and 0 to all 'no' answers. It is particularly important to use standard codes for 'unknown' and 'not applicable'—for example, 'unknown' might be entered as 9, 99, or 999 (choosing a number that is outside the range of possible data) and 'not applicable' as 8, 88, etc. This is advisable for numerical as well as categorical data, to reduce errors during data entry or analysis. Distinctive codes are sometimes used for 'unknown' values of different kinds, especially those resulting from refusal or failure to answer a question, explicit 'don't know' responses, and errors in the recording or handling of data.

A specimen portion of an imaginary coding key, incorporating coding instructions, is shown in Table 23.1. When coding is complicated, as for relative weight in this example, errors can be avoided by having it done by a computer; the coding key might then include the relevant computer instructions (algorithm).

Table 23.1 Code

Variable	Code	Coding instructions
Sex	1. Male 2. Female 9. Unknown	Precoded (question 1). If not shown, look at subject's name, and see whether questions 3–5 (for females only) have been asked. If sex is still uncertain, code 9
Marital status	1. Single 2. Married 3. Widowed 4. Divorced 9. Unknown	Precoded (question 2). If not shown, code 9
Social class	1. SC I 2. SC II 3. SC III 4. SC IV 5. SC V 8. Unclassifiable 9. No data on occupation	Code occupation stated in answer to question 6, using attached instructions. If occupation not stated, code 9
Height	999. Unknown	Centimetres (ignore fractions or decimals). If not measured, code 999
Relative weight	888. Unclassified 999. Unknown	Consult appended weight-for-height tables to find standard weight for a person of the subject's sex and height. Divide subject's weight by this standard weight, multiply by 100, round off downwards, and enter. Code 999 if sex, height or weight is unknown. Code 888 if height falls outside range shown in tables

A more ambitious codebook may be prepared, including additional information such as operational definitions (see Table 10.1, p. 120) and other relevant explanations (to what subgroups of study subjects the variable is applicable, how the data have been edited or manipulated, ranges of values regarded as acceptable, the variables' positions in the electronic record, etc.).

New *derived variables* are often created by manipulating the original data; this may be done during data entry (with appropriate software and programming) or afterwards. If their creation is planned in advance, they can be included in the coding key or codebook from the outset; otherwise, they should be added later. Their method of production should be explained, with (if necessary) details of the computer process by which they were produced. A *recoded variable*, for example, is created by altering the coding of a variable—age in years might be recoded by five-year age groups, or data on the number of cigarettes smoked might be used to categorize subjects as nonsmokers or light, moderate or heavy smokers. The new variable may also be based on *numeric transformation* of the original value, e.g. using its square or logarithm, or adding or subtracting a constant. A *constructed variable* is derived from two or more other variables. like the relative weight shown in Table 23.1; diagnostic criteria may be brought together so as to categorize subjects in terms of the presence or absence of a disease.

Coding is less important if the data are to be processed by hand. But even then, it may be convenient to make use of symbols or standard abbreviations such as + (present), – (absent), ? (unknown), M (male) and F (female).

Coding errors are not infrequent. In one study in which coding was done by the interviewers, half the mistakes made by interviewers (detected by comparing replicate interviews) were coding errors.[1] Coding by the examiner or interviewer at the time data are collected is obviously a cheap and fast method, and if the coding is simple it does not impose a burden. But coding errors can be detected and rectified only if the record forms make provision for the full data as well as the codes.

DECISIONS ABOUT CHECKING OF DATA

Data should be checked both when they are collected and at later stages. The procedures to be used during the data collection process obviously require to be planned before the collection of data starts; decisions concerning checks to be performed after data collection (see Ch. 26) are less urgent.

Early planning is especially important if the transfer of data to an electronic medium is to be an intrinsic part of the data collection process, as in computer-assisted interviewing. With appropriate software and programming, checks can be done on the fly—the computer can display a warning or refuse to accept the entry if an impermissible entry is made. For a coded categorical variable, a *wild code* not included in the coding key would be illegal. For an interval-scale or ratio-scale entry, a range of acceptable values can be defined in advance so that *out-of-range values* can be identified.

With suitable programming the computer can also perform *consistency checks* (*logical checks*), comparing entries for different variables and provide warnings when obvious errors are found, e.g. a man who immigrated before his date of birth or a woman who has given up smoking but smokes a pack a day.

DECISIONS ABOUT DATA PROCESSING

Data processing may be done by a personal computer or a mainframe computer (usually accessed through a personal computer), or (if the study is a small one) the data may be processed manually.[2] Use of a personal computer facilitates interaction, permitting decisions to be made in an ongoing way during the course of a statistical analysis session; also, personal computer software is generally more 'user-friendly' (providing on-screen explanations, warnings and instructions) than mainframe computer programs.

A few words of caution about computer use are not out of place. First, there is still a belief (especially among people with little experience of computers) that 'the computer is never wrong'. The computer is no mental giant, but a moron that slavishly follows instructions. It cannot be accurate if the humans who operate it make errors, and to err is human. Data may be inaccurate or entered inaccurately ('garbage in, garbage out'), errors may be made in giving instructions, or the programs may have unknown bugs. 'Because of the faith that is placed in computers, the possibility of undetected human error may be greater when computers are used.'[3] Secondly, analysis by computer is so easy that there may be a temptation to examine trivial hypotheses, or hypotheses based on 'data snooping' (i.e. constructed only after examining the findings)—which may lead to unwarranted conclusions (see p. 295).

Thirdly, complex statistical procedures have become so readily available that they are often used even if they are inappropriate for the data or for answering the questions that the study asks. One statistician laments that 'in the past we have had misgivings about "cook book" statistics, and now what has evolved would have to be termed the "TV dinner" ... Previously, we could believe that the user would at least have to read the recipe!'[4] Others observe that 'it is not hard to do a bad analysis ... All that is needed is a canned computer program ... and a lack of competence in biostatistics. These resources are widely available'.[5] 'Output from commercial computer programs, with their beautifully formatted tables, graphs, and matrices, can make garbage look like roses.'[6]

If computer processing is envisaged, decisions are required about the electronic data set required for this purpose. This data set and its preparation will be discussed in Chapter 26.

However processing is to be done, during the planning stage the investigator should decide, at least in broad outline, how the data will be analyzed in order to meet the specific objectives of the study. It is often helpful to draw up a number of specimen skeleton tables, with column and row headings but containing no figures, and to consider how different kinds of result will be interpreted. This process of 'thinking forward' to the analysis often reveals gaps in the data (variables omitted, no information on the denominator population, etc.), defects in scales of measurement, or the superfluity of certain data. It provides a further opportunity for second thoughts as to whether the study, as planned, is likely to meet its objectives.

Consideration should be given not only to the format of the tables, but to the statistical techniques to be used in the analysis (see p. 288), the general lines of which should always be decided in advance. Sometimes a detailed plan can be prepared (this may be demanded if an application is made for research funds), but options should be left open—the findings, as they emerge, may call for new or different analyses.

A statistician's help is often needed, although it is a consoling thought that the analysis of a well planned study sometimes requires only the simplest of statistical techniques. It is foolhardy to decide to use complex procedures without adequate statistical knowledge or expert guidance. If a statistician is to be consulted, this should be done during the planning phase, when the design of the investigation can still be influenced, and not after the data have been collected, when they may be found unsuitable for analysis.

When consulting a statistician it must be remembered that a silly question gets a silly answer. Unless the investigator can explain very precisely and specifically what is hoped to learn from the study, the advice received, however erudite and well meaning, may be inadequate and even misleading.

The remainder of this chapter deals with *manual data-processing methods* (hand tallying and hand sorting). These methods are appropriate for small-scale studies only and may be tedious, but are favoured by some investigators on the grounds that they keep them 'close to their data'. 'The figures that we are analyzing represent the patients, animals, things or processes that we are studying, and the more familiar we become with them, the more likely we are to know about their interrelationships, oddities and defects; and the more likely we are to catch hints of explanations and clues for further research.'[7]

Hand tallying is the most primitive method. A tally sheet is prepared in the form of a skeleton table, and a tally mark is made in the requisite cell for each individual. The usual method is to make a vertical mark for each individual. Every fifth individual in a cell is indicated by a diagonal line drawn through the preceding four: Ⅲ́

This facilitates subsequent counting. An alternative method[8] is to make dots (arranged in a square) for the first four, then to draw a line (joining two dots) for each of the next four, so that a square means 8 individuals. A diagonal is then drawn for each of the next two, so that a complete set of 10 looks like a little flag: ⊠

When a tabulation is done directly from lists (containing information on different individuals on the same page) or from unwieldy records (e.g. voluminous clinical files), hand tallying may be a convenient method. Its disadvantages are that it is laborious and time-consuming, and errors are prone to creep in, especially if a complicated cross-tabulation is being used. If an error is detected (e.g. if it is found that the total number shown in the table is one less than the actual number of individuals), this requires the repetition of the entire process, unless differently coloured inks have been used for different batches of records to help in the localization of errors.

Hand sorting is usually preferable to hand tallying. This requires a separate and easily handled record for each individual. The records are sorted and physically separated into piles conforming with the cells in the skeleton table, and the numbers in each pile are then counted, recounted, and entered. If an error is detected, it is usually necessary to repeat only part of the procedure. To prepare a cross-classification, the records are usually sorted 'hierarchically'; i.e. they are sorted into piles according to one variable, then each pile is sorted according to a second variable, and so on until the cross-classification is complete; each pile is then counted. Sorting is relatively easy if small cards are used, information on each variable is written in a standard position, and heavy lines or different colours are used to facilitate the visual identification of data.

NOTES AND REFERENCES

1. Horwitz R I, Yu E C 1985 Assessing the reliability of epidemiologic data obtained from medical records. International Journal of Epidemiology 14: 463.
2. *Peripheral punch cards* and *mechanical sorting* (which have become obsolete) and their coding requirements, are described in previous editions of this book.
3. Blum M L, Foos P W 1986 Data gathering: experimental methods plus. Harper & Row, New York, p. 80.
4. Schucany W R 1978 Comment. Journal of the American Statistical Association 73: 92.
5. Bross I D J 1981 Scientific strategies to save your life: a statistical approach to primary prevention. Marcel Dekker, New York, pp 42–43.
6. Tabachnick G B, Fidell L S 1989 try throughout their book (Using multivariate statistics, 2nd edn. Harper & Row, New York) 'to suggest clues for when the true message in the output more closely resembles the fertilizer than the flowers'.
7. Mainland D 1964 Elementary medical statistics. Saunders, Philadelphia, p. 168.
8. Tukey J W 1977 Exploratory data analysis. Addison-Wesley, Reading, Mass. pp 16–17.

24 Pretests and other practical preparations

Before the collection of data can be started, it is usually necessary to test the methods and to make various practical preparations. If the planning phase was the gestation period, this is the stage of parturition. It may not be free of pain, and if there are practical problems that cannot be overcome the study may yet be stillborn.

PRETESTS

Pretests, or prior tests of methods, vary in their scope. A pretest may consist of a single visit to a clinic to see whether patients' weights or other items of information are routinely recorded on their cards, or may take the form of a large and well planned methodological study or a full-scale 'pilot study', a dress rehearsal of the main investigation. Pretests may be required in order to examine the practicability, reliability or validity of methods of study, and their planning varies according to their purposes. A pretest may be a well constructed study aimed at yielding definitive results, or it may be designed to provide only a 'feel' of the suitability of a method. Pretests of examination schedules and questionnaires are usually of the latter type. If a data-entry program is to be used, it is wise to pretest it on a number of cases; this may reveal unexpected difficulties.

In a typical small-scale pretest of a questionnaire, 10–30 subjects are interviewed.[1] These may be chosen haphazardly, but should not be potential members of the study sample, since participation in the pretest interview may reduce willingness to be interviewed in the study proper, or may affect the responses given in the study proper. Subjects are usually chosen who are similar in their characteristics to the members of the study population. Sometimes, in order to highlight possible flaws in the questionnaire, 'difficult customers'—such as persons with an especially low or high educational level—are purposely chosen. The interviewer may be asked to record not only the responses for which the questionnaire makes provision but also maybe the respondent's reactions (boredom, irritation, impatience, antagonism—or even interest!), to make verbatim notes of the respondent's comments, to record the time taken by the interview, and to make criticisms and suggestions concerning the questions, their sequence, and skip patterns ('If no, go to …'). The interviewer (or another interviewer, in a special call-back visit) may be requested to discuss the questions with the respondent after they have been answered, asking whether they seemed clear, what the answers meant, why a 'Don't know' response was made, etc. This may be done informally, or a formal procedure may be used: after explaining that this is a test of some of the questions, the interviewer reads out each question with its response, and requests an explanation of exactly how the answer was arrived at; this is followed by preplanned questions designed to find out how particular terms were understood by the respondent.[2]

The best strategy is often to begin with a small-scale pretest that includes detailed questioning of the respondents about their reactions (a *participating pretest*[1]). This may require hand-picked respondents: 'investigators may find themselves relying on that familiar source of forced labor—colleagues, friends and family'.[1]

On the basis of all this information, it is often possible to identify 'difficult' questions—those that are offensive, hard to understand, or do not seem to elicit the information they are intended to get—and awkward sequences of items. If a question elicits many 'Don't know' answers, it is probably unsatisfactory; if it produces many qualifying comments, the response categories are probably not suitable. Inconsistencies between the answers to related questions, or uniform answers by all respondents ('all-or-none' responses) may also point to flaws. If questions were omitted or asked when they should not have been, the questionnaire's arrangement or provision of instructions is probably defective.

The pretest usually points to a need for changes in the questionnaire and the interviewing instructions. These changes are made, and a new version is available for pretesting.

Participation in pretesting can be a valuable component of the training of interviewers, and can also help to give interviewers a feeling of identification with the study.

The Internet can be used for easy and rapid pretests of questionnaires,[3] especially to see which questions often remain unanswered, presumably because they are not good ones. But the results may be of limited applicability—the sample (motivated Internet users) may not resemble the study population in which the questionnaire is to be used, and the problems that are revealed may differ from those that are likely to arise when the questionnaire is used in a different way.

ENLISTING CO-OPERATION

It is particularly important to enlist the good will of people who will be involved in the study (subjects who will be examined or interviewed, administrators and others who can provide access to records or various facilities and services, etc.), those who *think* they are involved in the study (such as physicians who feel that they own their patients), and those (such as some colleagues) who feel they *should* have been involved in the study. In a community study, co-operation can be enhanced by suitable public relations and preparatory educational work in the community. The best results are provided by contacts with key individuals and organizations in the community, but use may also be made of mass media, such as local television channels, radio talks, newspaper articles, pamphlets and posters. In such contacts, people should be told what they can expect to 'get out of' the study, but no false promises should be made; in medical surveys 'the two most generally effective motivations are the desire to contribute to the community effort to benefit health through science, and the subject's own interest in a free medical examination'.[4] Many investigators dislike the idea of offering financial incentives (cash, vouchers, lottery tickets or gifts), but a review of randomized trials of their use showed improved compliance in 10 of 11 studies.[5]

It may be decided to send out letters telling prospective respondents about the study and the impending visit or phone call by an interviewer (it is usually unwise to make the initial contact by telephone—this invites refusals). It may also be decided to prepare 'reminder' and 'thank you' letters. In studies in which access to confidential medical records is necessary, people may be required to give their approval in writing, and consent forms should be printed for this purpose.

OTHER PRACTICAL PREPARATIONS

A budget may have to be prepared, funds found, and arrangements made for administering them. Some few lucky people are experts in grantsmanship. Others should seek help from such an expert or from the numerous Internet sources that provide lists of funding opportunities and hints on the writing of grant applications.[6]

There may be many other practical preparations to be made before data can be collected. Approval may have to be obtained from an ethical committee. Accommodation, equipment and its maintenance, supplies, transportation, and access to laboratory, data processing, or other facilities may have to be arranged. Personnel may have to be found or trained. Record forms must be printed. Maps may have to be found or prepared, or a census of the study population may have to be performed. Sampling frames may have to be prepared, cases of a disease identified, and samples or controls selected. In a blind or double-blind experiment, complicated practical preparations may be needed to ensure secrecy (dummy medicinal preparations, containers identified by symbols, etc.). In a study involving a sequence of procedures performed by different examiners, logistic problems may require solution. An inspired researcher is not necessarily a good administrator (and vice versa, as the activities of many public health departments, hospitals and other medical services eloquently testify), and in a large investigation it is often wise to appoint a study co-ordinator or field-work director with a bent for practical matters.

If observational methods of data collection are to be used (by persons other than the investigator who has planned them), they should be carefully explained and demonstrated, and 'running in' exercises should be arranged. An 'examiner's manual' may be required, both for training purposes and for subsequent consultation. If necessary, reference standards should be made available, such as standard photographs of skin abnormalities or (for laboratory tests) solutions of known chemical composition.

If interviewers have to be found, they should be carefully selected, the main requirements being that they should be capable, personable, honest, interested, able to establish rapport, and good listeners. Interviewers who are new to the job should be given a general training[7] in interview methods (see p. 214), and all interviewers should receive an explanation of the objectives and methods of the study, should be told or shown, unhurriedly and in detail, what they are expected to do, and should conduct 'trial interviews' before starting work on the study proper.[8] An interviewer's manual should be prepared if it is thought this will be helpful.

If documentary sources are to be used, steps should be taken to ensure that there is access to them—confidentiality and poor systems of record storage and retrieval often pose problems—and that they contain the desired types of information. The persons who are to extract the data should receive detailed instructions.

Whatever methods are to be used, arrangements should now be made for 'quality control' during the stage of data collection. (This will be discussed in Ch. 25.)

If the data are to be coded, practical preparations for coding should be made, although these may sometimes be delayed until a later stage. Coding keys and coding instructions should be prepared, coders trained, and arrangements made for the testing and control of coding reliability.

Finally, a word of advice from Cochran[9]—when the study plan is near completion, find a 'devil's advocate'—a colleague who is willing to examine the plan and find its methodological weaknesses (not recommended for sensitive souls).

NOTES AND REFERENCES

1. Converse J M, Presser S 1986 (Survey questions: handcrafting the standardized questionnaire, 2nd edn. Sage Publications, Beverly Hills, CaL) who provide detailed advice on pretests of questionnaires, write: 'The Magic N for a pretest is of course as many as you can get. We see 25–75 as a valuable pretest range'.
2. Belson W A 1981 The design and understanding of survey questions. Gower, Aldershot, Hants.
3. Suchard M A, Adamson S, Kennedy S 1997 Netpoints: Piloting patient attitudinal surveys on the web. British Medical Journal 315: 529.
   A message sent to an Internet discussion group for epidemiologists (see note 3, p. 122) read 'I am composing a short questionnaire for a project about SCUBA divers ... I need to validate the questionnaire. I am looking for anyone who is a recreational SCUBA diver that will be willing to fill out the questionnaire twice (Test-Retest approach)...'. This pretest would presumably lead to the development of a superb questionnaire for a study of cooperative scuba divers who use the Internet and are happy to be epidemiologists.
   See note 19. p. 77 (use of the Internet for surveys).
4. Rose G A, Blackburn H 1968 Cardiovascular survey methods, WHO, Geneva, p. 58.
5. Giuffrida A, Torgerson D J 1997 Should we pay the patient? Review of

financial incentives to enhance patient compliance. British Medical Journal 315: 7110.

If a prize is to be raffled among participants, it should probably be big; in a controlled trial in England, small prizes had no effect on response rates (Mortagy A K, Howell J B L, Waters W E 1985 A useless raffle. Journal of Epidemiology and Community Health 39: 183). Financial incentives may deter well-off people from participating (Campanelli P 1995 Minimising non-response before it happens: what can be done. Survey Methods Bulletin 37: 35).

6. For a list of Internet resources that may be helpful in the quest for funds (tips on 'grant-writing', information on sources of funds, and application forms for downloading), visit biomednet.com/hmsbeagle/1998/28/webres/insitu.htm

   Simple tips on writing an application—the first of which, and possibly the most useful, is 'Ask a successfully funded researcher to critique your grant proposal before you submit it'—are provided by Hopkin K 1998 (How to wow a study section: a grantsmanship lesson. The Scientist 12[5]: 11; on the Internet: www.the-scientist.library.upenn.edu/yr1998/mar/prof_980302.html).

   Databases with information on sources of funds include www.grantsnet.org/, fundingopps.cos.com/, and (for the UK) wisdom.wellcome.ac.uk/wisdom/fundhome.html.

7. For fuller advice on the training of interviewers, see Bowling A 1997 (Research methods in health: investigating health and health services. Open University Press, Buckingham, Ch 13).

8. Preparations for a household survey in a disadvantaged community in South Africa, including the selection and training of community members as interviewers, are described by Hildebrandt E 1996 (Survey data collection: operationalizing the research design. Public Health Nursing 13: 135). She points out that 'surveys are conceived and designed in offices at desks by people who are concerned about validity, reliability, randomization, sample size and research rigor. These same surveys are carried out by people who have agreed to walk miles of city streets or dusty roads, knock on door after door, develop trusting relationships with absolute strangers, and subsequently probe these strangers' lives. It is a vulnerability of survey research that it is difficult to control the data-collection process in this "living test tube"'.

9. Cochran W G 1983 Planning and analysis of observational studies. Moses L E, Mosteller F (eds) Wiley, New York, p. 71.

25 Collecting the data

After the intellectual stimulation of the planning phase, the investigator now comes to a rather dull period when data are collected in a routine and predetermined manner. The greater the forethought and effort that were put into the planning and preparation, the more uneventful this new phase is likely to be.

However, the best-laid plans of good and bad researchers gang aft agley.[1] All kinds of unexpected contingencies may arise, and the investigator must be prepared to make running repairs as they become necessary.

Apart from this kind of troubleshooting, the investigator should take positive steps to test whether the collection of the data is in fact proceeding as it should. This may be done by instituting 'spot checks' (in Carl Becker's words, 'we need, from time to time, to take a look at the things that go without saying to see if they are still going') or, preferably, by regular periodic or ongoing surveillance.

This surveillance has two main aspects. *Quality control* measures should be instituted,[2] and ongoing records should be maintained of the performance of procedures—how many people have been examined? how many have refused to be interviewed? etc.

In a study where the investigator himself collects the data, all that may be required for quality control is that he should check each record form as he completes it, to make sure that it has been filled in properly. Coding may be done at the same time. In a study where the data are collected by others, each record form should, if possible, be similarly checked as it is handed in. Sometimes omissions and errors can be corrected on the spot by editing; at other times, it may be necessary to refer to the person who completed the form, or even, if the omission or error is an important one, to repeat part of the examination or interview. If it is not possible to check each form as it is handed in, a sample of forms should be scrutinized. Regular meetings with examiners or interviewers are advisable, to share problems and maintain interest, as well as reviewing completed forms. Quality control is an inbuilt feature of computer-assisted questionnaire programs (see p. 208).

Checks on reliability (see p. 176) form an important part of quality control. It is not often possible to conduct repeated examinations or interviews of the same persons, but sometimes the reliability of examinations is tested by having the same subjects examined simultaneously by two examiners. Sometimes, limited analyses of the findings are performed, to permit comparisons of the data obtained (for different individuals) by different examiners or interviewers, or at different times by the same examiners or interviewers. If, for example, one examiner finds a far higher rate of varicose veins than others, it is worth exploring the possibility that this is due not to a difference in the subjects, but to his method of diagnosing varicose veins. Similarly, if the hypertension rate springs up in a specific month, this may be due to a defect in the instrument used. All measuring equipment should be checked periodically. If laboratory procedures are used, reliability should be checked by periodic comparisons with standards and by the examination of replicate specimens ('blinded duplicates' with different labels). In addition, systematic differences between laboratories, or in the same laboratory at different times, may sometimes be detected by comparing the results of determinations (of different batches), in terms of their average values or the proportions of determinations falling above or below predetermined cutting points.

If these tests lead to substantive mid-study changes in methods or operational definitions it is important to ensure that the subjects affected by the changes can subsequently be identified, or to use the new method in parallel with the old, so that the effect of the change can be appraised.

Throughout this stage, detailed records should be kept of people who are omitted from the study—subjects who are replaced, nonrespondents, persons who drop out or are excluded because of side-effects, etc.—so as to permit possible selection bias to be taken into account in the analysis (see p. 298). A record should be kept of their demographic characteristics and any other relevant information that can be easily obtained. Sometimes it is feasible to concentrate resources upon an attempt to obtain full information about a sample of nonrespondents.

Identifying the subjects, finding them and persuading them to co-operate may require hard work, patience and ingenuity. In a case-control study, the identification of cases may involve tedious searches through clinical records, disease registers, diagnostic indexes of hospitals, or other sources. The selection of controls too may be far from easy, especially if they are matched. If the subjects were identified from old or incorrect records, it may be difficult to locate them. Names change—especially those of nubile females—and are often wrongly spelt. Recorded addresses may be incomplete, incorrect, or out-of-date. People who have moved may be difficult to trace, especially those who were living alone or as lodgers and the divorced and widowed.[3] With luck, the present residents at the previous address may know where the subjects went, or a letter may be forwarded by the post office. In other cases, intensive detective work may be needed, including contacts with ex-neighbours, known relatives and friends, local shopkeepers, the postman, the local doctor or public health nurse and so on.

Even in a simple household survey, it may not be easy to make contact, especially if the family is childless or all its members go out to work. The only solution, of course, is to try, try, try again, sometimes in the morning, sometimes in the late afternoon or evening, sometimes at weekends. Once contact has been made, obtaining co-operation usually presents little difficulty in an interview survey. More nonresponse is to be expected if medical examinations or blood samples are needed. The examination process should be made as painless as possible—flexible schedules, no waiting around, and above all a pleasant atmosphere—but broken appointments and frank refusals can be expected, however convenient the arrangements. Here too, perseverance is needed. Response rates can be boosted by establishing rapport, by repeated contacts and patient persuasion, by a judicious unreadiness to take 'no' for an answer (at least the first or second time it is said)—and, often, by a readiness to call for the help of a more irresistible member of the study team.

The longer these efforts go on, the more subjects will be traced and the more nonrespondents will turn into respondents. But a line has to be drawn, and it is important to know where to draw it. A time comes when the added benefits fall far short of keeping pace with the added investment of effort, and the investigator should not hesitate to cry halt. This law of diminishing returns has been rephrased as the Ninety-Ninety Rule—'The first 90 per cent of the task takes 90 per cent of the time, and the last 10 per cent takes the other 90 per cent'.[4]

NOTES AND REFERENCES

1. Some readers have complained that this phrase is Greek to them. It is not, it is Scottish—'gang aft agley' means 'often go wrong'.
   The following Will Rogers quotation may be substituted: 'There ain't but one place that a plan is any good and that's on paper. But the minute you get it off the sheet of paper and get it out in the air, it blows away, that's all' (Sterling B R, Sterling F N 1996 Will Rogers speaks. Evans, New York, p. 221).
   In an account of the day-to-day working of a cohort study in a family practice, a nurse and two doctors describe little things that can go wrong. When patients are asked to sign a consent form before blood-taking 'a few are illiterate, others arrive without their reading glasses ...'. The date of starting prophylactic aspirin therapy 'might be dated from a hospital summary provided the patient had not neglected to bring it ... [or] from an entry by the regular physician ... or by the nurse ... Sometimes all three sources are available but do not agree ... the information may be tucked away in a thick file containing tens of pages ... the energy with which the abstracter pursues the search is also a factor in determining what figure will ultimately be entered ... banal mistakes such as neglecting to rotate a test tube containing anticoagulants or a misplaced sticker ... A worm's-eye view has afforded us some sobering insights into what can go wrong with a project after issues of method have been decided' (Naveh P, Yaphe J, Herman J 1996 Research in primary care: a worm's-eye view. Journal of Clinical Epidemiology 49: 1323).
2. For a detailed account of the quality control measures used in a large-scale health examination survey, see National Center for Health Statistics 1972 (Quality control in a national health examination survey. Vital and Health Statistics, series 2, no 44. Public Health Service, Washington, D C).
3. For descriptions of methods used to trace hard-to-find subjects, see Skeels H M, Skodak M 1965 (Techniques of a high-yield follow-up study in the field. Public Health Reports 80: 249); Modan B 1966 (Some methodological aspects of a retrospective follow-up study. American Journal of Epidemiology 82: 297); Bright M 1967 (A follow-up study of the Commission on Chronic Illness Morbidity survey in Baltimore: I. Tracing a large population sample over time. Journal of Chronic Diseases 20: 707) and 1969 (A follow-up study of the Commission on Chronic Illness Morbidity survey in Baltimore: III. Residential mobility and prospective studies. Journal of Chronic Diseases 21: 749).
4. Wallechinsky D, Wallace I, Wallace A 1977 The book of lists. Cassell, London, p. 300.

26 Processing the data

This chapter deals with the preparation of a *data set* (or *database*) containing the data to be used in the analysis, and then gives consideration to the statistical analysis of the data. A distinction is made between the statistical analysis and the interpretation of results, which is dealt with in later chapters. Analysis and interpretation are in fact interdependent, and should be seen as activities that go hand in hand rather than as separate stages. Except in the simplest of investigations, the investigator produces or obtains a set of analytic results, then carefully considers them, sees what inferences may be drawn from them and what further questions they open up, decides what further facts are needed in order to test the inferences or answer the questions, produces or obtains the new tabulations or calculations that are required, thinks about the new facts, does more analyses if necessary, and so on.

Computers are today used in almost all studies. Most investigators can themselves run statistical analysis programs, but in large studies the creation, maintenance and management of the data set are often left to experts. This is best done by giving detailed explanations of the objectives and study plan to an expert early in the planning phase, in order to obtain the best possible aid and advice with regard not only to data processing, but to the planning of forms and record systems.

PREPARING THE DATA SET

'Getting from a questionnaire or an interview to an actual data record', it has been said, 'is a perilous journey with many potential accidents waiting to happen'.[1]

If the data are collected by a computer-assisted process, they go into the database automatically; results of chemical, electrocardiographic and other instrumental examinations can also be put straight into the electronic record, as can data read by optical scanning. Usually, however, data are coded manually (if not precoded) and then entered manually, using a computer keyboard.

Accurate manual coding may not be easy to achieve, even with detailed written instructions (see p. 267). Careful training and monitoring may be needed; as a check on coding reliability, double coding (by the same or different coders) may be done for all records, a sample of records, or selected hard-to-code variables. The codes may be written or marked on the original data sheets, or may be copied to code sheets. Unnecessary transcription should be avoided, to avoid errors; if the codes are copied, this process too may need checking. The process is simplified if coding is done at the time the data are collected, by the person who collects the data. But later checks and corrections are then possible only if the original data are recorded, as well as the codes.

Before data are entered, the structure[2] and content of the data set must be decided—what variables will be entered, in what order, whether entries will be treated as numbers or as strings of text ('alphanumerical)', how many decimal places, and so on. The data for each individual are entered into a separate *record* (or series of records), with the variables in a preset sequence and each variable in a separate *field* (which can accommodate one or more numbers, letters or other characters) in the record. Use may be made of a *freefield format*, in which the variables are recorded in fields without preset lengths but separated by blank spaces, commas, carriage returns, or other delimiters, or a *fixed format*, in which the length of the fields (and hence their locations in the record) are decided in advance.

The coded data are best entered with data-entry software,[3] which can check for errors (see p. 270) and may also be able to incorporate 'skip patterns' (conditional jumps that bypass irrelevant variables), insert 'missing data' codes and 'not applicable' codes consistent with the skip patterns, create derived variables (see p. 269), and offer a 'verification' procedure whereby the data can be re-entered ('double keying') and discrepancies identified. It is usually easy to get the program to provide a screen image of the record form, so that during data entry the items appear on the screen in the same order and with the same spatial arrangement as on the record form. Spreadsheet programs can also be used for data entry, and can usually conduct checks and create new variables. Word-processing programs too can be used (but not for checks) by simply typing strings of digits or other characters, with or without delimiters to separate the variables.

One trial of methods of data entry showed that use of a word processor was more than adequate for short record forms. For longer forms, a simple program using a screen image of the form was fastest and most liked. A more sophisticated program, with inbuilt logical checks and skip patterns, did not realize its theoretical advantages; it was slower, and identified only 10% of errors. Most errors caused by incorrect key-punching (at least 1% of all digits entered can be expected to be wrong)[4] are not detected by these checks. The recommended method was the simple one using a screen image of the record form, followed by re-entry for verification.[5]

A good data set does not present surprises when it is used. Measures that may be taken to reduce errors[1] include: use of a data-entry program that can catch impossible values; double entry for verification; careful checking of the first records created, and then of a sample throughout the process; separation of the coding and data-entry processes, to permit concentration on one task at a time; letting the computer do complex recoding tasks; and further checks when data entry has been completed.

Data sets should always be checked before use. The minimal check —one that should never be forgotten—is a simple count; data forms have a nasty habit of going astray. A 'machine edit' can identify such obvious errors as a person aged 342 years, a woman who was married before she was born, or a man who is still menstruating. The errors, which may arise from inaccuracies in the original data or in coding or data entry, are corrected if this is possible. Otherwise the unacceptable values may be changed to 'unknown', and the individuals concerned may be excluded from specific analyses or from the analysis as a whole. Erroneous and missing values are also sometimes changed to 'imputed'[6] ones.

Data set management tasks may persist throughout the process of analysis—new needs may arise for derived variables, for work files confined to a subgroup of the sample or selected variables, or for files appropriate for use with specific statistical software.

It is important to have a backup copy of the data set, kept elsewhere for safety.

STATISTICAL ANALYSIS

The detailed analysis plan must obviously depend on the objectives of the study. We will deal with general strategy, not detailed tactics, and will not attempt to explain statistical techniques.

Many statistical programs for computers are available.[7] Even if the investigator is not personally involved in running the program, it is important to read the documentation and know what the program does and what options are available, and to be able to understand the printout and check for blatant errors in the instructions or output.

The investigator should start with a clear conception of the main kinds of result required to meet the specific objectives of the study. We have previously discussed the use of skeleton tables as an aid in planning the analysis (p. 271). At this stage, such tables not only help to crystallize ideas about the analysis, they are a basis for the instructions to be given to the computer, or can be used as frameworks (work sheets) for the manual entry of results.

Adequate documentation of the analysis should be kept, whether processing is done by computer or manually. Tables and other results should be fully labelled, even if they are only for one's own use; it is amazing how much one can forget as time goes on. There should be a record of the categories of individuals who were included or excluded and how 'missing values' were handled, and the variables and their categories should be explicitly spelt out. All this information may come ready-printed in computer outputs; but the investigator should make sure he can decode it.

If there are many tables they should be numbered, and an index may be a good idea. This makes it easy to record the source of findings used when drafting the report, and may obviate a tedious search if confirmation or additional facts are needed.

Figures should be checked and cross-checked whenever possible, even if they come from a computer. Totals and marginal totals[8] can usually be compared with numbers known from previous tables. Sometimes errors are shown by the fact that the figures just 'don't make sense' (the interocular traumatic test).[9]

No hard and fast rules can be laid down for the sequence of the analysis, but the inexperienced investigator is advised to keep to the following order:

1. Examine each variable separately
2. Examine pairs of variables
3. Examine sets of three or more variables

Multivariate methods of analysis, which permit the simultaneous examination of relationships involving a number of variables, are today easily available, and it is tempting to start with them. Many experts consider this unwise:

> We regard this approach as unsound, and instead recommend a more orderly application of analytic methods, beginning with simple descriptive statistical displays and summaries. Gaps, patterns and inconsistencies in the data can be discovered and further analyses suggested by this examination. Next, relationships between variables can be explored by means of simple cross-tabulations, scatter plans, and measures of association ... Once again, patterns and inconsistencies are sought and, when found, lead to additional tabulations. Finally, multivariate methods may be applied to the data after a full exploration has been conducted using simpler techniques.[10]

A textbook on multivariate statistics stresses that detailed prior screening of the data—'cleaning up your act'—is fundamental to an honest multivariate analysis.[11]

It is usually advisable to start the analysis by *examining the frequency distributions* of all variables. That is, a separate table is prepared for each variable, showing how many individuals fall into each category or at each value of the variable. It is best to use detailed scales of measurement at this stage—i.e. narrow categories, with little or no 'collapsing'—so that the distributions can provide a basis for decisions about the categories to be used in subsequent stages.

The frequency distributions may influence decisions about subsequent steps in the analysis. Plans for detailed studies of relationships between social class and illnesses, for example, may have to be abandoned if the study population turns out to be very homogeneous in social class. ('Make sure your variables vary.'[12]) If there are only three cases of gout, there is little point in planning complicated tables on the epidemiology of this disease. If there are an excessive number of individuals in an 'unknown' category, it may be decided that the variable cannot be studied. Moreover, peculiarities in a distribution may throw doubt on the accuracy of the data (low face validity). *Outliers* may be found—specific values that differ very markedly from the others. These isolated values can have an unduly large effect on statistics, and may need special handling;[13] even if there is no reason to doubt the correctness of the extreme values, their presence may make it difficult to draw conclusions that can be applied more generally than to the particular sample studied.

Simple indices that summarize frequency distributions,[14] such as means, percentages and rates, may be calculated at this time or later. They may of course come ready-made from a computer together with the frequency distributions.

A major part of the analysis usually involves pairs or sets of variables—a dependent variable and one or more independent variables—rather than single variables. Even in the simplest descriptive survey the investigator will probably want to look separately at the findings in the two sexes and in various age groups; in a simple programme review he may want to see whether the performance of care procedures varied for different categories of patients or at different times of the year. In epidemiological studies aimed at testing causal hypotheses and in clinical and programme trials, the examination of *associations between variables*—putative causes and putative effects—is the main focus of the analysis.

In seeking evidence of associations, emphasis is given to those the study was designed to investigate—that is, the associations that are specified or implied in the stated objectives of the study—and to other possibly important relationships with the dependent variables. In most community medicine studies it is helpful if associations between the dependent variables and age, sex, and other selected 'universal' variables (see p. 117) are explored early in the analysis. The process of examining a body of data in order to determine which variables are associated with one another may be referred to as 'screening for associations'.

Simple methods may suffice to reveal associations between pairs of variables. A relationship between pregnancy and anaemia, for example, may be revealed by a *contingency table* (cross-tabulation) in which each woman is simultaneously classified according to her pregnancy status and the presence or absence of anaemia. For an example of such a table, see page 306; but note that a different format[15] is called for if *paired data* are used—that is, if pairs of individually matched cases and controls were studied, or if 'before' and 'after' measurements were made of the same subjects. An association may be revealed by simple scrutiny of the figures in the table or elementary summarizing statistics[14] based on them, by various measures of the strength of an association (see p. 306), or by simple diagrams, such as the scattergrams (or scatter plots) produced by some computer programs. Once identified, the associations can be studied more intensively (see Ch 27 and 28).

The next step is to consider a number of variables at the same time. The simplest way of doing this is by *stratification (subclassification)*, i.e. the construction of multiple contingency tables that allow for simultaneous cross-classification by three or more variables; for an example, see Table 28.2 on page 309. Multiple linear regression analysis, multiple logistic regression analysis, the proportional hazards model, and other techniques of multivariate analysis may also be used. These techniques permit the simultaneous examination of relationships involving a number of variables, and can be used to examine *modifying effects* (does a variable modify the relationship between other variables?) and control for *confounding effects* (see p. 311). Since the mathematical models on which they are based may or may not be appropriate in a specific situation, their results should be used only if there is evidence suggesting a good fit between the facts and the model, e.g. a goodness-of-fit test if logistic regression is used. It is often helpful to do an analysis by stratification techniques first, so as to identify and get some understanding of important interrelationships.

Age, sex and other 'universal' variables are among those most frequently introduced into the analysis. In addition, consideration is usually given to other variables known or suspected to be associated with the dependent variable. No set rules can be laid down. Decisions depend on the aims of the study, on feasibility, and above all on the imaginativeness and ingenuity of the investigator.

It is of course not essential to follow the above sequence. Instead, other variables may be built into the analysis from the outset. This applies especially to 'universal' variables; tables are often broken down by age and sex[16] from a very early stage of the analysis. When there are two or more study populations, e.g. cases and controls, they are often analyzed separately from the outset.

NOTES AND REFERENCES

1. Inter-university Consortium for Political and Social Research 1997 ICPSR guide to social science data preparation and archiving. On the Internet: www.icpsr.umich.edu/ICPSR/Archive/Deposit/dpm.html#variable
2. *Structure of the data set.* The data set may contain one or more data files, stored on disk, tape, or other medium. A data file is a collection of data records, which may be of any length, but are often 'card-images' each containing 80 'columns' (i.e. accommodating 80 characters, like the old IBM punch card). Each record stores a predecided sequence of fields; the fields

may have a predecided size (fixed format) or be separated by predecided characters (freefield format). In the former instance the data file is 'rectangular' (the records are of the same length).

The guide cited in note 1 provides useful advice on file formats and file structure, codes and codebooks, and other aspects of data set preparation, and contains a useful glossary of technical terms.

3. *Epi Info* is a public-domain program that streamlines data entry. All you need do is type the questionnaire or data entry form, using certain conventions for numeric, yes/no and other fields. This is subsequently shown on the screen so that each subject's data can be entered and stored. The program allocates variable names, field lengths, etc., using information derived from the form. Data entry constraints (acceptable ranges, etc.) and skip patterns can be built in. The program can convert the data to formats appropriate for various statistical programs. The questionnaires can be used in computer-assisted interviews.

The program can be obtained from the Epidemiology Program Office, Centers for Disease Control, Atlanta, Georgia or (on the Internet) from www.cdc.gov/epo/epi/downepi6.htm or ftp.demon.co.uk/pub/ibmpc/dos/apps/epi6. (If and when Version 7 is issued, 'epi6' will presumably change to 'epi7'.)

4. Martin J N T, Morton J, Ottley P 1977 Experiments on copying digit strings. Ergonomics 20: 409.

5. Crombie I K, Irving J M 1986 An investigation of data entry methods with a personal computer. Computers and Biomedical Research 19: 543.

6. Erroneous and missing values are sometimes replaced by *imputed* ones, especially if exclusion of the subjects from the analysis is likely to cause bias. Use may be made of the mean or usual value of the variable in the total study population or in people similar to the subject who has a wrong or missing value.

For other methods, see Brick J M, Kalton G 1996 (Handling missing data in survey research. Statistical Methods in Medical Research 5: 215) or Kelsey J L, Thompson W D, Evans A S 1986 (Methods in observational epidemiology. Oxford University Press, New York, pp 269–271).

The best method is probably multiple imputation, a complicated procedure that uses several imputed values, producing different data sets requiring separate analyses and subsequent averaging of results. See: Greenland S, Finkle W D 1995 (A critical look at methods for handling missing covariates in epidemiologic regression analysis. American Journal of Epidemiology 142: 1255); Heitjan D F 1997 (Annotation: What can be done about missing data? Approaches to imputation. American Journal of Public Health 87: 548); and Rubin D B 1987 (Multiple imputation for nonresponse in surveys. John Wiley, New York).

Imputation is particularly difficult if the probability of being missing depends on the value itself (*nonignorable*, as opposed to *missing at random*).

Whatever method is used, it is often wise to do the analysis without as well as with the 'guessed' values, so that the effect of their inclusion can be observed and (if necessary) taken into account.

7. Apart from the well-known commercial *statistical packages*, there are many free and shareware programs, some of which can be downloaded from the Internet. To find them, useful starting-points are www.statserv.com/softwares.html, www.utexas.edu/cc/stat/world/softwaresites.html, and www-personal.umich.edu/~dronis/statfaq.htm

The *PEPI* package contains over 40 statistical programs (for DOS or Windows) for use in epidemiological studies. The programs can be downloaded free (contact www.shareware.com and search for 'pepi' in the 'DOS' category, or can be acquired (with their manual and installation and menu programs) from Brixton Books Unit K, Station Building, Llanidloes, Powys SY18 6EB, Wales, UK (e-mail tracey@brixtonbooks.demon.co.uk) or USD Inc. 2075A West Park Place, Stone Mountain, GA 30087, US (e-mail usd@usd-inc.com).

The programs are described by Abramson J H and Gahlinger P M (1999 Computer books for epidemiologists: PEPI Version 3. Brixton Books, London). For information, visit www.usd-inc.com/pepi.html or www.brixtonbooks.demon.co.uk

The strengths and weaknesses of *Epi Info* and other programmes are reviewed by Oster R A 1988 (An examination of five statistical software programs for epidemiology. The American Statistician 52: 267).

8. In a table showing a cross-classification, the totals of the figures in each column and row are referred to as 'marginal totals'. These are the totals in each category of the variables shown, i.e. simple frequency distributions. When one inspects the frequency distributions of variables (see p. 289) one can puzzle the uninitiated by saying that one is looking at the marginals.

9. It hits you between the eyes.

10. Stolley P D, Schlesselman J J 1982 Planning and conducting a study. In: Schlesselman J J (ed) Case-control studies: design, conduct, analysis. Oxford University Press, New York, pp 69–104.

11. Tabachnick B G, Fidell L S 1989 Using multivariate statistics, 2nd edn. Harper and Row, New York. This book is a methodical guide to the use of BMDP, MYSTAT, SAS and SPSS for multivariate analyses.

12. 'If the heart of research is to compare cases which fall in different categories, the research worker must have plenty of cases which differ in their classification. It is hard to argue with such a truism, but it is easy to forget it' (Davis J A 1971 Elementary survey analysis. Prentice Hall, Englewood Cliff, N J).

13. There is no simple solution to the problem of *outliers*. The least that should be done is to be aware of their presence, and it is generally worth seeing how their exclusion affects the findings. It may be decided to modify the scale of measurement (e.g. by collapsing categories) so that they are grouped together with less extreme values, or to exclude them, or to change them to less extreme values. See Tabachnick & Fidell 1989 (see note 11), pp 66–70.

14. Indices that may be used to describe frequency distributions include measures of central tendency, measures of dispersion, and proportions.

The commonest *measures of central tendency* are the arithmetic *mean* (used for interval or ratio scales) and the *median* or *50th percentile*, which is the value of the middle observation when all the observations are arranged in ascending order (for ordinal, interval or ratio scales). Using a mean, the average human being has one testis.

The commonest *measure of dispersion* around the mean is the *standard deviation* (not to be confused with the standard error of the mean). *Quartiles* (the values below which fall one quarter, one half, and three quarters, respectively, of all values) or the *interquartile range* between the upper and lower quartiles may be used to measure dispersion around a median. Use is frequently made of percentiles (the values below which fall 3%, 10% etc. of the observations), especially to summarize anthropometric data.

The number of individuals in a category may be expressed as a *relative frequency*, i.e. as a *proportion* (e.g. a *percentage*) of the total. The data may be combined to show what proportions of individuals have values that lie above (or below) successive levels (*cumulative frequencies*).

Rates are briefly discussed in note 1 on p. 121.

15. *Paired data*, such as those derived from pairs of individually matched cases and controls, or matched pairs of persons exposed and not exposed to a putative causative factor, or from pairs of observations made on the same

| | Cases | |
	Factor absent	Factor present
Controls		
Factor absent	a	b
Factor present	c	d

persons before and after exposure to some factor, need special attention. Pairs and not individuals should be classified, using a contingency table of the following kind:

A disparity in size between b and c provides evidence of an association. A measure of the strength of the association is described in note 3, p. 322.

16. Hopefully, unlike the investigator.

27 Interpreting the findings

Now has come the time to reap the fruits of the study, by considering its findings and using them to answer the questions that were specified as study objectives.

There may also be fringe benefits—interest is sometimes extended to finding answers to questions that were not posed at the outset. This exploration can be useful, provided that it is done with reservations—since the study was not designed to answer these other questions, the answers may be inadequate or misleading. The testing of hypotheses that the study was not designed to test, but that are suggested by the data, has been referred to as 'data dredging'.[1] Any large set of variables is likely to show some associations that have occurred only by chance, and misleading conclusions may be reached if the possibility is ignored that this is the reason for some or all of the associations detected.[2] An association brought to the surface by data dredging is best treated not as evidence that the relationship exists—that is, that it is likely to be found in other data sets also—but only as a clue suggesting that it *may* exist. Other studies can then be designed to test this hypothesis.

The interpretation of findings may be child's play,[3] or may present formidable difficulties. Usually the task is more exacting than it seems on the surface. In one investigator's words of warning:

> An eminent British biostatistician, Major Greenwood, remarked that
> once the proper questions are asked and the relevant facts collected,
> any sensible person can reach the correct conclusions. There are two
> limitations. The facts are never quite complete nor completely
> accurate, and, as Voltaire pointed out in his *Dictionnaire Philosophique*,
> 'Common sense is not so common'.[4]

When interpreting the findings, the first and main task is to 'make sense' of them, with reference to the population that was studied or sampled. Consideration should be given to the possible effects of random sampling variation and bias, both of which will be discussed in this chapter. What is the *internal validity* of the study, i.e. can it yield sound conclusions relating to the study population? Interpreting the findings is generally more difficult in analytic studies, which investigate associations between variables, than in simple descriptive ones; the appraisal of associations will be discussed in the next chapter (Ch. 28).

The second task is to draw inferences that go beyond the specific findings in the specific study population. This has two aspects, both of which are discussed in Chapter 29. First, is it possible to make generalizations to a broader population?—what is the *external validity* of the study? (its capacity to yield sound generalizations going outside the study population); internal validity is a prerequisite for, but does not guarantee, external validity. Second, what are the practical implications of the results?—do the findings point to a need for changes in the provision of medical care, for public health action, for further studies, for the development of new investigative tools, etc.?

We have previously emphasized the interdependence of the analysis and interpretation of findings. Throughout the process of interpretation, a need may arise for new analyses, and sometimes for supplementary data.

RANDOM SAMPLING VARIATION

Caution is required in drawing inferences from findings in samples, even if the samples are representative ones, since chance differences may be expected between different samples drawn randomly from the same population. Chance differences may similarly arise in a trial in which subjects are randomly assigned to experimental and control groups.

One of the advantages of random sampling and random assignment, however, is that it is easy to estimate the findings in the sampled population. Using formulae, tables, or a computer program, we can estimate, with a specified degree of certainty (usually 95 or 99%—this is the *confidence level*), within what range (*confidence interval*) the value in the sampled population probably lies.[5] The narrower this range, the greater the *precision* of the estimate. If a prevalence of 10% is detected in a simple random sample containing 200 individuals, there is an exact 95% probability that the rate in the population is between 6.2 and 15.0% (the *lower* and *upper* *confidence limits*). If the sample contains only 30 individuals the interval is much wider, from 2.1 to 26.5%. Confidence intervals can also be calculated for means and other measures of a distribution, and for rate ratios, odds ratios, and other measures of the strength of an association.

BIAS

Bias is defined as 'any trend in the collection, analysis, interpretation, publication, or review of data that can lead to conclusions that are systematically [i.e. one-sidedly] different from the truth'.[6]

'Bias' is not used here as a synonym for 'prejudice'. The investigator's preconceived opinions and preferences are, of course, among the factors that may lead—as a result, it may be hoped, of unconscious processes only—to biased findings or to distortions in the interpretation and use of findings. A selective blindness to awkward facts, a failure to look for contrary evidence, and a too-easy acceptance of incomplete proof may lead to conclusions that happen to coincide with what the investigator wanted ('wish bias') or expected. This is part of the 'self-fulfilling prophecy' syndrome.[7] The investigator should seek insight into his or her motivations—how strong is the felt need to 'prove a case' or come up with a 'discovery'? Some journals require authors of study reports to report all relationships that may pose a conflict of interest.[8] An investigator aware of being prejudiced, or of a possible conflict of interests, should take special pains to interpret findings objectively and fairly, should use every opportunity to discuss the interpretation with colleagues, and should then not only hear but listen to what they have to say.

Avoiding bias is an important element in the planning and performance of a study, as stressed in previous chapters, where many specific sources of bias are mentioned. At the present stage, before interpreting the findings, the investigator should systematically consider the possibility that they may be biased, as a result of shortcomings either in the study plan or (by the ineluctable operation of Murphy's Law)[9] in its execution. It may not be too hard, if the study's imperfections are not yet known, to find a colleague who will gladly point them out.

We will here consider two kinds of bias—*selection bias* and *information bias*. (*Confounding*, which may also be regarded as a kind of bias, will be discussed on p. 311.)

Selection bias

Selection bias is defined as an error due to a systematic difference between the characteristics of the individuals studied and not studied. If the individuals for whom data are available are not representative of the study population, this may obviously impair the study's validity with respect to whatever the investigator wants to know about the study population—the prevalence of a disease, the strength of an association with a disease, etc.—as well as the capacity to make valid generalizations.

Selection bias may be caused by failure to choose an appropriate sample (*sample bias*) or by losses or exclusions of study subjects, e.g. *nonresponse* or (in a trial) *nonconsent bias*, or (in all analyses or only specific ones) *missing data bias*. In a cohort study or trial there may be *follow-up* or *drop-out bias*; i.e. the risk of developing the outcome condition (the dependent variable) may differ for subjects who are *censored* (withdrawn from the analysis because of loss of contact, refusal to continue, death, etc., before development of the outcome condition) and for subjects who remain in the analysis. In the analysis of a trial, bias may be caused by excluding subjects who stopped their treatment (see 'intention-to-treat analysis', p. 366). Failure to select appropriate controls is a common cause of bias in cohort and case-control studies and in trials; Greenland[10] reserves the term 'selection bias' for bias resulting from the manner of selection of cases or controls in case-control studies (see Ch. 9).

The ability to generalize findings from the study population to a reference population (should the investigator wish to do so) may obviously be affected by the above sources of bias, which can hence impair both internal and external validity. There are also kinds of selection bias that may affect external validity without necessarily affecting internal validity, as a result of the choice of a study population that is not representative of the population to whom the investigator wishes to apply the results. A study of hospital patients, for example, may yield completely sound conclusions about factors associated with a given disease in the study population, but these may not be applicable in the population at large (*referral filter bias*, *Berksonian bias*, etc.). This kind of problem may arise in any study performed in a 'special' or 'different' study population. This may result from selective admission to the study population, as in a study of volunteers (*self-selection bias*) or of bus drivers, vegetarians, or other groups defined by their occupations or behaviour; examples are listed on pages 73–76. It may also result from *selective migration* into or out of a population, or from *selective survival*. The 'special' nature of a study population of course does not lead to bias if interest is limited to this population.

Selection bias can have a marked impact on a study's results.[11] While selectivity can seldom be completely avoided, its degree should always be appraised. To do this, the way in which the sample or samples were chosen should be critically reviewed. Special attention should be paid to substitutions (see p. 96), nonrespondents, nonparticipants, patients who were removed from a clinical trial because of side-effects, and drop-outs. How numerous were these, and what were the reasons? Bias is particularly likely if the selective factors were illness, death, or other reasons that might be connected with the variables under study. Unless the rates of substitutions, nonresponse and drop-outs were negligible, the individuals included in the study should be compared with those who were omitted, using any demographic and other relevant information available; in a study in which repeated efforts are made to enlist response, it may be helpful to compare early and late respondents to obtain insights into factors affecting response (but it cannot be assumed that nonrespondents necessarily resemble late respondents).[12] The use of multivariate analysis may simplify these tasks.[13] Even at this stage, it may not be too late to collect further data to make these comparisons possible. Any differences that are found, such as an under-representation of working mothers among the respondents, may be helpful in the interpretation of the findings. An absence of such differences increases the likelihood that there is no important selection bias, but unfortunately it can never guarantee this, especially if nonresponse or drop-out rates are high.

Sometimes it is possible to control selection bias by statistical manipulations during the analysis.[14] If there was a low response or follow-up rate in some age groups, for example, the findings can be weighted in accordance with the age composition of the total study population, to obtain an estimate that compensates for this selectivity.[15] This method of adjustment becomes complicated if many variables (age, sex, social class, etc.) are taken into account, and is especially unwieldy if stratified sampling was used, so that different weights are needed in each stratum; multivariate procedures can simplify the computation. Alternatively, the findings in separate groups (age-specific rates, etc.) might suffice, without using the global finding in the total study population. A disadvantage is that these methods are based on the assumption that, within each defined category of the population, respondents and nonrespondents are similar, which is not necessarily true. Weighting may actually increase bias, if a greater weight happens to be given to a stratum where the respondents are especially unrepresentative.

Adjustments may also be based on assumed dissimilarities between the individuals for whom data are and are not available. In a study of causes of death, for example, the data were adjusted to compensate for the fact that (in different years) between 4 and 16% of deaths were not medically certified. Two alternative assumptions were made: (1) that the proportion of deaths from each cause (in a given age–sex stratum and in a given year) was twice as high among the uncertified as among the certified cases; and (2) that it was half as high. The two sets of alternative estimates yielded similar conclusions concerning trends of mortality from specific causes.[16] Extreme assumptions are sometimes made—e.g. that all or no nonresponders smoke—so as to obtain maximal and minimal estimates.

Probably the best way of handling nonresponse bias, although seldom a practicable one, is to invest intensive efforts in an attempt to obtain full information about a sufficiently large and representative sample of nonrespondents. These can then be compared with respondents with respect to the characteristics the investigator wishes to study.

Information bias

Information bias is bias caused by shortcomings in the collecting, recording, coding or processing of data. Its origins include the people who collected information (*observer bias, interviewer bias*), the use of defective questionnaires or other instruments (*measurement procedure bias, insensitive measure bias, instrument bias*, etc.), the use of proxy variables (e.g. date of diagnosis instead of date of onset, or current diet to represent previous diet), and one-sided responses by the people studied (*recall bias, response bias, social undesirability bias*). It may arise because 'blind' procedures (see p. 165) were not used, or because of deviations in compliance with experimental or other study procedures.

Information bias is particularly troublesome when its presence, degree or direction varies in different groups of subjects. Differential validity (see p. 188) of this kind may occur if (among other possibilities) the data for the various groups under comparison were not collected in a standard way—there may have been different observers or interviewers, or different operational definitions or criteria may have been used, or different instruments or techniques, or different follow-up periods.

In a case-control or cross-sectional study of a supposed cause of a disease, bias may be produced by the fact that information about the supposed cause is collected after the occurrence of the disease; this may result in *exposure suspicion bias* (knowledge of the subject's disease status may influence the intensity of a search for exposure to the cause), *rumination bias*[17] (a form of recall bias: cases may ruminate about causes for their illnesses and thus report different prior exposures than controls), or *obseqiousness bias*[17] (subjects may alter their responses to fit what they think the investigator wants). Conversely, if there is a known history of exposure (in a cohort or cross-sectional study or a trial) there may be a more energetic hunt for the disease (*diagnostic suspicion bias*, a form of *detection bias*).

When possible bias is suspected, evidence of its presence should be sought. In a study in which people with and without cancer were interviewed, for example, the presence of bias caused by awareness that respondents had cancer was tested by examining data for patients whose cancer diagnoses were subsequently disproved.[18]

When possible, the direction and magnitude of the bias should be appraised, so that allowances can be made when inferences are drawn. The effects of the bias can sometimes be controlled or corrected. If, for example, there is a constant bias in laboratory results, due to a mistake in the preparation of a standard solution, it may be rectified by applying a correction factor to the results. Special analyses may be required, as in a case-control study of a form of cancer, where there was a suspicion that the differences observed between patients and controls might be partly due to the fact that proxy informants had been far more often used for patients (many of whom had died) than for controls. Special analyses were therefore conducted, restricted to data with a high face validity. When parity was investigated, attention was confined to cases and controls who themselves reported their parity. When the subjects' home circumstances in their childhood were investigated, use was made of information provided by subjects or their parents or siblings, not by other informants.[19] Computations may be used to assess the effects of misclassification.[20]

NOTES AND REFERENCES

1. Finding an association by *data dredging* and then using the same data to test its significance may lead to unwarranted conclusions; this has been termed '*post hoc bias*' (Feinleib M, Breslow N E, Detels R 1997 Cohort studies. In: Detels R, Holland W W, McEwen J, Omenn G S, eds. 1997 Oxford Textbook of public health, 3rd edn, vol 2. The practice of public health. Oxford University Press, New York, pp 557–570). See also: Selvin H C, Stuart A 1966 (Data-dredging procedures in data analysis. American Statistician 20[3]: 20).

   On the other hand, there are proponents of data dredging, who stress 'the important danger of not studying an association when it actually exists', which they call a 'type zero error' (Michels K B, Rosner B A 1996 Data trawling: to fish or not to fish. Lancet 348: 1152). The noteworthiness of an association (or its absence) depends on whether it provides new knowledge and on the quality of the data, and not on its statistical significance or whether the hypothesis was formulated a priori, says Marshall J R 1990 (Data dredging and noteworthiness. Epidemiology 1: 5).

2. *Multiple comparison* or *simultaneous inference* procedures, which yield adjusted P values, can be used to reduce the danger that associations found by dredging will be reported as significant when they have arisen by chance (Armitage P, Berry G 1994 Statistical methods in medical research, 3rd edn. Blackwell Scientific Oxford, pp 226–227).

   Opinions on the use of these procedures vary. 'It is to be hoped that they will become as much a part of accepted statistical practice as unadjusted P values are now,' says Wright P S 1992 (Adjusted P-values for simultaneous inference. Biometrics 48: 1005). Others oppose them: 'every association should be evaluated on its own merits; its prior credibility and its features in the study at hand' (Cole P 1979 The evolving case-control study. Journal of Chronic Diseases 32: 15); see also: Rothman K J, Greenland S 1998 (Modern epidemiology, 2nd edn. Lippincott-Raven, Philadelphia, pp 227–228). Perneger T V 1998 concludes that while these procedures make sense in only a few situations, one of these is 'when searching for significant associations without pre-established hypotheses' (What's wrong with Bonferroni adjustments. British Medical Journal 316: 1236).

   ADJUSTP, in the PEPI package, computes 'safe' P values based on these procedures (see note 7, p. 292).

3. See Abramson J H 1994 (Making sense of data: a self-instruction manual on the interpretation of epidemiological data, 2nd edn. Oxford University Press, New York).

4. Mann G V 1977 Diet-heart: end of an era. New England Journal of Medicine 297: 644.

5. More strictly, the 95% *confidence interval* for a value is the interval calculated from a random sample by a procedure which, if applied to an infinite number of random samples of the same size, would, in 95% of instances, contain the true value in the population. To unravel this and find formulae, see a statistics textbook.

   It would seem pointless to estimate a confidence interval if the whole of the study population was studied; but the study population can be visualized as a sample of an imaginary larger population (see note 9, p. 322).

   Methods of calculating commonly used confidence intervals are explained in a series of papers in the British Medical Journal: Gardner M J, Altman D G 1986 (Confidence intervals rather than P values: estimation rather than hypothesis testing. 292: 747); Campbell M J, Gardner M J 1988 (Calculating confidence intervals for some non-parametric analyses. 296: 1454); Altman

D G, Gardner M J 1988 (Calculating confidence intervals for correlation and regression. 296: 1238); and Machin D, Gardner M J 1988 (Calculating confidence intervals for survival time analyses. 292: 1369).

The PEPI package (see note 7, p. 292) computes confidence intervals for most commonly used indices; the manual provides formulae and references.

6. Definition of *bias* from Last J M, Abramson J H, Friedman G D, Porta M, Spasoff R A, Thuriaux M 1995 (A dictionary of epidemiology, 3rd edn. Oxford University Press, New York).

For a detailed discussion of bias, with special reference to the study of associations between two dichotomous variables, see Kleinbaum D G, Kupper L L, Morgenstern H 1982 (Epidemiologic research, part II. LifeTime Learning Publications, Belmont, Cal.) Sources of bias in case-control studies are reviewed by Schlesselman J J, Stolley P D 1982 (Sources of bias. In: Schlesselman J J, ed. Case-control studies: design, conduct analysis. Oxford University Press, New York, Ch 5).

7. 'This is the bias a researcher is inclined to project into his methodology and treatment that subtly shapes the data in the direction of his foregone conclusions.' (Isaac S, Michael W B 1977 Handbook in research and evaluation for education and the behavioral sciences. EdITS, San Diego, p. 58). Maier's Law is relevant here: 'If the facts do not conform to the theory, they must be disposed of'. If the investigator's prejudice is a reflection of a conventional or fashionable belief, his findings may tend to confirm this belief. This is the 'Self-perpetuating Myth' syndrome; see Fleiss 1981 (Statistical methods for rates and proportions, 2nd edn. John Wiley, New York, p. 208).

8. Investigators submitting manuscripts to journals may be requested to specify relationships that may pose a conflict of interest. These exist when an author 'has ties to activities that could inappropriately influence his or her judgment, whether or not judgment is in fact affected. Financial relationships with industry ... either directly or through immediate family, are usually considered to be the most important conflicts of interest. However, conflicts can occur for other reasons, such as personal relationships, academic competition, and intellectual passion' (International Committee of Medical Journal Editors 1997 Uniform requirements for manuscripts submitted to biomedical journals. Annals of Internal Medicine 126: 36).

9. Murphy's Law: 'If anything can go wrong, it will'. Murphy's corollary: 'If nothing can go wrong, it will anyway'. O'Toole's commentary: 'Murphy was an optimist'.

10. Greenland S 1997 Concepts of validity in epidemiological research. In: Detels R, Holland W W, McEwen J, Omenn G S (eds) 1997 (see note 1), pp 597–615.

11. Examples showing how *selection bias* can lead to misleading or entirely incorrect results are presented by Ellenberg J H 1994, who would like studies with selection bias to be considered 'scientifically "politically incorrect"', so that the scientific community will 'just say no' to them (Selection bias in observational and experimental studies. Statistics in Medicine 13: 557).

12. Sheikh H 1998 Late response vs. non-response to mail questionnaire. Annals of Epidemiology 8: 75.

13. McNeill D 1996 Epidemiological research methods. John Wiley, New York, p. 167.

14. The effect of selection bias can be examined if external information about the selective factors is available. See Greenland S 1996 (Basic methods for sensitivity analysis of biases. International Journal of Epidemiology 25: 1107); and Rowland M L, Forthofer R N 1993 (Adjusting for nonresponse bias in a health examination survey. Public Health Reports 108: 380).

15. For a numerical example of this method of adjusting for nonresponse bias,

see Moser C A, Kalton G 1972 (Survey methods in social investigation, 2nd edn. Heinemann, London, pp 181–184).

This book also describes the Politz–Simmons technique for dealing with the 'not-at-home' problem in household interview surveys (pp 178–181). The results are weighted in accordance with the proportion of days the respondent is ordinarily at home at the time of the interview. Most weight is given to respondents who are seldom at home, who represent a group with a high nonresponse rate.

16. Abramson J H, Gofin R 1979 Mortality and its causes among Moslems, Druze and Christians in Israel. Israel Journal of Medical Sciences 15: 965.
17. An annotated catalogue of biases is provided by Sackett D L 1979 (Bias in analytic research. Journal of Chronic Diseases 32: 51). It includes 'hot stuff bias', 'looking for the pony bias', 'tidying-up bias', etc.
18. Lilienfeld A M, Lilienfeld D E 1980 Foundations of epidemiology, 2nd edn. Oxford University Press, New York, pp 208–209.
19. Abramson J H, Pridan H, Sacks M I, Avitzour M, Peritz E 1978 A case-control study of Hodgkin's disease. Journal of the National Cancer Institute 61: 307.
20. The arithmetical control of *misclassification* errors is explained by Greenland S 1996 (Basic methods for sensitivity analysis of biases. International Journal of Epidemiology 25: 1107) and by Fleiss J L 1981 (Statistical methods for rates and proportions, 2nd edn. John Wiley, New York, Ch 12) and Kleinbaum et al 1982 ([see note 6], Ch 12).

MISCLASS, in the PEPI package (see note 7, p. 292), uses estimates of sensitivity and specificity to correct for misclassification in a 2 × 2 table.

28 Making sense of associations

The exploration of associations[1] between variables is usually the most challenging and rewarding part of the analysis. This is especially true in analytic epidemiological studies in which causal hypotheses are tested, and in clinical and programme trials, which aim at testing hypotheses about the effects of health care.

Simple methods of detecting associations are listed on page 290. Whenever an association is found, there are six basic questions that may be asked.

QUESTIONS ABOUT AN ASSOCIATION

1. Actual or artifactual? (Influence of bias?)
2. How strong?
3. Nonfortuitous?
4. Consistent? (Influence of modifying factors?)
5. Influence of confounding factors?
6. Causal?

Questions 1, 2 and 4 should usually be asked, in any kind of study, and 3, 5 and 6 are important if the investigator wants to explain his findings and not only describe them.

As will be pointed out, some of these questions may also be asked about the *absence* of an association.

ARTIFACTS

The first question, always worth asking, is whether the finding actually exists, or whether it may be an artifact, i.e. ask *whether* before asking *why* there is an association.

Artifactual ('spurious'[2]) associations may be produced by flaws in the design or execution of the study, that result in bias (see Ch. 27). The prevalence of anaemia may appear to be higher in one town or one group of patients than in another because of selection bias or the use of different sources of data, different definitions of anaemia, different methods of measuring haemoglobin, etc. Artifactual associations may be caused by errors, often remediable ones, in the handling of data. Not uncommonly they result from mistakes in arithmetic or computer programming.

Flawed methods may of course not only produce an artifactual association, they may also weaken, obscure, strengthen, or change the direction of an actual association.

If marked bias is strongly suspected and there is no way of correcting or controlling its effects, further examination of the association is usually pointless.

STRENGTH

The strength of an association is a measure of its importance. If anaemia is found among 30% of pregnant women and 2% of non-pregnant women (see Table 28.1), this marked disparity (a difference of 28%, or a ratio of 15) indicates a strong and important relationship between anaemia and pregnancy.

Table 28.1 Contingency table showing relationship between pregnancy and anaemia among 10 000 women (imaginary data)

	No anaemia	Anaemia	Total
Pregnant	a: 1400 (70%)	b: 600 (30%)	2000 (100%)
Not pregnant	c: 7840 (98%)	d: 160 (2%)	8000 (100%)

How strong an association must be if it is to be regarded as important is a matter of judgement. A difference of 2% in anaemia rates would probably be considered trivial, but a similar difference in infant mortality rates—i.e. 20 extra infant deaths per 1000 live births—would be more likely to be regarded as important.

As will be seen below, conclusions about the strength of an association may sometimes be modified when additional variables are incorporated into the analysis. An association should therefore not be prematurely discarded as unimportant. This, it must be said, is not easy advice to follow; it is very tempting to restrict further analysis to associations that 'come through loud and clear' from the beginning.

Measures of the strength of an association include the *difference between rates or proportions*, their *ratio* (both used in the above example), the *odds ratio*,[3] the *difference between means* (e.g. of haemoglobin values), and *correlation and regression coefficients*.[4] Ratios (rate ratios or odds ratios) are generally appropriate in studies of causal processes or the influence of interventions, and absolute differences between rates are suitable if there is interest in the magnitude of a public health problem. *Attributable (aetiological)*, *prevented and preventable fractions* (which are based on differences between rates) measure the *impact* of a harmful or protective factor on the health of people exposed to it, or on the total community; the *attributable fraction in the population*, for example, is the percentage of the disease in the population that can be attributed to a given cause.

Whatever measure is used, a confidence interval may be informative. This is the range within which we can assume the true value (in the population from which the study sample was drawn) to lie, with a specified degree of confidence.[5]

NONFORTUITOUSNESS

Anything[6] may happen by chance. However strong the association that is observed between two variables, it may be fortuitous, unlikely though this may be. 'The "one chance in a million" will undoubtedly occur, with no less and no more than its appropriate frequency, however surprised we may be that it should occur to *us*.'[7] The absence of an association may also be a fortuitous occurrence.

The question is not whether the association observed in the study may have occurred by chance—the answer to which is almost always 'yes'—but whether we are prepared to regard it as nonfortuitous. Occasionally—e.g. if there is a big difference between the rates observed in two groups, and the groups are large—just looking at the results may enable us to decide whether to regard the association as nonfortuitous. When this 'eye test'[8] is not enough, a test of statistical significance[9] may be used to enable us to make this decision.

Significance tests should not be done when they are not needed.

In some studies, especially in simple descriptive surveys and programme reviews in which probability sampling was not used, the issue of fortuitousness may have little importance. For practical purposes it may be enough to know that housebound patients are concentrated in certain neighbourhoods of a city or that the proportion of women given postnatal guidance on family planning is lower in one clinic than in others, without worrying about deciding whether these associations occurred by chance. There is little point in doing a significance test on an association that is likely to be an artifact, or one that is so weak that it would be of no consequence even if it were regarded as nonfortuitous.

An association is adjudged to be statistically significant if the test yields a P value that is less than an arbitrarily chosen *significance level* (*alpha*). Critical levels often selected are 5% (0.05) and 1% (0.01). Whatever level is chosen, it must be remembered that significance tests have 'built-in errors'. Using a significance level of 5%, purely random processes will produce a verdict of 'statistically significant' in about five of every hundred significance tests performed, even if no real associations exist ('making a fool of yourself five times out of every 100'[10]). This is an important consideration if many tests are performed. The chance of such errors may be reduced by lowering the critical level, but can never be eliminated.

If the association is statistically significant we may regard it as nonfortuitous, without forgetting that, because of the 'built-in errors', we have not proved beyond doubt that the difference is not due to chance. A 'statistically significant' result does not mean that the relationship is necessarily strong, and it tells us nothing about the importance of the relationship. If the prevalence of anaemia is 30% in one group of pregnant women and 32% in another, this difference would be considered negligible even if it were statistically significant, which it would be if each group contained 5000 women.

If the result is 'not statistically significant' this does not necessarily mean that the association is fortuitous (any more than a negative sputum test for the tubercle bacillus necessarily means that a patient does not have tuberculosis). The verdict is 'not proven'. If the samples are large such a result may, however, be taken to mean that there is unlikely to be a nonfortuitous association of any great strength.

It is generally more useful to know in what range the true value of a measure of association probably lies, i.e. its confidence interval (see p. 296), than merely to know whether the difference is statistically significant. This was illustrated by a review of 71 randomized controlled clinical trials that yielded 'negative' results, i.e. there was no statistically significant difference between the outcomes in the experimental and control groups; when 90% confidence intervals were calculated, however, it was found that in half the studies the interval included a 50% reduction in mortality or whatever other endpoint was used in the study, so that an appreciable favourable effect of the therapy could not be ruled out.[11]

Confidence intervals provide an indication of statistical significance. If, for example, the 95% confidence interval for a difference between two rates or means does not include 0, or if the 95% confidence interval for the rate ratio or odds ratio does not include 1, this means a significant difference (by most two-tailed tests) at the 5% level.

CONSISTENCY OF THE ASSOCIATION

An association may vary in different parts of the population or in different circumstances. The simplest way of detecting this is to stratify the data in accordance with the categories of another variable, and then inspect the findings in each stratum separately. In Table 28.1, for example, we saw an association between pregnancy and anaemia. In Table 28.2 the same data are additionally subclassified according to educational level, so that education can be 'held constant' in the analysis. (This could of course be done better by using more than two educational categories, so as to ensure greater homogeneity within each educational stratum.) This table shows a much stronger association between pregnancy and anaemia among the poorly educated (where the relative risk, i.e. the ratio of the proportions, is 50% ÷ 2%, i.e. 25) than among the

Table 28.2 Multiple contingency table showing relationship between pregnancy and anaemia among 10 000 women, by educational level (imaginary data)

	No anaemia	Anaemia	Total
High educational level			
Pregnant	900 (90%)	100 (10%)	1000 (100%)
Not pregnant	3960 (99%)	40 (1%)	4000 (100%)
Low educational level			
Pregnant	500 (50%)	500 (50%)	1000 (100%)
Not pregnant	3920 (98%)	80 (2%)	4000 (100%)

better educated (relative risk = 10% ÷ 1%, i.e. 10). If odds ratios are used, the respective values are 49 and 11. The difference between the associations is statistically significant: P = 0.00002 (a test that compares the associations in two or more strata is called a test of heterogeneity[12]).

In such analyses the additional variable (education) may be called a *modifier variable*,[12] since it 'modifies' the relationship between pregnancy and anaemia. In statistical parlance, there is *statistical interaction*[12] between education and pregnancy. This means that the association between pregnancy and anaemia differs when educational level varies, and also (check this in the table) that the association between poor education and anaemia is different in pregnant women (relative risk = 50% ÷ 10%, i.e. 5) and non-pregnant women (relative risk = 2% ÷ 1%, i.e. 2).

Effect modification always refers to a specific measure of association. In the above calculations we used the ratio of the proportions with anaemia. We would also find evidence of interaction if we used the difference between the proportions, which is 50 minus 2, i.e. 48%, among the poorly educated, and only 10 minus 1, i.e. 9%, among the better educated. With different data the results using different measures of association might not coincide: if the proportions were 40 and 20% in one stratum, and 4 and 2% in another, the ratio would be identical (2) in each stratum, but the differences would be 20 and 2 respectively. It is also possible for rate ratios to be consistent and odds ratios inconsistent.[13]

If multiple regression analysis is used, modifying effects can be appraised by including appropriate interaction terms in the model (logistic regression analysis uses odds ratios, linear regression analysis uses differences).

The findings in Table 28.2 can be usefully looked at in a different way, by comparing the prevalence of anaemia when both risk factors—pregnancy and low educational level—are present with the prevalence when only one is present, using the women with neither risk factor as a reference group when calculating ratios and differences (Table 28.3).

We can now compare the *joint effect* of the risk factors with their combined separate effects. The two factors multiply the anaemia prevalence by 10 and 2 respectively, so that their expected combined effect is a 20-fold prevalence. The observed joint effect is much stronger—a 50-fold prevalence, with a 95% confidence interval (37–68) that does not include 20. This is *positive interaction* (or *synergism*) on a multiplicative scale. We could instead look at

Table 28.3 Prevalence of anaemia, in relation to presence of two risk factors

	Anaemia prevalence	Ratio	Difference
No risk factors (reference group)	1%	1	—
Pregnancy only	10%	10	9%
Low educational level only	2%	2	1%
Both risk factors (joint effect)	50%	50	49%

the differences: the two factors raise the anaemia prevalence by 9% and 1% respectively, so that their expected combined effect is a rise of 10%; the observed joint effect is a rise of 49%—positive interaction on an additive scale. If a joint effect is smaller than any single effect, this is *antagonism*.

The different findings in different strata are often of interest in their own right. They may have important practical implications. It may be possible, for example, to identify vulnerable 'high-risk' population groups who may require special health care. The presence of positive interaction (on the additive or multiplicative scale) may point to particularly vulnerable groups. In an evaluative study, a care procedure or programme may be found to be more effective among some categories of patients or population groups than among others.

The detection of effect modification is also a fruitful source of clues for the investigator who wishes not only to describe associations but to explain them. It often suggests what directions the subsequent analysis (or a subsequent study) should take—for example, can an explanation be found for a finding of synergism or antagonism?

Consistency may sometimes be worth investigating even when no association has been found, since an association that occurs only in a relatively small stratum can be drowned by the findings in other strata, so that no association is observed in the data as a whole. An association may also (less commonly) be concealed if there are positive and negative associations in different strata, so that they cancel each other out.

CONFOUNDING EFFECTS

An association between two variables is sometimes distorted by the influence of another variable. This is of obvious concern to an investigator who wants to understand his findings.

As an example, a survey in Massachusetts revealed that the children of fathers who smoked tended to have lower birth weights than those of fathers who did not smoke. This apparently occurred because smokers tended to have wives who smoked, and women who smoked during pregnancy tended to have light babies.[14] As another curious illustration:

> consider the association between storks and babies (which, depending on time and place, is almost always small but positive). Few people believe that storks bring babies, and the small positive relation is undoubtedly due to rural areas having both a large number of storks and a higher birth rate than urban areas.[15]

People who give up cigarettes have a high death rate in the next year or two. This occurs not because smoking is good for you, but because decisions to give up smoking are commonly due to the onset of diseases that carry a high fatality. Statistics show that the larger the number of fire engines that come to deal with a fire, the greater the fire damage. But does this necessarily mean that it is the fire engines that cause the damage?

Similarly, elderly people who live alone use chiropody services more than those who do not live alone. But this is a distorted finding, caused by the fact that those who live alone are older and include more women. When age and sex are held constant in the analysis, i.e. when people of the same age and sex are compared, it is found that those who live alone receive much *less* chiropody care.[16]

In each of these instances the association that was originally observed was a *secondary* one, resulting from the fact that both variables were related to a confounding[17] variable (or, in the chiropody example, two confounding variables). This may be portrayed as A—C→B, where A and B, the independent and dependent variables respectively, are both linked with C, the confounding factor. Variable A is a *passenger variable*[18] that C has carried into its association with B. It follows that the variables that should be investigated as possible confounders are those with known or suspected associations with both the dependent and independent variables.

As a numerical illustration, we can use the findings in the subgroup of 2000 pregnant women in our fictional sample. In these pregnant women there was an association (relative risk = 5) between anaemia and poor education (Table 28.2). In Table 28.4 these data are subclassified according to an additional variable, the presence of hookworm infestation. When separate attention is paid to women with hookworm and those without, no association

Table 28.4 Multiple contingency table showing relationship between education level and anaemia among 2000 pregnant women, by presence of hookworm infestation (imaginary data)

	No anaemia	Anaemia	Total
Hookworm infestation			
High educational level	36 (36%)	64 (64%)	100 (100%)
Low educational level	260 (35%)	490 (65%)	750 (100%)
No hookworm infestation			
High educational level	864 (96%)	36 (4%)	900 (100%)
Low educational level	240 (96%)	10 (4%)	250 (100%)
Total			
High educational level	900 (90%)	100 (10%)	1000 (100%)
Low educational level	500 (50%)	500 (50%)	1000 (100%)

between anaemia and poor education is found in either stratum, although in the total sample of pregnant women the relative risk was 5. The association observed in the total sample is a distortion of the true situation—hookworm infestation is apparently a confounding variable. This effect arises from the strong relationships (shown in the top four lines of figures in the table) of hookworm both with poor education (750 of the 1000 poorly educated women in this sample had hookworm, as compared with 100 of the 1000 better educated) and with anaemia (ratio of 64% ÷ 4% = 17 in the better educated and 65% ÷ 5% = 13 in the poorly educated).

It must be stressed that if an association disappears or is altered when another variable is controlled, this does not necessarily mean that there is a confounding effect. This could also happen if the pattern of associations was A→C→B, i.e. if A produces or affects C, and C produces or affects B. In this pattern, C is an *intermediate* or *intervening cause*; A is an *indirect cause* of B. In the present instance, the possibility must be considered that poor education, or some closely related factor for which poor education serves as a proxy, is a cause of hookworm infestation and hence, indirectly, of anaemia. To the extent that this is true, the relationship between education and anaemia may be causal. Even the association between fathers' smoking habits and their babies' birth weights may to an extent be causal, if men's smoking habits affect their wives'.

To confound an association between variables A and B, variable C must influence or be a cause of B (or be a closely associated stand-in for a variable that influences or causes B), and it must be associated with A in the study population, but not simply because it is caused or influenced by A. Only if its associations with A and B are strong can C have a confounding effect of any importance. The associations with A and B do not mean that C is a confounder, they only make it a *potential confounder*. Note that the associations with A and B may not be readily visible to the naked eye.[19]

The way that a confounding variable distorts an association depends on the strength and direction of its relationships with the other variables. Controlling a confounding variable may make an association disappear (as in the above example); it may weaken it, exaggerate it, or change its direction (from positive to negative or vice versa); and it may reveal an association not previously apparent.

Confounding effects can be detected and handled only if there was sufficient forethought in the planning stage of the study to ensure that possible confounders were selected as study variables (see p. 116), and hence measured. An endeavour to cope with confounding may have been made when planning the study design, by *restricting* the study to a homogeneous group (see p. 70) or by using *matching* (Ch. 7) or *randomization* (Ch. 32). If the latter methods were used it is wise to test their effectiveness by checking the similarity of the groups that are to be compared.

There are three main approaches to the detection or control of confounding effects during the analysis of the study:

1. The variable suspected of being a confounding factor can be held constant by *stratification*. The study population is divided into strata in accordance with the categories of the suspected confounder, and the association between the dependent and independent variables is measured separately in each stratum and compared with the association found in the data as a whole. If, as in the above example, this comparison reveals a difference large enough to be considered meaningful by the investigator (there are no statistical tests for this), and if the suspected confounder is not an intermediate cause, the difference is evidence of a confounding effect. The stratum-specific data provide estimates of the strength of the 'true' association when the confounding variable is controlled. As pointed out on page 309, stratification also permits the inspection of modifier effects.

2. The confounder can be *neutralized*. The strength of the association is measured by a statistical technique, such as standardization, multiple linear or logistic regression, the Mantel–Haenszel procedure, etc., that 'holds constant' and thus nullifies the effect

of the suspected confounder or confounders, and computes an *adjusted* measure of the strength of the association.[20] The difference between this adjusted measure and the corresponding *crude* measure (not controlling for confounding) is an indication of the degree of confounding. It should be remembered that 'over-adjustment' may have the same effects as overmatching (see p. 81): the association that the investigation was designed to study may be masked, and unnecessary adjustment (for variables that are not confounding) may impair the precision with which this association can be measured.[21]

3. Confounding factors can occasionally be *reasoned away*; that is, it may be possible to deduce that an observed association between A and B is unlikely to be a secondary one caused by their common association with C. The reasoning is based on known and assumed facts about the relationships between C and the other two variables. An appreciable confounding effect can be produced only if these relationships are very strong—'the spurious effect is only a relatively weak echo'. Also, the direction of these relationships (positive or negative) influences the direction of the confounding effect.[22]

Adjusted measures that control for confounding should be used with discretion. They may not be appropriate if the confounders have strong modifying effects; if, for example, a study in Guinea-Bissau shows that various risk factors have different associations with diarrhoea in older (weaned) and younger (breast-fed) children,[23] these conditional associations may provide a basis for appropriate intervention of different kinds in children of different ages, but controlling for age to obtain adjusted (overall) measures may not be very helpful. If regression models are used, they may provide misleading findings if they do not include interaction terms, or if there is a poor fit with the regression model. If the confounder is a strong effect modifier, standardization too can yield misleading results; in Britain, age-standardized mortality data show persistent differences between regions but obscure the fact that the differences have become small at younger ages, and persist only at middle to late ages.[24]

CAUSALITY

Finally, we come to the question of causality. How can we know whether the association between A and B (i.e. A—B) is a cause–

effect one? Does A, or a factor of which A is a proxy measure, produce or affect B (i.e. A → B)? (Or, of course, vice versa: A ← B.)

Let us pause to consider what we mean by causality.[25] For our purpose, a causal association may be defined as 'an association between two categories of events in which a change in the frequency or quality of one is observed to follow alteration in the other. In certain instances the possibility of alteration must be presumed and a presumptive classification of an association as causal may be justified'.[26] A cause may be defined, for example, as a factor that alters the probability of occurrence of a disease.[27]

Usually we wish to obtain information that can be put to practical use, now or in the long run. We want to identify factors that, if altered, would lead to a reduction in something we consider undesirable—premature deaths, disease, etc.—or to an improvement in something we regard as desirable, such as health care. For us, these factors are causes, even if manipulating them is unfeasible or unacceptable. In a clinical or programme trial, we want to know what effects, desirable and undesirable, can be attributed to intervention.

Not only do we want to know whether A causes B, we may also want to know what the mechanism is—by what process is this influence exerted? In the chain of causation A→X→Y→Z→B, we may be interested not only in A, but also in the intervening causes X, Y and Z. Having learned about X, Y and Z, we can endeavour to modify them as well as or instead of A, so as to modify B. In an evaluative study we may be interested not only in the achievement of changes in health and other desirable outcomes, but also in the chain of activities and intermediate outcomes that led to these end-results. What we may actually want (but can probably never attain) is a complete picture not only of all the links in the chain of causation, but also of the other variables that influence A, X, Y, Z and B or the processes by which they affect each other (Fig. 28.1).

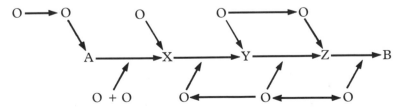

Fig. 28.1 The web of causation.

In fact, we may want to know the total nexus, the 'web of causation',[26] incorporating not only the A → B chain and its intervening causes and modifying factors, as shown in the figure, but also any other chains of causation that culminate in B, as well as the interactions between chains. From our immediate pragmatic viewpoint all these variables, A, X, Y, Z, the various Os shown in the diagram, and all those not shown, can be regarded as causes of B. Various micro-organisms, dirty feeding bottles, early weaning, poverty, malnutrition, respiratory infections, treatment by traditional practitioners, a lack of clinics or hospitals—all these, and more, are causes of deaths from gastroenteritis.

The web will include causes that operate at different levels (molecular, cellular, personal, familial, community, societal, etc.). Some few causes may be *sufficient* to produce or influence B without the participation of other causes (beheading is enough to produce death), but even they will have antecedent causes. Some causes may be *necessary* ones, without which B cannot occur or be modified, but on their own they will seldom be sufficient—exposure to the HIV virus is a necessary cause of AIDS, but not everyone who is exposed develops the disease. Clearly, causes are always multiple,[28] and effects are always the *joint effects* of multiple causes.

A sufficient cause can be defined as a set of minimal conditions and events that inevitably produces a given disease (or other effect) when an individual is exposed to them, 'minimal' meaning that there are no superfluous factors in the set.[29] Many alternative constellations of causes (known or unknown) may be involved in the aetiological process in different individuals, and no single constellation is therefore a necessary cause. But in each constellation, every component is a necessary element—i.e., without the interaction between the components, the effect will not occur. Following this line of thinking, the importance of any cause in a given population will depend on the prevalence of the other components of the constellations in which it features.

The better we understand the causal processes, the better the prospect of finding an effective way of prevention; but this does not mean that a complete picture is essential for this purpose—many effective preventive procedures have been based on data connecting a cause and effect[30] without knowledge of the contents of the mysterious 'black box' concealing the intermediate mechanism (the causal web and constellations are now in a box!). What we need is to identify causes that are always or frequently necessary, i.e. that feature in all constellations of causes or in many of the frequently operating constellations that lead to the effect. If we can remove or minify (or block the action of) even a single such cause we have a 'preventive broom'[31] that can sweep away the causal web or a good part of it, whether it is in a black box or not (or, stating this less ambitiously, we can break 'selected strands of this causal web'[32]). Immunization, for example, aims to control an always necessary cause (low level of immunity), and wearing of seat belts or the manufacture of vehicles with a low centre of gravity and a wide base[31] may prevent many severe road accident injuries. If we extend the model to include causes at different levels, ranging from the molecular to the societal, we may find preventive actions that operate at different levels; this replaces the black box with a nest of 'Chinese boxes, each containing a succession of smaller ones ... we envisage successive levels of organization, each of which encompasses the next and simpler level, all with intimate links between them'.[33]

The best evidence for a causal relationship comes from a well-designed and well-conducted randomized experiment (especially if the findings are replicated in other experiments). The value of evidence from a non-experimental study depends on how well the study was designed and conducted[34]—how close was it to a good experiment, with respect to the avoidance or control of selection and information bias and confounding? This is not easy to achieve, and it is not unusual for non-experimental studies to yield conflicting results, or findings that differ from those of experiments.[35]

Whatever kind of study the evidence comes from, four conditions must be met before we can seriously entertain the possibility that A may be a cause of B. First, A and B must be associated. Secondly, we must be sure that A preceded B, or at least that A *may* have come before B. This is essential, although a time sequence cannot by itself prove causation; 'if winter comes, can spring be far behind?'—but does winter cause spring? Thirdly, we must satisfy ourselves that there is little likelihood that the association is an artifact (see p. 305) caused by shortcomings in the study methods. And fourthly, we must decide that the association is probably not wholly attributable to confounding (see p. 311). We can of course never be quite sure that there are no confounding factors that were not taken into account in the design or analysis of the study, and that we may not even suspect. We can therefore never really 'prove' a causal relationship. What we want, however, is 'reasonable proof', strong enough to be used as a basis for decision and action. To this end, we should review the way that possible confounders were handled in the study. Can we think of any important factors that were not measured, in themselves or by proxy, or that were measured unsatisfactorily? How well were possible confounding influences explored and controlled in the analysis? Do the size of the sample and the nature and complexity of the findings permit a thoroughgoing analysis of these influences? If not, to what extent can confounding influences be 'reasoned away' (see p. 315)?

If these conditions are met, we can consider other evidence. Basically, we see how well the facts fit in with what we might expect to find if the association were causal. This is not quite the same thing as 'proving' a causal association, but it is the best we can do. For this purpose, use may be made of the following additional criteria,[36] which (taken together) may strengthen or weaken the case for causality, although none of them is essential or conclusive. These are:

1. *Statistical significance*—this supports the case for a causal association; its absence weakens the case, but only if the test is sufficiently powerful[9] (this usually means 'if the sample is large enough').
2. *Strength* of the association—the stronger it is, the more likely that it is causal, and not produced by bias or confounding; but a weak association may also be (weakly) causal.
3. *Dose-response relationship*—the case for causality is supported if there is a correlation between the amount, intensity or duration of exposure to the 'cause' and the amount or severity of the 'effect'. But there may also be a correlation with the dose of a placebo.[37] Also, there may be an 'all-or-none' response that appears only when the causative factor reaches a threshold level, or a relationship between cause and effect that is U- or J-shaped (or inverted U- or J-shaped) rather than linear.
4. *Time-response relationship*—if the incidence of the 'effect' (e.g. the rate of new cases of a disease) rises to a peak some time after a brief exposure to the 'cause' and then decreases, this supports the case.
5. *Predictive performance*—if surveys or experiments provide new knowledge supporting an a priori causal hypothesis, this supports the case; a failed prediction weakens the case.[38]
6. *Specificity*—the finding that the 'effect' is related to only one 'cause', or that the 'cause' is related to only one 'effect', may be regarded as supporting the case; but a lack of specificity in no way negates a causal relationship.

7. *Consistency* (in different populations or circumstances, and in studies by different investigators or methods)—if the same association is found repeatedly, this strongly supports the case. If results are inconsistent, and the variation cannot be attributed to modifying factors or differences in study methods, this weakens the case.

8. *Coherence* with current theory and knowledge—in particular, the availability of a satisfactory explanation of the *mechanism* by which A may affect B—supports the case; but the investigator who cannot think up *some* plausible explanation for his findings must indeed be a rare bird;[39] if *no* plausible explanation can be suggested, a cause–effect relationship may be difficult to accept,[39] but should probably not be ruled out. Incompatibility with known *facts* weakens the case.

The 'rules of evidence'[36] are not clear-cut, and the appraisal of causality is a matter of judgement. Experts often differ in their conclusions. Critics emphasize this heavy reliance on judgement, stating that 'epidemiological attribution of causation is not a science but an activity more akin to the arguing of a case in law: based on evidence but not dictated by the evidence'—epidemiology cannot produce predictions as reliable as those produced by some other disciplines, and 'cannot be regarded as a scientific discipline because it aims at concrete usefulness rather than abstract truth-fulness'.[40] There is no disagreement, however, about the usefulness of these judgements as a basis for decisions about health care in situations where (as almost always) there is no completely valid answer.

There is usually interest in knowing not only *whether* A is a cause of B, but also *how* it inter-relates with other causes in producing B. We have seen how even simple techniques of analysis can point to the role of an intervening cause (p. 313) and demonstrate modifying effects (p. 309), which often supply clues to the intricacies of causal processes.[41] Multivariate analysis can streamline the production of information about the inter-relationships among a series of factors. It does not, unfortunately, eliminate the need for causal interpretation of the findings.

The temporal characteristics of causes may be of interest. A cause of an infectious disease may influence the probability of infection, of subsequent pathogenesis, or of progression or recovery; and a cause of accidental injuries may influence the probability of accidents or the probability and severity of injury during the event, or it may affect the subsequent course. A distinction may be made between a *predisposing cause* or *precondition*, a *precipitating cause* or *initiator*, and a *promoter* (a later-acting cause in carcinogenesis); *concomitant causes* act simultaneously.

Before leaving the subject of causality, it must be stressed that things may be more complicated than they seem, since not only may one cause have many effects and one effect many causes, but variables may simultaneously have more than one kind of association with each other. For example, there may be a reciprocal causal relationship, where A affects B, and B affects A (A ↔ B). Poverty may be a cause of chronic illness, for example, and chronic illness may lead to poverty. At the same time there may be a secondary association between poverty and chronic illness, due to a common association with an identifiable factor such as ethnic group (A←C→B), or with unknown, possibly remote, common causes (A←?←?→?→B). The association between A and B may thus be partly causal and partly non-causal. A third variable may be both a confounding factor and an intervening cause; or it may have both confounding and modifying effects, and so on. 'O, what a tangled web we perceive.' Even Sir Isaac Newton observed that 'to myself I seem to have been only like a boy playing on the sea-shore, and diverting myself in now and then finding a smoother pebble, or a prettier shell than ordinary, whilst the great ocean of truth lay all undiscovered before me'.[42] But let us take heart—we don't have to find *all* the answers (not all at once, anyway), only *some* useful answers, and this we can do.

NOTES AND REFERENCES

1. *Associations* may be referred to nonspecifically as *relationships* or *concomitant variation* or by a variety of other terms. *Statistical dependence* is a nonspecific statistical term synonymous with 'association'.

    The variables that are associated are usually designated as *dependent* (generally a measure of health status, health behaviour, or health care) and *independent* (see p. 115). The terms *criterion variable* and *response variable* refer to a dependent variable, and independent variables may be called *predictor*, *explanatory*, *stimulus* or *exposure* variables.

    An association is *positive* if the two variables tend to 'go along' with one another. It is *negative*, or *inverse*, if the variables tend to go in opposite directions, e.g. if the presence of one characteristic is associated with the absence of another, or if high values of one variable are associated with low values of another.

    The *appraisal of associations* (epidemiologic inference) and the pros and cons of different measures are discussed in most epidemiology textbooks. They are treated in depth in many writings, including: Rothman K J, Greenland S 1998 (Modern epidemiology, 2nd edn. Lippincott-Raven,

Philadelphia); Kleinbaum D G, Kupper L L, Morgenstern H 1982
(Epidemiologic research: principles and quantitative methods. Lifetime
Learning Publications, Belmont, Cal.); and Greenland S 1997 (Concepts of
validity in epidemiological research. In: Detels R, Holland W W, McEwen J,
Omenn G S, eds. 1997 Oxford Textbook of public health, 3rd edn, vol 2.
The methods of public health. Oxford University Press, New York, pp
597–615).

For exercises in the appraisal of associations, see Abramson J H 1994
(Making sense of data: A self-instruction manual on the interpretation of
epidemiological data, 2nd edn. Oxford University Press, New York).

2. Authors writing about associations between variables vary in their
terminology and often use the same terms with different connotations.
'Spurious' for example, is variously used to refer to artifactual associations,
fortuitous ones, secondary ones, and non-causal associations as a whole. The
terms used in the text of this chapter were chosen because they are relatively
clear and unambiguous. Alternative terms are mentioned in footnotes.

3. Using the symbols shown in Table 28.1, the simplest formula for the *odds
ratio* (also called the *cross-ratio* or *cross-product ratio*) is $ad \div bc$. For the data in
the table this gives a value of 21.0. A slightly more elaborate formula, which
carries certain advantages, is

$$\frac{(a + 0.5)(d + 0.5)}{(a + 0.5)(c + 0.5)}$$

This gives a value of 20.9. The numerators and denominators in these
formulae may be transposed, giving a value of 0.048 (i.e. one twenty-first
instead of 21). These findings may be interpreted as meaning that in this
sample the odds in favour of having anaemia are 21 times higher among
pregnant than among non-pregnant women, or alternatively that the odds in
favour of being pregnant are 21 times higher among anaemic than among
non-anaemic women.

For *paired data* the formula is $(b \div d)$ or $(d \div b)$, using the symbols shown
in note 15, page 293.

Odds ratios (unlike ratios of rates and proportions) can be computed in
case-control studies as well as in cross-sectional and cohort studies. They
have useful properties, but opinions of their utility vary; see, for example:
Nurminen M 1995 (To use or not to use the odds ratio in epidemiologic
analyses? European Journal of Epidemiology 11: 365). For references and a
brief review of their advantages, see Abramson J H 1997 (Cross-sectional
studies. In: Detels R et al 1997 [see note 1], pp 517–535).

4. A *correlation coefficient* indicates the degree to which two variables have a
linear relationship, but does not indicate how much each variable changes
when the other changes; this requires regression analysis.

5. See note 5, page 302 and note 9 below. The 95% confidence interval for the
difference between rates (28%) shown in Table 28.1 is from 26 to 30%.

6. Well, almost anything.

7. Fisher R A 1966 The design of experiments, 8th edn. Oliver & Boyd,
Edinburgh, p. 13.

8. Mainland D 1963 Elementary medical statistics, 2nd edn. Saunders,
Philadelphia, p. 73.

9. *Significance tests* are usually concerned with random sampling variation (see
p. 296). At the risk of oversimplification, most tests can be said to measure
the probability (P) that an association that is as strong as or stronger than
that actually observed will occur in a random sample drawn from a wider
population in which this association does not exist (i.e. in which the null
hypothesis holds true). That is, if a large number of random samples were

drawn from this population, all of the same size as the sample actually studied, in what proportion of them could such an association be expected?

When these tests are used in non-random samples or total populations they are generally based on the notion that the study sample or population is drawn from 'a hypothetical population which would be generated if an indefinitely large number of observations showing the same sort of random variation as those at our disposal could be made'. (Armitage P, Berry G 1994 Statistical methods in medical research, 3rd edn. Blackwell Scientific, Oxford, p. 94). Many statisticians reject this use of what Feinstein 1977 (Clinical Biostatistics. C V Mosby, St Louis, p. 311) has called 'a great imaginary parent population out there somewhere in the sky', and they limit the use of the tests to situations where there is random sampling variation or another 'chance' process, such as random intrapersonal variation, random measurement error, and random permutation of the observations.

Two-tailed or *two-sided* significance tests test the null hypothesis (e.g. that there is no difference between the rates of anaemia in two groups) against the alternative that there is a difference, no matter in what direction. For a *one-tailed (one-sided)* test the alternative is that there is a difference in a prespecified direction (e.g. that there is a higher rate in group 1), and the null hypothesis is that there is not a difference in this direction. It is easier to obtain significance with a one-tailed test. Such a test should be used if, and only if, the null hypothesis and its alternative, stated before the analysis, are such as to warrant its use.

The *P* value is the probability of rejecting the null hypothesis when in fact it is true, i.e. of concluding that there is a real association when actually there is none. This is a type I error. A type II error is the erroneous missing of a true association; the power of a test is its capacity to avoid type II errors.

10. Hamilton M 1974 Lectures on the methodology of clinical research. Churchill Livingstone, Edinburgh, p. 43.
11. Freiman J A, Chalmers T C, Smith H Jr, Kuebler R R 1978 The importance of beta, the type II error and sample size in the design and interpretation of the randomized control trial: survey of 71 'negative' trials. New England Journal of Medicine 299: 690.
12. A *modifier variable* may also be termed an *effect-modifier* or a *moderator* or *qualifier variable*. It may also be called a specifier or conditional variable, terms which do not imply that the association is in fact inconsistent—the variable *specifies* the *conditions* in which the association will be examined. The form of analysis shown in Table 28.2 (subclassification or stratification) may also be termed *specification*.
The associations observed in the separate strata of analysis are *conditional relationships*. If these differ in their strength or direction, there is *statistical interaction* between the independent and modifier variables.
Tests of heterogeneity that compare the associations observed in three or more strata have a low power (they are not very good at determining that the difference is 'true'); to be on the safe side, a *P* value of over 0.1, over 0.2, or even more is generally demanded as reasonable evidence that there is no modifying effect.
13. Morabia A, Have T T, Landis J R 1997 Interaction fallacy. Journal of Clinical Epidemiology 50: 809.
14. MacMahon B, Alpert M, Salbert E J 1966 Infant weight and parental smoking habits. American Journal of Epidemiology 82: 247.
15. Labovitz S, Hagedorn S 1971 Introduction to social research. McGraw-Hill, New York, pp 80–81.
16. Harvey I, Frankel S, Marks R, Shalom D, Morgan M 1997 Foot morbidity and exposure to chiropody: population based study. British Medical Journal 315: 1054.

17. *Confounding* has diverse definitions. The working definition used here is that the measure of association has different values when the confounder is ignored and when its effects are held constant (by stratification, standardization or other methods). The presence and degree of confounding may vary, depending on what measure of association is used.

For a fuller simple description of confounding, see Rothman K J, Greenland S 1998 ([see note 1], pp 59–62, 120–126). Confounding is termed 'comparison bias' by Greenland S 1997 (see note 1).

A confounding variable may also be referred to as a *disturbing* or *nuisance* variable.

The term 'intervening variable' is best avoided, as it may be misinterpreted as meaning an intervening cause (see note 28, below). A secondary association may also be called an *indirect association*—which may be misconstrued as an indirect causal association (see note 28, below)—or a spurious association, a term which has several other connotations (see note 2).

18. A term suggested by Susser M 1973 (Causal thinking in the health sciences. Oxford University Press, New York).

19. Confounding may occur even when the crude data do not demonstrate associations between the suspected confounder (C) and variables A (independent) and B (dependent), since *conditional associations* that satisfy the requirements may be present. These are associations that exist under specified conditions—in this instance an association with A in the study population when B is held constant, and an association with B when A is held constant.

20. Several procedures that control for confounding effects (multiple logistic and Poisson regression, Mantel–Haenszel and random-effects procedures for rates and proportions, etc.) are provided by the PEPI package (see note 7, p. 292).

21. *Overadjustment:* see Day N E, Byar D P, Green S B 1980 (Overadjustment in case-control studies. American Journal of Epidemiology 112: 696), and subsequent correspondence in American Journal of Epidemiology 1982 115: 797 and 799.

22. Rules for deciding whether C's relationships with A and B are strong enough to account for the association observed between A and B are provided by Bross I D J 1966 (Spurious effects from an extraneous variable. Journal of Chronic Diseases 19: 637) and 1967 (Pertinency of an extraneous variable. Journal of Chronic Diseases 20: 487). For the 'direction rule', see Abramson 1994 ([see note 1], pp 210–211).

23. Molbak K, Jensen H, Ingholt L, Aaby P 1997 Risk factors for diarrhoeal disease incidence in early childhood: a community cohort study from Guinea-Bissau. American Journal of Epidemiology 146: 273.

24. Illsley R, Le Grand J 1993 Regional inequalities in mortality. Journal of Epidemiology and Community Health 47: 444.

25. For epidemiologists' views concerning *causality* and how to make judgements about causation, see collections assembled by Greenland S (ed) 1987 (Evolution of epidemiologic ideas: annotated readings on concepts and methods. Epidemiologic Resources, Chestnut Hill, Mass.) and Rothman K J (ed) 1988 (Causal inference. Epidemiologic Resources, Chestnut Hill, Mass.).

Also, see: Susser M 1973 (see note 18); Rothman K J, Greenland S 1997 (Causation and causal inference. In: Detels R, Holland W W, McEwen J, Omenn G S, eds. 1997 Oxford Textbook of public health, 3rd edn, vol 2. The methods of public health. Oxford University Press, New York, pp 617–629; also in: Rothman K J, Greenland S 1998 Modern epidemiology, 2nd edn. Lippincott-Raven, Philadelphia, pp 7–28); Charlton B G 1996 (Attribution of causation in epidemiology: chain or mosaic? Annals of

Epidemiology 49: 105); and Weed D L 1997 (On the use of causal criteria. International Journal of Epidemiology 26: 1137).
For papers stressing social and ecological processes, see note 11, p. 32.

26. MacMahon B, Pugh T F 1970 Epidemiology: principles and methods. Little, Brown, Boston, Mass., pp 17–27.

27. 'A causal relationship would be recognized to exist whenever evidence indicates that the factors form part of a complex of circumstances that increases the probability of occurrence of a disease and that a diminution of one or more of these factors decreases the frequency of that disease' (Lilienfeld A M, Lilienfeld D E 1980 Foundations of epidemiology, 2nd edn. Oxford University Press, New York, p. 295).

28. We can never speak of A as *the* cause of B. A always has its own determinants, and these are also causes of B. Moreover, as we learn more about the mechanism by which A affects B we can usually interpose *intervening (mediating) causes*, thereby changing A from a *direct* cause (A → B) to an *indirect* one (A → X → Y → Z → B). A cause is seldom *sufficient* to produce an effect without the participation of other causes—the outcome of exposure to pathogenic germs, for example, depends upon the susceptibility of the persons exposed. Sometimes A can be defined as a *necessary* cause of B, without which B cannot occur. But this need not mean that there are no other causes of importance; only a small fraction of people infected with the tubercle bacillus become ill with tuberculosis, indicating that factors other than the bacillus (the necessary cause) play a crucial role.
According to the 'constellations of causes' concept explained in the text, causes are components of various alternative constellations, each of which is sufficient to cause the effect in an individual, and all causes are necessary (in the specific constellations in which they feature).

29. Rothman K J 1976 Causes. American Journal of Epidemiology 104: 587.

30. There is an extreme view, which most epidemiologists do not share, that epidemiological evidence alone, without laboratory and clinical studies that support and explain a cause—effect relationship, can never be conclusive enough to warrant a preventive programme (Charlton B G 1995 A critique of Geoffrey Rose's 'population strategy' for preventive medicine. Journal of the Royal Society of Medicine 88: 607). In this view, a preventive strategy at the population level is justified only if the 'black box' concealing the mysteries of causal mechanisms has been opened (Skrabanek P 1994 The emptiness of the black box. Epidemiology 5: 553).
Examples that refute this view include: the link between a dearth of fresh fruit and scurvy, demonstrated in 1753, long before vitamins were thought of; between exposure to soot and scrotal cancer, in 1775, when the carcinogenic role of polycyclic aromatic hydrocarbons was undreamt of; between polluted water and cholera, in 1855, before bacteria had been discovered; between a poor diet and pellagra at the beginning of the 20th century, when this was thought to be a communicable disease; between smoking and lung cancer and other diseases before the pathogenetic mechanisms were understood; and, more recently, between putting babies to sleep on their tummies and the sudden infant death syndrome.

31. Robertson L S 1998 Causal webs, preventive brooms, and housekeepers. Social Science and Medicine 46: 53.

32. Krieger N 1994 Epidemiology and the web of causation: has anyone seen the spider? Social Science and Medicine 39: 887.

33. The 'Chinese box' metaphor was suggested by Susser M, Susser E 1996 (Choosing a future for epidemiology: II. From black box to Chinese boxes and eco-epidemiology. American Journal of Public Health 86: 674).
Metaphors suggested by Krieger 1994 (see note 32) are a web spun by two spiders (one social and one biologic) or, preferably, a fractal structure—a

'branching bush' pattern repeated indefinitely at every level, subcellular to societal.

34. For papers on the *use of experimental principles in non-experimental studies*, see Horwitz R I, Feinstein A R 1981 (The application of therapeutic-trial principles to improve the design of epidemiologic research: a case-control study suggesting that anticoagulants reduce mortality in patients with myocardial infarction. Journal of Chronic Diseases 34: 575); and Esdaile J M, Horwitz R I 1986 (Observational studies of cause–effect relationships: an analysis of methodologic problems as illustrated by the conflicting data for the role of oral contraceptives in the etiology of rheumatoid arthritis. Journal of Chronic Diseases 39: 841).

35. Contradictory results from case-control studies are listed by Mayes L C, Horwitz R O, Feinstein A R 1988 (A collection of 56 topics with contradictory results in case-control research. International Journal of Epidemiology 17: 680).

    In a prospective survey in which precautions were taken to control bias and confounding, Gray-Donald K and Kramer M S 1988 (Causality inference in observational vs. experimental studies: an empirical comparison. American Journal of Epidemiology 127: 885) found a clear association between formula supplementation of newborn babies in hospital, and a low breast-feeding rate at 9 weeks; but a controlled trial conducted in the same hospital demonstrated no association at all. This discrepancy was probably mainly attributable to confounders that were controlled in the trial but not measured (and therefore not controllable) in the survey (mothers' motivation to breast-feed and the occurrence of sore nipples or other indications for formula feeding).

36. These *criteria for the appraisal of causality*, or similar ones, are explained in all epidemiology textbooks. Their resemblance to the *Rules by which to judge of causes and effects* written by the philosopher Hume in 1740 has been pointed out by Morabia A 1991 (On the origins of Hill's causal criteria. Epidemiology 2: 367).

    The list in the text is based in part on Susser M 1986 (The logic of Sir Karl Popper and the practice of epidemiology. American Journal of Epidemiology 124: 711). See also: Hill A B 1965 (The environment and disease: association or causation? Proceedings of the Royal Society of Medicine 58: 296); Surgeon-General's Advisory Committee on Smoking and Health 1964 (Smoking and health. Public Health Service Publication no 1103, Department of Health, Education and Welfare, Rockville, Md); and Susser M 1973 and the other references cited in note 25.

    For an illustration of how judgements using the same criteria may differ, see a debate by Burch P R J and Lilienfeld A M on the evidence concerning smoking and lung cancer: Journal of Chronic Diseases 1983 36: 821, 837 and 1984 37: 148.

37. Coronary Drug Project Research Group 1980 Influence of adherence to treatment and response of cholesterol to mortality in the Coronary Drug Project. New England Journal of Medicine 303: 1038.

38. Susser M 1985 Falsification, verification, and causal inference in epidemiology: reconsiderations in the light of Sir Karl Popper's philosophy. In: Susser M 1987 Epidemiology, health, and society. Oxford University Press, New York, pp 82–93. Also in: Rothman K J (ed) 1988 (see note 25), pp 33–57.

39. The story (possibly true) is told of a trial comparing two treatments. When the statistician announced that one drug was superior, the researchers explained why this result could have been predicted, on the basis of prior knowledge about absorption, metabolism, tolerance, etc. When the statistician announced that he had confused the drugs, and it was the other

that was superior, there was a short silence, and then a discussion that explained why the new result was consistent with expectations (Park C B 1981 Attributable risk for recurrent events: an extension of Levin's measure. American Journal of Epidemiology 113: 491).

A paper on the 'biological plausibility' criterion points out that associations between smoking and subsequent suicide and between smoking and subsequent murder, detected in a large US risk factor study, are unlikely to be causal because they are biologically implausible (although they are strong, show clear dose-response relationships, and remain apparent when obvious confounders are controlled). 'It is likely that many more such associations ... are equally spurious, but are protected by their lack of obvious implausibility' (Smith G D, Phillips A N, Neaton J D 1992 Smoking as 'independent' risk factor for suicide: illustration of an artifact from observational epidemiology? Lancet 340: 709).

When a study of Kenyan prostitutes showed that oral contraceptive use was related to risk of future HIV infection, several hypothetical mechanisms were forthcoming (Plummer F A, Simonsen J N, Cameron D W et al 1991 Cofactors in male–female sexual transmission of human immunodeficiency virus type 1. Journal of Infectious Diseases 163: 233), but when a later study in Italians found that oral contraceptive use apparently protected against HIV infection, a plausible biological explanation was again available (Lazzarin A, Saracco A, Musicco M, Nicolosi A 1991 Man-to-woman sexual transmission of the human immunodeficiency virus. Risk factors related to sexual behavior, man's infectiousness, and woman's susceptibility. Archives of Internal Medicine 151: 2411).

40. Charlton B G 1996 (see note 25).
41. *Effect modification.* All effect modifiers are causes. Causes that have the same effect (i.e. that act on a common intermediate factor or process) may complement each other and manifest synergism (a more-than-multiplicative joint effect). Causes that operate along the same pathway (one cause setting the stage for another) may have a multiplicative joint effect. Causes that operate in different pathways can have an almost additive joint effect. In each of these instances the joint effects may be less marked if other pathways are involved. If a cause–effect association is positive in some strata and negative in others, the cause is both a risk factor and a preventive factor, with a varying balance between these actions.

For an in-depth discussion of joint effects (take your bathyscaphe with you!) see Koopman J S, Weed D L 1990 (Epigenesis theory: a mathematical model relating causal concepts of pathogenesis in individuals to disease patterns in populations. American Journal of Epidemiology 132: 366); or (if they are still accessible on the Internet) find a lecture given by Koopman in 1997 (www.sph.umich.edu/group/epid/epid655/1997/lecmr19a.htm and lecmr19b.htm) and the 77 slides used in a lecture in 1998 (http://www.sph.umich.edu/group/epid/epid655/ThirdVar/index.htm).
42. Brewster D 1885 Memoirs of the life of Sir Isaac Newton, vol 2, Ch. 27.

29 Application of the study findings

As part of the process of interpreting the study findings, thought should be given to the ways in which they can be applied. This chapter deals with two aspects: generalizations to a broader or different population, and the practical implications of the results.

GENERALIZATION FROM THE FINDINGS

We will often want to generalize from our findings. We may in fact have chosen the population we studied or sampled because we believed it was typical of a broader 'reference population' or an 'external population' to which we wished to generalize the findings. Even if the study population was not chosen on these grounds, every population may be regarded as a part of a wider population, and we are often tempted to make generalizations. Having studied varicose veins in a single study neighbourhood, we may want to draw conclusions about their prevalence in the population at large, or to arrive at generalities, going beyond the population that was studied, about the strength of the association of varicose veins with fatness or leanness, the importance of occupation or tight garments as causal factors, and so on.

Consideration must therefore be given to the study's *generalizability* (external validity, 'representativeness'), unless interest is limited to the specific population studied. The study may be of solely local interest if it was performed in a practical setting as an aid in the planning, monitoring or evaluation of a specific health care programme—in, for example, community-oriented primary health care (see Ch. 34), health care in a school or workplace, or district health care. Even in such instances, possible applications of the findings in other contexts may be contemplated.

Generalization from a sample to the study population requires allowance for random sampling variation, by computing confidence intervals (see p. 296). Confidence intervals are sometimes computed even when generalizations are made to a reference population from which the sample was *not* randomly chosen (e.g. to 'patients with peptic ulcer' or 'Canadian men');[1] this use of confidence intervals is open to debate.

The main issue is whether the external population is sufficiently similar to the study population to warrant extrapolation of the findings. Are the people similar, and are their circumstances (including health care) similar? Can the findings in one neighbourhood be applied to another? Can they be applied to the general population? Are the results of a study in one sex applicable to the other? Are the results applicable to other ethnic or age groups? Such questions may be difficult to answer. Populations and population groups differ in their health status, in the occurrence of risk and protective factors, and in their health care and other circumstances and exposures that may affect their health or the effectiveness of interventions. Causal processes that are important in one population may be unimportant in another; not only may the prevalence of anaemia differ in a slum and a well-off neighbourhood, but different causes may operate in the two areas, or the modifying factors affecting their operation may vary—so that the risk associated with dietary iron deficiency may differ, and so may the effectiveness of routine administration of iron or other supplements to pregnant women.

All this may seem obvious, yet how often do we read a statement like 'Conflicting findings are reported in the literature; A and B found something or other, C and D found something quite different, and E found something else again, which was not confirmed by F et al', without any designation or description of the populations studied by these investigators, let alone any effort to explain the discrepancies?

Although wide use was made of the results of the Framingham Heart Study concerning risk factors for heart disease, for many years there was uncertainty about the generalizability of the results; the study started with a set of volunteers, who were then supplemented by a random sample of the town's population—with a response rate of 69%. Only in 1987, almost 40 years after the inception of the study, was it possible to compare the findings with those of a cohort study of a national probability sample and confirm that the Framingham risk model predicted coronary deaths in the national sample 'remarkably well'.[2]

A decision to beware of generalization may be easy if there is sufficient selection bias to impair a study's internal validity (see p. 296), since this will obviously also impair its external validity. Also, if the study was done in a very 'special' population (see p. 73) application of the findings to the general population may clearly be problematic; some study populations are representative of nothing but themselves. A common instance is the application of strict eligibility and exclusion criteria when selecting subjects for a clinical trial; this raises obvious doubts about general clinical relevance—in two recent drug trials, for example, only 17% and 9% of patients could be included in the study.[3] Usually there is no simple foolproof way of deciding on generalizability. What is often done is to compare the demographic and other known characteristics of the study and reference populations, or of the patients included and excluded, so as to see whether there are obvious differences that may affect comparability. It may then be possible to try to compensate for these differences by making adjustments like those described on page 299.

Three questions that may not be obvious but are often worth asking are:

1. *Why was this study population chosen?* The reasons for the choice may be reflected in the findings—was the population chosen because of a high prevalence of a disease or drug addiction or broken homes, or because of its ethnic heterogeneity or residential stability, or a local community's special interest in a health problem, etc.? In an evaluative study, reasons with a possible bearing on health care are of particular importance. The study population may have been 'chosen' simply because the investigator was responsible for its health care, or because the staff of a particular clinic or health centre were motivated to perform or join in a study. Might this interest in research be a symptom of a high general standard of care? Was there special enthusiasm about the treatment or programme that was evaluated? And may this have influenced effectiveness? Was the study population chosen because there were especially good clinical records, or because special facilities were available? Was it chosen because a high level of co-operation or compliance was expected? Or was a captive population selected, whose diet or medical treatment

could be manipulated with ease? If the population was selected because it was exposed to a novel health programme, *why* was this programme provided in this particular setting?

2. *May the study itself have produced an effect?* One distinctive feature of every study population is that a study was performed in it. Sometimes the performance of the study may in itself affect the results. Interviews and examinations, and especially the 'feedback' of examination findings to subjects, may lead to changes in health practices and health care. This possibility should be considered in longitudinal studies, particularly if investigations were repeated frequently; weekly weighing of infants, or weekly interviews about their diet, may modify the growth pattern. The effect of the study itself is especially important in evaluative studies, where the subjects may be affected by their awareness that they are participating in an experiment, as well as by the experimental situation as a whole (see p. 84).

3. *Do operational definitions or other features of the study limit its applicability?* A study of the prognosis of diabetes may have limited relevance to diabetics diagnosed by other criteria, and the results of an evaluation of a diagnostic or surgical procedure performed by experts may not be applicable if the procedure is performed by people less skilled.

PRACTICAL IMPLICATIONS

It is arguable that just as every one of Aesop's fables has its moral ('Be content with your lot', 'Do not count your chickens before they are hatched', etc.), so should every study's findings be complemented by a statement of practical implications—what (if anything) ought to be done, and what are the expected consequences of doing or not doing it. Remember Will Rogers' salutary epigram 'The more we find out about anything the less we ever do about it'.

A clear-cut message concerning practical implications may reduce the likelihood that the findings will be ignored or misapplied. Decision makers, health workers and the public at large often exhibit two opposing tendencies: on the one hand, to disregard research findings or unnecessarily delay their application; and, on the other, to be unduly credulous and rush into injudicious action. The latter—and probably more regrettable—propensity generally results from undue reliance on a single study, ignoring the fact that different studies of the same topic often produce different results,[4,5] as a result of chance variation, differences in methods or circumstances, or differences between study populations. There is insufficient realization that 'what medical journals publish is not received wisdom, but rather working papers ... Each study becomes a piece of a puzzle that, when assembled, will help either to confirm or to refute a hypothesis'.[4] Also, associations are too readily taken to mean causation, methodological shortcomings are too readily overlooked, and the specific circumstances in which the results may be applicable, as well as contraindications, may be ignored.

The minimal requirement is to specify whatever reservations there may be about the validity of the findings, to say whether there is a need to confirm conclusions by replicating the study or conducting other research, and (if relevant) to present the findings in a manner that facilitates decisions concerning possible changes in the provision of medical care, public health action, health behaviour, or other spheres. Many feel that this not enough and that the investigator should *always* go further and make recommendations on whether and how the study's results should be used, not just 'light the touch paper and then stand back'.[6] Whether this kind of advocacy is an ethical obligation is open to discussion,[7] but it is probably a good thing to do, provided that the recommendations are based on an unbiased consideration of all the available objective evidence and are presented only as opinions. A reasonable role is that of the 'thoughtful advocate', who 'acknowledges uncertainties, anticipates policy option consequences, and balances consequences of intervention versus no intervention'.[8]

In other words, after reviewing the findings the investigator should always ask 'So what?', should supply facts that can form a useful basis for an answer to this question, and should consider providing a thoughtful answer based on the available information. Needs for further research and new investigative tools should be spelled out in detail, unless the conclusions can be regarded as definitive, with no need for confirmation. Even then there may be suggestions for new lines of study, or new hypotheses to be tested.

To help in formulating recommendations about practical applications and, subsequently, in decisions about their implementation, 'action-oriented' indices[9] (based on ancillary data when necessary as well as on the study findings) may be desirable; these may necessitate new analyses. For example, if intervention directed at a risk factor is under consideration, the attributable fraction in the population[10] would be a useful measure; this is an estimate of the proportion of cases in a given population that (under certain assumptions)[10] can be attributed to the risk factor and would be prevented if the risk factor were eliminated. It is a much more helpful basis for decisions than (say) a rate ratio or odds ratio. A large case-control study in New York revealed a weak association between breast cancer and ever taking alcoholic drinks, with an odds ratio (controlling for numerous confounders) of only 1.4, but because of the high prevalence (83%) of drinking, the attributable fraction was appreciable: '25% of breast cancer among these women ... is attributable to ever drinking alcohol'.[11] The absolute number of cases caused is often of more interest than any ratio. At the level of lifestyle changes by the individual, it is less useful to know that there is a statistically significant dose-response relationship between the consumption of fruit and vegetables and cancer, than to know by how much the risk decreases per serving.[12] As a guide to clinical practice, answers to specific questions like 'What is the risk of cardiovascular disease among healthy non-smoking young women who use combined oral contraceptives?'[13] are more useful than overall findings controlling for effects related to health, smoking and age.

If the introduction of a specific preventive procedure is being considered, the preventable fraction in the population (what proportion of cases would be prevented?) can be estimated and translated into terms of (for example) doctor visits, hospital beds, disability, or deaths. Also, it is very easy to estimate the number of people to whom the procedure must be applied in order to prevent one case,[14] and this can be converted to economic terms. Similar indices can be used to express the expected impact of therapeutic procedures. If screening is under consideration, useful indices include the numbers of tests and positive tests required in a given population to identify one case; measures of gain in certainty[15] may be helpful with respect to decisions about diagnostic tests.

If recommendations are made, it may be necessary to qualify them by specifying the conditions necessary for their application, and by limiting them to specific populations or circumstances.

NOTES AND REFERENCES

1. See citation from Armitage and Berry 1994 in note 9, page 323.
2. Leaverton P E, Sorlie P D, Kleinman J C, Dannenberg A L, Ingster-Moore L, Kannel W B, Cornoni-Huntley J C 1987 Representativeness of the Framingham risk model for coronary heart disease mortality: a comparison with a national cohort study. Journal of Chronic Diseases 40: 775.

3. In a trial of antimanic treatment, only 17% of consecutively admitted patients meeting the inclusion criteria (area of residence, age, diagnosis, severity of illness) could be included in the study. There were substantial differences between the included and excluded patients (Licht R W, Gouliaev G, Vestergaard P, Frydenberg M 1997 Generalisability of results from randomised drug trials: a trial on antimanic treatment. British Journal of Psychiatry 170: 264).

   In a trial of schizophrenia treatment, on the other hand, the authors concluded that the selection bias had little clinical relevance (except for inferences relating to some small subgroups of patients), although only 22% of diagnostically appropriate patients met the eligibility criteria and only 9% entered the study (Robinson D, Woerner M G, Pollack S, Lerner G 1996 Subject selection biases in clinical trials: data from a multicenter schizophrenia treatment study. Journal of Clinical Psychopharmacology 16: 170).

4. Angell M, Kassirer J P 1994 Clinical research—what should the public believe? New England Journal of Medicine 331: 189–190.

5. Taubes G 1995 Epidemiology faces its limits. Science 269: 164–169.

6. Pharaoh P 1996 Bed-sharing and sudden infant death. Lancet 347: 2.

7. Weed D L 1994 Science, ethics guidelines, and advocacy in epidemiology. Annals of Epidemiology 4: 166.

8. Savitz D A, Greenland S, Stolley P D, Kelsey J L 1990 Scientific standards of criticism: a reaction to 'Scientific standards in epidemiologic studies of the menace of daily life' by A. R. Feinstein. Epidemiology 1: 78.

9. PEPI programs (see note 7, p. 292) can compute the indices mentioned in the text.

10. The simplest formula for the attributable fraction in the population is $(R_p - R_u)/R_p$, where R_p is the rate in the population and R_u is the rate in people unexposed to the causal factor. An alternative formula is $P_e(RR - 1)/[1 + P_e (RR - 1]$, where P_e is the proportion of the population exposed to the factor and RR is the ratio R_e/R_u, where R_e is the rate in people exposed to the causal factor.

    This measure assumes that the risk factor is causal. Its use to indicate the proportion of preventable cases is meaningful only if the factor can be eliminated and it can be assumed that this would reduce the risk. See Rockhill B, Newman B, Weinberg C 1998 (Use and misuse of population attributable fractions. American Journal of Public Health 88: 15).

11. Bowlin S J, Leske M C, Varma A, Nasca P, Weinstein A, Caplan L 1997 Breast cancer risk and alcohol consumption: results from a large case-control study. International Journal of Epidemiology 26: 915.

12. Colditz G A 1997 Epidemiology—future directions. International Journal of Epidemiology 26: 693.

13. A review of 74 studies about combined oral contraceptives and cardiovascular disease revealed only five that addressed the cited question, and 14 others that did not, although they probably had the necessary data (Hannaford P C, Owen-Smith V 1998 Using epidemiological data to guide clinical practice: review of studies on cardiovascular disease and use of combined oral contraceptives. British Medical Journal 316: 984).

14. The number of people to whom a procedure (preventive or therapeutic) must be applied in order to prevent one case, complication or death is the reciprocal of the difference between the rates or proportions (incidence or mortality) in the study samples exposed and not exposed to the procedure. For example, if the rates are 5 and 3 per 1000 respectively (i.e. 0.005 and 0.003), this number is 1:(0.005–0.003), or 500. If the calculation is based on person-year rates the number obtained is the required number of person-years of exposure.

15. See note 33, page 203.

30 Writing a report

' "Ouch! Have a heart, Doc!" spluttered shapely Dolores X, the last of my hundred age and sex-matched controls, as I struggled to find her vein. "Do you really *have* to have my blood to find out whether people with malignant lymphogranuloma have a lot of antibody to some silly old virus?" ' may be overdoing it somewhat as an introductory paragraph in a scientific report. But it serves to draw attention to the need for readability—a report should be written so as to attract, or at all events not repel, potential readers. To do this, it need not be written as a farce, a whodunit, or a lyric poem, but it should fulfil the following criteria:

1. The title should clearly explain what the report is about; if necessary, a subtitle can be added for extra clarity. A prospective reader usually looks first at the contents page of a journal, to see which titles 'tickle his fancy'. A journal is 'an open market where each salesman must cry his goods if he wishes to get an audience at his stall'.[1]

2. The abstract should be informative. A reader who has been attracted by the title will usually look at the abstract next, to decide whether the report is worth reading. 'The summary is your advertisement',[2] and should provide a picture in miniature of the whole report. It should include the objectives, specify the study population, and summarize the findings and discussion. Salient numerical details may—even should—be included. Many journals request structured abstracts, with subheadings such as Background, Objectives, Methods (or Design, Setting, Sample, Measures), Results, and Conclusions.

3. The report should be easily intelligible.[3] This requires clarity of language (this is preferable to elegance of style), a logical presentation of facts and inferences, the use of easily understood tables and charts, and an orderly arrangement of the report as a whole. A scientific report may be Greek to the layman, but it should be easily understood by the readers for whom it is written. A report's style and content should be appropriate for its expected readers; a report written for the general public or political decision makers would obviously differ from one aimed at a professional public.

4. The report should be no longer than is necessary. Unnecessary verbiage should be removed, and the report pruned to the minimum required for clearly communicating what has to be communicated. This process of pruning and condensing is not an easy one (who was it who apologized for sending a long letter by saying that he had not had the time to write a short one?).

Writing a good report may take much time and effort. The most difficult task is usually the preparation of the first draft, since this requires a crystallization of the investigator's ideas on how best to express his facts and inferences; subsequent revisions are usually easier. Comments from colleagues are often useful. Many writers find it helpful to tuck a draft in a drawer—or let it rest in peace on a computer disk—and bring it out for a fresh look after a few weeks.

No investigation is complete until a report has been written. Even if the results are of interest only to the investigator, they should be placed on record, albeit in a short and even handwritten form. If they are of wider interest, they should be made available to a wider audience. Whether they should be published in print is a question for the investigator (and later, of course, an editor or publisher) to decide. Particularly in academic fields, there is a tendency to publish whenever possible, because of the stress laid on the number or weight of publications when decisions are made about hiring, firing, promotion and tenure.

This 'Publish or perish!'[4] motivation apart, publication may often be seen as an obligation. The investigator may feel a duty to communicate his results, 'positive' or 'negative', to others who may be able to replicate his findings, build their own research efforts upon them, or apply them in action. An editorial in the *British Medical Journal* relates that Kocher's method of reducing dislocations of the shoulder was regarded as an innovation when it was described in a German medical journal in 1870. His method had been portrayed 3000 years earlier, however, in a wall painting in a tomb in the Nile Valley. 'The moral of this episode,' says the editorialist, 'is clear. Recognition of original work can be ensured only by publication in a reputable journal'.[5]

Succinct advice on the writing of a paper is to be found in a document describing 'uniform requirements for manuscripts submitted to biomedical journals (the Vancouver style)', prepared by a committee of editors.[6] Over 500 journals have sanctioned these guidelines. Some journals, however, have their own requirements, particularly for the format of references; consult the journal's 'advice to contributors'.

To be useful, a report should not only give the results of the study and the inferences that have been drawn from them, but also enough information about the methods to enable a critical reader to appraise the validity of the findings and conclusions or (ideally) to check the findings by replicating the study. The report should include a description of the study population and its characteristics and information (if relevant) about methods and criteria used for choosing subjects or groups, sampling and randomization procedures, response rates, representativeness of samples, comparability of groups, reasons for non-participation and withdrawals, etc. Operational definitions (including diagnostic criteria) should be specified. Ideally, the description of the methods should be a detailed one. Unfortunately (or fortunately?) this is usually practicable only in books or dissertations required for university degrees, and as a rule only the highlights can be described. The rest has to be taken on trust.

To help the reader to make his judgement, the investigator should himself offer an honest and critical appraisal of the study, and point out and discuss the main sources of possible error. Possible biases should be stated and not left for others to reveal.

Where possible, facts should be presented in a form that may be useful to other investigators who prefer to use different categories or indices when measuring variables, e.g. by presenting full frequency distributions rather than 'collapsed' scales and combinations of categories.

Tables and figures should be well enough titled and captioned and (if necessary) have enough footnotes to be reasonably intelligible without reference to the text.

The tables should be well constructed, and without anomalies such as totals that do not tally, percentages that do not add up to about 100% (say between 99.8 and 100.2%), and the use of too many decimal places. If percentages are used, no doubt should be left as to what the denominator is (it is often helpful to add '100%' in the requisite place).

Diagrams should clarify and not complicate, and care should be taken that they do not mislead.[7] They should serve to explain tables and should not replace them, unless the investigator is sure the reader will not require numerical data. If curves have been 'smoothed', the method used should be stated. There are many computer programs that can draw diagrams.

The results of statistical procedures should be given in numbers and not just words (and preferably not only in pictures). Until lately, many writers and some editors felt that a sprinkling of P values lent a report an aura of scientific respectability, but the pendulum has now swung away from significance tests towards confidence intervals. The advice in the 'Vancouver style' guidelines is:

> When possible, quantify findings and present them with appropriate indicators of measurement error or uncertainty (such as confidence intervals). Avoid relying solely on statistical hypothesis testing, such as the use of P values, which fails to convey important quantitative information.[6]

References should be carefully checked. A few small errors are probably inevitable; but an examination of a random sample of references in three public health journals found that in 15% the cited reference 'failed to substantiate, was unrelated to, or even contradicted the author's assertation', and 3% had major citation errors ('reference not locatable'). Minor citation errors were rife.[8]

The report should include a clear statement of the author's views about whether further research is needed (and if so, what); recommendations (if any) about the practical application of the results—i.e. whether and how they should be applied, and any cautions about their application—should be very explicit. This may not only be helpful to readers who may wish to extend or apply the research, but it may help journalists, assiduously hunting for 'news' in the columns of scientific journals, to avoid exaggerating the importance of findings, overstating health hazards, or suggesting unwarranted changes in lifestyle or health care.

ORAL REPORTS

Study findings are often reported orally, especially to colleagues or students and at scientific meetings. Oral reports are generally very different from written ones; they are much less complete and are often accompanied by more (but simplified) tabular or graphic material, and the sequence of presentation may be altered to maintain interest or stimulate discussion. Just as much care should be taken, however, to present the methods and findings accurately, to point out possible sources of error in the data and the inferences, and if there are recommendations, to make them even-handed.

Especial care is needed in reports to journalists. Investigators sometimes make exaggerated claims or statements to reporters (as do their research institutions in press releases), going beyond what is said or will be said in the published study report. 'Preliminary' announcements of results, prior to the study's completion, may be hazardous.

NOTES AND REFERENCES

1. Asher R 1958 Why are medical journals so dull? British Medical Journal ii: 502.
2. Dart R A, Galloway A 1934 Memorandum on writing a scientific paper. Department of Anatomy, University of the Witwatersrand (Roneo), Johannesburg.
3. The need for intelligibility was realized by Geoffrey Chaucer in the 14th century when he departed from tradition and wrote a scientific treatise in simple English rather than in Latin, in order to explain the astrolabe to his son: 'This tretis, divided in fyve parties, wole I shewe thee under ful lighte rewles and naked wordes in English; for Latin ne canstow yit but small, my lyte sone. But natheles, suffyse to thee thise trewe conclusiouns in English, as wel as suffyseth to thise noble clerkes Grekes thise same conclusiouns in Greek, and to Arabiens in Arabik, and to Jewes in Ebrew, and to the Latin folk in Latin' (Chaucer G A Treatise on the astrolabe. Cited by Gordon I S, Sorkin S 1959 The Armchair Science Reader. Simon & Schuster, New York, p. 294).
4. The pressure to publish is so strong that some investigators are led to falsify data or to pirate papers. *Scientific fraud* is usually undiscovered or (if unmasked) unreported. From the little evidence available, 'the best estimate today is perhaps that the prevalence of fraud is between 0.25% and 0.5% of research projects' (Lock S 1997 Fraud in medical research. Journal of the Royal College of Physicians of London 31: 90). For examples, see: Broad W J 1981 (Fraud and the structure of science. Science 212: 137, 264); Broad W J, Wade N 1982 (Betrayers of the truth. Simon & Schuster, New York); Stewart W W, Feder N 1987 (The integrity of the scientific literature. Nature 325: 207). One researcher who submitted reports containing repeated falsifications received nearly $1 million in cancer research funds.
5. Editorial 1968 Where to publish? British Medical Journal 4: 344.
6. The *Vancouver style* guidelines (5th edn) are published by several journals. See, for example, International Committee of Medical Journal Editors 1997 (Uniform requirements for manuscripts submitted to biomedical journals. Annals of Internal Medicine 126: 36). They are also available from several sources on the Internet, e.g. www.acponline.org/journals/resource/resortoc.htm
7. For misuses of diagrams, see Huff D, Geis I 1993 (How to lie with statistics. W W Norton, New York).

8. Eichorn P, Yankauer A 1987 Do authors check their references? A survey of accuracy in three public health journals. American Journal of Public Health 77: 1011.

Similar levels of inaccuracy of quotations and citations of references have been reported in numerous medical, dental and nursing journals. The following advice, given towards the beginning of the 20th century, is apparently not yet followed: 'Take no reference for granted. Verify the reference that your best friend gives you. Verify the reference that your revered chief gives you. Verify, most of all, the references that you yourself found and jotted down. To err is human, to verify is necessary' (Place F Jr 1916 Verify your references: a word to medical writers. New York Medical Journal 104: 697). We borrowed this reference from Putterman C, Lossos I S 1991 (Author, verify your references! or, The accuracy of references in Israeli medical journals. Israel Journal of Medical Sciences 27: 109), who apparently copied it from Roland C G 1976 (Thoughts about medical writing. XXXVII. Verify your references. Anesthesia and Analgesia 55: 717). Readers are advised to verify it!

31 Rapid epidemiological methods

The terms 'rapid epidemiological methods', 'rapid appraisal', and 'rapid assessment' usually refer to simplified procedures that can speed up a study, providing real-time results as a basis for programme decisions.[1] In a district of Uganda, only 10 days were required to collect, analyze and publish information on the utilization of health services, health-seeking behaviour, immunization coverage, and the nutritional status of children;[2] a 50-page report of the findings of a health survey of children in a town in Burma was also issued 10 days after the commencement of field work, as was a 70-page report on surveys of antenatal care and family planning in Thailand.[3]

Since these rapid methods are relatively undemanding and inexpensive, they are usually advocated for use in developing countries. They may, however, be useful wherever manpower, finances or other research resources are limited, as in many studies carried out by practitioners in the context of community health services in developed countries. Some rapid methods (not discussed in this chapter) involve the use of sophisticated and expensive electronic communication and processing techniques.

Simplified methods may provide less detailed or valid information than would be provided by more rigorous methods. They are to an extent 'quick and dirty', and the key question to be asked before using them is whether their results can adequately meet the study's purpose. Can the direction and degree of inaccuracy be estimated, and are the results likely to be useful despite their margin of error? If so, there is no reason not to use simple procedures, particularly if the alternative is to obtain no information at all. Care must be taken of course to avoid unnecessary inaccuracy, e.g. by giving due attention to the training of data collectors and by checking completed questionnaires and the coding of data.

We will give separate consideration to four aspects: simplified sampling procedures (especially the use of two-stage cluster samples), simple data collection (including rapid qualitative appraisal), rapid processing, and rapid evaluation methods (especially the use of case-control methods for evaluation).

SIMPLIFIED SAMPLING PROCEDURES

The easiest way to simplify sampling is, of course, to use a sample of convenience instead of a probability sample. But the disadvantages are obvious, and this short cut should be taken only if rough 'ballpark figures' will suffice, or for some qualitative research procedures.

Purposive sampling will often satisfy a study's needs. It may be decided, for example, that patients attending a health facility are sufficiently representative of the total community to warrant their use (with reservations) as a study sample for a specific purpose, or that tests and interviews of antenatal clinic attenders and men attending outpatient clinics will provide useful information on the prevalence of sexually transmitted diseases in refugee camps,[4] or that surveillance of influenza can be carried out by watching 'sentinel' populations (e.g. by recording sick absenteeism in selected schools or workplaces).

In developed countries the selection of subjects and controls for telephone interviews can be simplified by random digit dialling (see p. 92), but this is not necessarily cheap or time-saving.

Two-stage cluster sampling

The EPI cluster sampling technique was initially advocated by WHO's Expanded Programme on Immunization as a rapid, cheap and accurate basis for surveys of immunization coverage, and has since been widely used for descriptive surveys of specific diseases, service coverage, health service needs, blindness, and other topics.[5] Cluster surveys of this kind should be considered not only when resources are limited, but whenever rapid results are required, especially in emergency situations.[6]

The EPI technique has four advantages: it does not require a detailed sampling frame; it uses clusters of subjects who live close to one another; subjects are selected in the field by a procedure so simple it can be used by health workers with minimal technical support; and it can provide reasonably representative data.

The selection process has two stages. First, communities (villages, urban blocks, neighbourhoods of a city, etc.) are chosen, using a random procedure requiring reasonably accurate estimates of population size. Then clusters are selected in the chosen communities, by a method that provides a 'self-weighted' sample. The sample falls short of being a true probability sample, since the second stage does not use random sampling, which would require a census or detailed map for use as a sampling frame. The basic method is simple:

1. *Decide on the number of clusters and determine their size.* The number of clusters will depend on the manpower and time available; the more clusters, the more valid the results—30 is probably a minimum. Calculate the size of the required sample[7] and divide it by the number of clusters (and round the answer up, to make it a whole number) to determine how many subjects are needed in each cluster. The original EPI recommendation (for surveys of vaccination status) was 30 clusters with 7 children in each; 30 clusters of 30 individuals have been suggested for nutritional surveys.

2. *Randomly select the communities where clusters will be sought.* Make a list of the communities (in any order), with their population sizes, and calculate the cumulative population size, as shown in Table 31.1 which displays the communities in an imaginary

Table 31.1 List of communities, showing cumulative population size

Community	Population size	Cumulative population size
D	1100	1100
F	2800	3900
P	5000	8900
S	600	9500
H	9400	18 900
E	3200	22 100
A	3500	25 600
Q	1200	26 800
C	4300	31 100
M	4900	36 000
G	3900	39 900
etc.	—	120 300

region. Compute a sampling interval by dividing the total population size by the required number of clusters. In this instance, if 30 clusters are wanted, the sampling interval is 120 300 ÷ 30 = 4010. Choose a random number between 1 and 4010, and fit it into position in the list to identify a community. If the random number is 1946, which lies between 1100 and 3900, the first community chosen is F. Now add the sampling interval to 1946 (1946 + 4010 = 5956) and use the result (5956) to select the second community (P). Repeat this (5956 + 4010 = 9966) and select community H. Again repeat it (9966 + 4010 = 13 976) and select H again—meaning that two separate clusters are required from community H. And so on. This procedure selects communities with a probability proportional to their size.

3. *Select clusters.* For each cluster, randomly select one household to be the starting point, and then use a systematic procedure to select other households. To choose the starting point, go to a central place and randomly choose a direction, e.g. by spinning a bottle or throwing up a pencil and seeing how it lands; then count the number of households between the central point and the edge of the community in that direction, choose one of them at random, and visit it. For subsequent choices, take the unvisited household whose door is closest to the household last visited. Visit each of the chosen households in turn until the number of subjects (say, children of the right age) required in a cluster has been found.

In a survey of a very large region a multistage design may be used, by selecting communities in two (or more) stages, each using the systematic probability-proportional-to-size method described above: that is, first select subregions, and then communities.

Computer simulations have shown that the EPI sampling method is usually satisfactory for the rapid appraisal of immunization status or the prevalence of a disease, although the results may be biased and less precise than those based on random sampling, and its accuracy for different diseases varies. The method is less satisfactory if the survey covers a wide range of topics, so that different-sized clusters are required for measuring different characteristics, or if associations (e.g. with nutritional status) are under study. The results in different clusters or subsets of clusters can be compared only if the samples are large. The main deficiencies of the EPI design arise from its failure to use random methods when selecting clusters, and from the use for this purpose of quota sampling; results may be misleading if subjects with similar characteristics tend to live close to one another.

The use of random selection would of course mitigate the deficiencies. If a list or map of households in each chosen community is available or can be constructed, the households to be visited can be selected randomly from this sampling frame; but then this is not a 'rapid' method. Simpler suggested remedies are the use of the fifth nearest household instead of the nearest one, and splitting the community into quadrants and selecting a quarter of each cluster from each quadrant, starting at the centre point of the quadrant.

A suggested 'not quite as quick but much cleaner alternative'[8] to the EPI cluster survey design, aimed at retaining the advantages of ease and cheapness but making the procedure more rigorous and appropriate even for surveys that make multiple measurements, is based on the preselection of a 'target segment size'—the number of households to be surveyed for each cluster—instead of fixing the number of subjects needed in each cluster. This number is reached by first calculating the required sample size,[7] then (using the best available data) estimating how many households will have to be contacted in order to locate this number of subjects (e.g. children aged under five, or children with diarrhoea in the previous fortnight), and dividing this total number of households by the number of clusters (at least 30). Communities are selected randomly (as in the basic EPI method), and the chosen communities are divided into equal segments, each containing (approximately) the required number of households; this requires a rough sketch map showing the dwellings (households) in the community. A segment of the community is then chosen at random, and *all* eligible individuals in *all* the dwellings in the chosen segment are included in the sample. This method ensures that all households in the study population have approximately the same probability of being selected.

SIMPLE DATA-COLLECTION METHODS

Data collection may be simplified in various ways. The most obvious ones are to restrict the variables to those that are essential to meet the study's purposes (resulting in very short questionnaires or examinations) and to choose sources that are easily accessible (available records may, despite their deficiencies, contain enough information to obviate the need for a more demanding survey).

If available, simpler procedures can be chosen rather than more accurate but elaborate ones, e.g. a rapid urine test for use in surveys of iodine deficiency[9] or a simple test card for identifying people with low vision.[10] Household food inventories or brief dietary questionnaires may supply enough information on dietary practices, rendering detailed dietary interviews unnecessary.[11] In countries without well-developed death certification, *verbal autopsies*[12]—structured interviews administered by lay personnel to relatives or friends of the deceased—may provide a degree of information on mortality from gastroenteritis, measles, accidents, HIV-associated conditions and other causes.

It may be decided to use simple proxy measures, e.g. arm circumference or weight-for-height as easy and cheap indices of malnutrition in children,[13] night blindness as a relatively easily measured surrogate for vitamin A deficiency,[14] or a characteristic depigmentation pattern ('leopard skin') as an index of the endemicity of onchocerciasis;[15] or to appraise the burden of lymphatic filariasis by measuring the rate of infection of insect vectors[16] or by examining a small sample of men for hydroceles.[17]

If the measures are simple, it is easy to train health workers or others in their use. Schoolteachers can measure weight and height with adequate precision, assistants can be taught simple cataract recognition,[18] and traditional midwives have been taught to identify low birth weight babies by using a hand-held scale that shows a coloured signal if the weight is below 2.5 kg.[19] In Tanzania, a simple questionnaire on diseases and symptoms was administered to children by teachers; a comparison with urine tests showed that reports of haematuria or schistosomiasis had a high validity.[20]

Cross-sectional methods, e.g. for appraising child growth in a community, are obviously faster than longitudinal ones. Simple data on current infant feeding practices can, if appropriately analyzed, rapidly provide a picture of the average duration of breast-feeding and the age at introduction of supplements.[21]

Rapid qualitative appraisal

Simple qualitative methods (see p. 166) permit rapid appraisal of knowledge, attitudes and practices relevant to health and health care (*'rapid ethnographic assessment' 'rapid assessment procedures'*) using procedures for which 'one does not need an advanced degree in anthropology ... One *does* need ... the ability to develop rapport with people and to accurately record and transmit their views, beliefs and behaviours'.[22]

The basic methods[23] are conversations and informal interviews with members of the public and key informants, focused discussions with small groups of people whose opinions and ideas are of interest, the nominal group technique (described in Ch. 20), and unstructured observations, e.g. of housing conditions or sanitary arrangements or the manner in which mothers prepare infant foods or oral rehydration solutions. Simple guides and checklists are available for use in collecting data on various aspects of health and health care.[22]

Confirmation of validity by 'triangulation' (comparing what different methods reveal, to determine their common findings) is an important feature of this approach.

The participation of community leaders, members of the public and providers of health services in qualitative research activities can often be developed into partnerships in the ongoing development of services and improvements in their delivery and utilization.[24]

RAPID PROCESSING

The keys to rapid processing are good planning, prompt entry of data into a computer—preferably at the time of obtaining the data—and appropriate statistical software.

The use of computers as survey tools is no longer unusual even in developing countries, although special courses and customized programs may be required.[25] As demonstrated in a malaria survey in the Gambia, use of a hand-held computer for collecting and checking questionnaire data can significantly increase both speed and accuracy.[26] In Burma, initially computer-illiterate survey personnel learned to operate a spreadsheet program in order to estimate sample sizes and select communities for a two-stage cluster design, and calculate and graphically display confidence intervals.[27]

RAPID EVALUATION METHODS

A rapid evaluation method developed by WHO in order to provide timely information on the population's health status and the performance and quality of health care services, as a basis for immediate adjustments to care programmes, generally provides critical tables required by health service managers within 7–10 days, and a draft report in a few weeks. In essence it consists of a set of cross-sectional studies using rapid methods, carried out mainly in health care facilities, with the aim of identifying and solving operational problems. Depending on the issues studied, information may be obtained from the community, e.g. leaders, mothers, or people attending for care (clinic exit interviews), or from health workers, using interviews or focus group discussions, as well as from direct observations of activities in clinics, checks on clinic facilities and supplies, and (rarely) household interviews.[28]

The *lot quality technique*, a method developed to assess the acceptability of lots (batches) of manufactured parts coming off an industrial production line, is a promising rapid technique for monitoring the quality of health care. It has been used (especially in developing countries) to assess immunization coverage, family planning, antenatal care, the use of oral rehydration therapy, and health worker performance.[29]

A simple way of testing the effectiveness of a health programme is to compare the status of people who have and have not been exposed to the programme. In clinics in Lesotho, for example, a children's growth monitoring and nutrition education programme was evaluated by means of a cross-sectional study in which maternal knowledge about infant feeding was measured, and mothers were classified according to whether or not they had previously attended the clinic. Women who had attended were found to be more knowledgeable about the introduction of animal protein foods, the use of oral rehydration salts, and the method of weaning.[30] But an evaluative study based on simple comparison of the findings or changes seen in people who voluntarily or perforce participate or do not participate in a programme is generally not convincing, as the comparison may be confounded by differences (not all of which may be controlled in the analysis) other than the difference in exposure to the programme. The authors correctly limited their conclusion to the statement that previous clinic attendance 'appeared to be' beneficial.

Case-control studies to evaluate procedures or programmes

A relatively simple and rapid way of evaluating preventive and therapeutic procedures or programmes is to compare people who have experienced an unfavourable outcome (cases) with controls, to see whether they differ in their prior exposure to the procedure or programme. The unfavourable outcome is generally one that the procedure or programme aims to prevent, as in case-control studies[31] to evaluate immunization procedures, PAP testing, breast cancer screening, aspirin to protect against myocardial infarction, family planning, prenatal and intrapartum care, child health services, and improvements in water supply and sanitation, but it may also be a suspected undesirable side-effect, as in studies comparing the neonatal exposure to vitamin K prophylaxis of children who do and do not develop cancer.[32]

Like all case-control studies, these pose problems, with particular reference to the appropriateness of the controls. It is not easy to exclude the possibility that the cases and controls may have initially had differences in characteristics affecting their prognosis, maybe related to their eligibility, preparedness or ability to undergo the procedure or participate in the programme. There may also be bias due to differences in the recall or reporting of exposure. Care is therefore required to control for confounding and other biases. But the information required for properly appraising or controlling these biases is generally difficult to obtain, and the conclusions are often equivocal. An inbuilt limitation of this method is its capacity to examine only the outcome used to define cases.

NOTES AND REFERENCES

1. The evolution and use of rapid methods are reviewed by Smith G S 1989 (Development of rapid epidemiologic assessment methods to evaluate health status and delivery of health services. International Journal of Epidemiology 18 [suppl 2]: S1), who points out that their introduction was a major factor in the worldwide eradication of smallpox.
   For symposia on the use of rapid methods, see special issues of the International Journal of Epidemiology (Rapid epidemiologic assessment. 18[suppl 2], 1989: S1) and Health Policy and Planning (Rapid assessment methods for the control of tropical diseases. 7[1], 1992: 1). Also, see Scrimshaw S C M, Hurtado E 1987 (Rapid assessment procedures for nutrition and primary health care: anthropological approaches to improving programme effectiveness. UCLA Latin American Center Publications, Los Angeles).
   Rapid assessment is especially important in mass emergencies, where health needs should be appraised within 24–48 hours (Guha-Sapir D 1991 Rapid assessment of health needs in mass emergencies: review of current concepts and methods. World Health Statistics Quarterly 44: 171).
2. Materia E, Imoko J, Berhe G, Dawuda C, Omar M A, Pinto A, Guerra R 1995 Rapid surveys in support of district health information systems: an experience from Uganda. East African Medical Journal 72: 15.
3. Frerichs R R, Tar K T 1989 Computer-assisted rapid surveys in developing countries. Public Health Reports 104: 14.
4. Mayaud P, Msuya W, Todd J et al 1992 STD rapid assessment in Rwandan refugee camps in Tanzania. Genitourinary Medicine 73: 33.

5. For fuller descriptions of *EPI cluster sampling* see Lemeshow S, Robinson D
1985 (Surveys to measure programme coverage and impact: a review of the
methodology used by the Expanded Programme on Immunization. World
Health Statistics Quarterly 38: 65) and Bennett S, Woods T, Liyanage W M,
Smith D L 1991 (A simplified general method for cluster-sample surveys of
health in developing countries. World Health Statistics Quarterly 44: 98).

Examples: Legetic B, Jakovljevic D, Marinkovic J, Niciforovic O,
Stanisavljevic D 1996 (Health care delivery and the status of the population's
health in the current crises in former Yugoslavia using EPI-design
methodology. International Journal of Epidemiology 25: 341); Katz J 1995
(Sample-size implications for population-based cluster surveys of nutritional
status. American Journal of Clinical Nutrition 61: 155); Rothenberg R B,
Lobanov A, Singh K B, Stroh G Jr 1985 (Observations on the application of
EPI cluster survey methods for estimating disease incidence. Bulletin of the
World Health Organization 63: 93); Materia E et al 1995 (see note 2).

Bias and precision vary for prevalence studies of different diseases (Katz J,
Yoon S S, Brendel K, West K P Jr 1997 Sampling designs for xerophthalmia
prevalence surveys. International Journal of Epidemiology 26: 1041).

The degree of clustering of a disease within the sample clusters may be of
interest; a survey in Tanzania, for example, revealed clustering of trachoma
within neighbourhoods in villages, not explained by known risk factors
(West S K, Munoz B, Turner V M, Mmbaga B B O, Taylor H R 1991 The
epidemiology of trachoma in Central Tanzania. International Journal of
Epidemiology 20: 1088).

Approximate incidence rates can sometimes be derived from prevalence
findings based on cluster studies. For example, approximate poliomyelitis
incidence rates have been computed from the prevalence of lameness and
other symptoms (LaForce F M, Lichnevski M S, Keja J, Henderson R H
1980 Clinical survey techniques to estimate prevalence and annual incidence
of poliomyelitis in developing countries. Bulletin of the World Health
Organization 58: 609; Babaniyi O, Parakoyi B 1991 Cluster survey for
poliomyelitis and neonatal tetanus in Ilorin, Nigeria. International Journal of
Epidemiology 20:515; Schwoebel V, Dauvisis A-V, Helynck B et al 1992.
Community-based evaluation survey of immunizations in Burkino Faso.
Bulletin of the World Health Organization 70: 583).

Computer simulations to test the accuracy of EPI cluster sampling are
described by (among others) Bennett S, Radalowicz A, Vella V, Tomkins A
1994 (A computer simulation of household sampling schemes for health
surveys in developing countries. International Journal of Epidemiology 23:
1282) and Harris D R, Lemeshow S 1991 (Evaluation of the EPI survey
methodology for estimating relative risk. World Health Statistics Quarterly
44: 107).

6. Cluster surveys have a special role in emergency situations. In the public
health disaster that followed civil disturbances in Rwanda in 1994, for
example, when over half a million Rwandans fled to Zaire, such surveys,
combined with morbidity surveillance, provided a basis for a well co-
ordinated programme that was associated with a steep decline in deaths of
refugees by the second month of the crisis (Goma Epidemiology Group 1995
Public health impact of Rwandan refugee crisis: what happened in Goma,
Zaire, in July, 1994? Lancet 345: 339). After Yugoslavia's civil war and
disintegration it took only two months to obtain a picture of health services
use and related problems (Legetic B et al 1996; see note 5).

7. See note 17, page 103.

8. Turner A G, Magnani R R J, Shuaib M 1996 A not quite as quick but much
cleaner alternative to the Expanded Programme on Immunization (EPI)
cluster survey design. International Journal of Epidemiology 25: 198.

9. Rendl J, Bier D, Groh T, Reiners C 1998 Rapid urinary iodide test. Journal of Clinical Endocrinology and Metabolism 83: 1007.
10. Keeffe J E, Lovie-Kitchin J E, Maclean H, Taylor H R 1996 A simplified screening test for identifying people with low vision in developing countries. Bulletin of the World Health Organization 74: 525.
11. Patterson R E, Kristl A R, Shannon J, Hunt J R, White E 1997 Using a brief household food inventory as an environmental indicator of individual dietary practices. American Journal of Public Health 87: 272.
    Examples of short dietary questionnaires: Dobson A J, Blijlevens R, Alexander H M et al 1993 (Short fat questionnaire: a self-administered measure of fat-intake behaviour. Australian Journal of Public Health 17: 1144); Retzlaff B M, Dowdy A A, Walden C E, Bovbjerg V E, Knopp R H 1997 (The Northwest Lipid Research Clinic Fat Intake Scale: validation and utility. American Journal of Public Health 87: 181).
12. *Verbal autopsies.* See: Quigley M A, Schellenberg J R M A, Snow R W 1996 (Algorithms for verbal autopsies: a validation study in Kenyan children. Bulletin of the World Health Organization 74: 147); Anker M 1997 (The effect of misclassification error on reported cause-specific mortality fractions from verbal autopsy. International Journal of Epidemiology 26: 1090); Kamali A, Wagner H-U, Nakiyingi J, Sabiiti I, Kengeya-Kayondo J F, Mulder D W 1996 (Verbal autopsy as a tool for diagnosing HIV-related adult deaths in rural Uganda. International Journal of Epidemiology 25: 679).
13. Arm circumference: see Velzeboer M I, Selwyn B J, Sargent F, Pollitt E, Delgado H 1983a (Evaluation of arm circumference as a public health index of protein energy malnutrition in early childhood. Journal of Tropical Pediatrics 29: 135) and 1983b (The use of arm circumference in simplified screening for acute malnutrition by minimally-trained health workers. Journal of Tropical Pediatrics 29: 159). Weight-for-height may be more useful than arm circumference (Bern C, Nathanail L 1995 Is mid-upper-arm circumference a useful tool for screening in emergency settings? British Medical Journal 345: 631).
14. Sommer A, Hussaini G, Muhilal T I, Susanto D, Saroso J S 1980 History of nightblindness: a simple tool for xerophthalmia screening. American Journal of Clinical Nutrition 33: 887.
15. Edungbola L D, Alabi T O, Oni G A, Asaolu S O, Ogunbanjo B O, Parakoyi B D 1987 'Leopard skin' as a rapid diagnostic index for estimating the endemicity of African onchocerciasis. International Journal of Epidemiology 16: 590.
16. Pani S P, Srividya A, Krisknamoorthy K, Das P K, Dhanda V 1997 Rapid assessment procedures (RAP) for lymphatic filariasis. National Medical Journal of India 10: 19.
17. Gyapong J O, Adjei S, Gyapong M, Asamoah G 1996 Rapid community diagnosis of lymphatic filariasis. Acta Tropica 61: 65.
18. Venkataswamy G, Lepkowski J M, Ravilla T, Shanmugham C A K, Vaidyanathan K, Tilden R L and the Aravind rapid epidemiologic assessment staff 1989. Rapid epidemiologic assessment of cataract blindness. International Journal of Epidemiology 18: S60.
19. Ritenbaugh C K, Said A K, Gaslal O M, Harrison G G 1989 Development and evaluation of a colour-coded scale for birthweight surveillance in rural Egypt. International Journal of Epidemiology 18: S54.
20. Lengeler C, Mshinda H, de Savigny D, Kilima P, Morona D, Tanner M 1991. The value of questionnaires aimed at key informants, and distributed through an existing administrative system, for rapid and cost-effective health assessment. World Health Statistics Quarterly 44: 150.
21. Ferreira M U, Cardoso M A, Santos A L, Ferreira C S, Szarfarc S C 1996 Rapid epidemiologic assessment of breastfeeding practices: probit analysis of current status data. Journal of Tropical Pediatrics 42: 50.
22. Scrimshaw S C M, Hurtado E 1987 (see note 1).

23. For descriptions and illustrations of *rapid qualitative assessment* methods, see Scrimshaw S C M, Hurtado E 1987 (note 1), the symposia cited in note 1, and Ong B N, Humphris G 1994 (Prioritising needs with communities: rapid appraisal methodologies in health. In: Popay J, Williams G, eds. Researching the people's health. Routledge, London).

24. See, for example, Dale J, Shipman C, Lacock L, Davies M 1996 (Creating a shared vision of out of hours care: using rapid appraisal methods to create an interagency, community oriented, approach to service development. British Medical Journal 312: 1206).

25. The use of computers in surveys in *developing countries* is illustrated by Forster D, Snow B 1982 (Using microcomputers for rapid data collection in developing countries. Health Policy and Planning 7: 67); Bertrand W E 1985 (Microcomputer applications in health population surveys: experience and potential in developing countries. World Health Statistics Quarterly 38: 91); Gould J B, Frerichs R R 1986 (Training faculty in Bangladesh to use a microcomputer for public health: followup report. Public Health Reports 101: 616); Forster D, Behrens R H, Campbell H, Byass P 1991 (Evaluation of a computerized field data collection system for health surveys. Bulletin of the World Health Organization 69: 107); Frerichs R R 1989 (Simple analytic procedures for rapid microcomputer-assisted cluster surveys in developing countries. Public Health Reports 104: 24); Frerichs R R, Tar K T 1989 (see note 3); and Blignaut P J, McDonald T 1997 (A computerised implementation of a minimum set of health indicators. Methods of Information in Medicine 36: 122).

   However helpful a computer may be, it cannot work magic. A description of one computer program claims that it 'is designed to allow anyone, no matter how knowledgeable or ignorant of statistical and survey methods, to conduct a useful and correctly designed survey. It has everything you need ...' (PC Magazine 1989, 8: 254). (Throw away this book!)

26. Forster D et al 1991 (see note 25).

27. Frerichs R R 1989 (see note 25).

28. Division of Epidemiological Surveillance and Health Situation and Trend Analysis, WHO 1993 Rapid evaluation methods in health services. International Journal of Epidemiology 22: 578. Anker M, Guidotti R J, Orzeszyna S, Sapirie S A, Thuriaux M C 1993 Rapid evaluation methods (REM) of health services performance: methodological observations. Bulletin of the World Health Organization 711: 15.

29. Robertson S E, Anker M, Roisin A J, Macklai N, Engstrom K, LaForce F M 1997 The lot quality technique: a global review of applications in the assessment of health services and disease surveillance. World Health Statistics Quarterly 50: 199.

30. Ruel M T, Habicht J-P, Olson C 1992 Impact of a clinic-based growth monitoring programme on maternal nutrition knowledge in Lesotho. International Journal of Epidemiology 21: 59.

31. Most of these case-control studies are cited by Baltazar J C 1991 (The potential of the case-control method for rapid epidemiological assessment. World Health Statistics Quarterly 44: 140) and Smith G S 1989 (see note 1).

32. Conflicting results are presented by McKinney P A, Juszczak E, Findlay E, Smith K 1998 (Case-control study of childhood leukaemia and cancer in Scotland: findings for neonatal intramuscular vitamin K. British Medical Journal 316: 173) and Passmore S J, Draper G, Brownbill P, Kroll M 1998 (Case-control studies of relation between childhood cancer and neonatal vitamin K administration: retrospective case-control study. British Medical Journal 316: 178) and discussed by von Kries R 1998 (Editorial: Neonatal vitamin K prophylaxis: the Gordian knot still awaits untying. British Medical Journal 316: 161).

32 Clinical trials

Clinical trials are experiments or quasi-experiments that test hypotheses concerning the effects (favourable or unfavourable) of intervention techniques applied to individuals. They may be tests of therapeutic agents, devices, regimens or procedures (*therapeutic trials*), preventive ones (*prophylactic trials*), or rehabilitative, educational, etc. (trials of screening and diagnostic tests were discussed on pp. 197–199). The main objectives are usually to measure the efficacy and safety of the procedure, and their variation among patients with different characteristics. Attention may also be focused on efficiency, e.g. by comparing the costs of different ways of achieving a similar benefit. Other questions (concerning compliance, satisfaction, etc.—see p. 56) may also be asked, but are usually seen as subsidiary, serving only to explain why the outcome is or is not satisfactory; they may, however, be dominant features if the study centres on the feasibility or acceptability of a procedure.

A distinction has been made between *explanatory* clinical trials, whose purpose is mainly to provide biological information (e.g. about the way drugs act and the way the body reacts to them) and *pragmatic* ones, which aim to test procedures under the conditions in which they would be applied in practice.[1]

Clinical trials may be set up not only to appraise the effects of individual-focused procedures, but (in some instances) to evaluate programmes. The latter use of clinical trials will be discussed in the next chapter.

The use of case-control studies (instead of trials) to appraise the effects of treatments and other procedures is discussed on pages 350–351.

Here are six examples of trials. In the first four the subjects were randomly allocated to the groups that were compared. (For the findings, refer to the notes; no prizes.) The study objectives were:

1. To compare the incidence of stroke in elderly people with systolic hypertension (and normal diastolic blood pressure) who received medicinal treatment or indistinguishable placebos.[2]
2. To compare the prevalence of symptoms of adenoidal hypertrophy, before and after operation, in children who had only their tonsils removed or who had their adenoids out too.[3]
3. To compare the proportions of people with common colds who were cured or improved 2 days after starting treatment with antihistaminic tablets or indistinguishable dummy placebo tablets.[4]
4. To compare the relief of symptoms in patients with angina pectoris after ligation of the internal mammary arteries (an operation designed to increase blood flow to the heart) or a sham operation (in which only a skin incision was made.)[5]
5. To compare the occurrence of complications in soldiers whose wounds were treated with boiling oil or with a mixture of egg yolks, oil of roses and turpentine.[6]
6. To compare the countenances of four children fed on legumes and water for 10 days (Daniel, Shadrach, Meshach and Abednego) with those of children fed on King Nebuchadnezzar's meat and wine.[7]

STUDY DESIGNS

The following are the basic study designs.[8] If the intervention is not under the investigator's control—i.e. if decisions on who gets what, and when, are not made by the investigator—the study is a quasi-experiment. (As noted on p. 16, some writers refer to any unrandomized trial as a quasi-experiment; the terminology used is less important than an awareness that careful consideration must be given to the possible biases in all experiments, whether 'true' or 'quasi'.)

1. *Parallel studies*, in which two or more independent groups are studied prospectively and compared.
2. *Externally controlled studies*, in which a single experimental group is studied and the findings are compared with data obtained from other sources.

3. *'Self-controlled'* studies, in which the subjects are their own controls. These may be based on observations before and after a single treatment (*before—after studies*), or *crossover studies*, in which two or more treatments are applied in sequence to the same subjects.

These designs may be combined. Other designs (e.g. factorial, Latin squares) may also be used.[9] A factorial design permits appraisal of the effects of two or more factors, and also of their joint effects. A simple example is the Physicians' Health Study, which examined the effect of aspirin on cardiovascular mortality and the effect of beta-carotene on cancer incidence; participants were randomly divided into four groups, who were respectively given aspirin and a placebo, beta-carotene and a placebo, aspirin and beta-carotene, or two placebos.[10]

Types of clinical trials

1. Parallel (concurrent controls)
2. Externally controlled
3. 'Self-controlled'

Parallel studies, or trials with *concurrent controls*, compare groups exposed to different interventions. A treated group may be compared with a control group that receives no treatment (or a placebo), or two or more groups who are having different treatments may be compared with each other or with an untreated group. If the allocation of subjects to the groups is random, the study is a *randomized controlled trial (RCT)*. A well done RCT provides more convincing evidence and more precise estimates of the effect of an intervention than any other study method, and is generally regarded as the standard with which other methods should be compared.

Parallel comparisons require information about the subjects before as well as after the intervention (i.e. they should be 'premeasure—postmeasure' or 'pretest—post-test' studies). This not only permits a check on the comparability of the groups before the intervention, it also makes it possible to take proper account of possible confounders and modifiers in the analysis. Many studies are based on a comparison of the changes observed in different groups; the measurement of change, e.g. in blood pressure or other characteristics, requires base-line data. Trials with no information about prior status ('postmeasure only' trials or 'post-test trials') have unknown and possibly serious biases; Daniel's biblical trial (see p. 356) is an example.

In *externally controlled studies* the findings in the experimental group are compared with control data obtained from other sources, e.g. with statistics reported by other medical agencies that did not use the experimental procedure. In a therapeutic trial of this sort the comparison is usually with cases treated in the past (*historical controls*). This approach may sometimes be of unquestioned validity, for example if the disease being treated is one that, according to previous experience, never disappears or is always fatal. Ethical constraints may compel the use of historical controls; a physician who is convinced of the merit of a new treatment and therefore cannot ethically use randomization may decide to perform a pilot trial using historical controls, in the hope of convincing sceptical colleagues to do a randomized trial. There may, however, be serious bias in externally controlled studies; the results of treatment may differ because the controls differed from the experimental subjects, or were treated by other clinicians, or at another time (when circumstances affecting the prognosis, such as other components of patient management, were different), or were appraised differently, etc. Even patients treated in the same centre and in the same way, but at different times, may have very different outcomes.[11] Trials with historical controls may provide the first clues to real breakthroughs in medical science; on the other hand, results may be misleading, and yet make a subsequent RCT ethically unacceptable. Historical controls are sometimes used as a check on the results of a trial using concurrent controls; if the randomized controls fared worse than previous experience would lead one to expect, this needs explaining.

In *self-controlled studies*, use of the subjects as their own controls prevents confounding by many characteristics that may influence the outcome. But there are possible biases in a simple 'before—after' study—those connected with extraneous events or changes that occur with time, non-specific effects caused by the performance of the experiment itself, changes in methods of measurement, and regression to the mean (see p. 85); in a parallel study, comparison is made with a control group that is subject to the same effects. However, such studies may be appropriate in some circumstances (e.g. testing a treatment in patients with refractory disease, or appraising the value of supplementary feeding for children in refugee camps[12]).

In a *crossover study* each subject is given the different treatments (or treatment and placebo) under comparison, one after another. Each subject is his own control. The sequence of assignment is generally randomized, so that this is a kind of RCT. A 'washing-out period' may be required between treatments, to permit the effects of the previous treatment to disappear, and the method is not feasible if a treatment has protracted 'carry-over' effects. The *'N of 1'* *clinical trial* or 'single-case experiment' is a special kind of crossover study aimed at determining the efficacy of a treatment (or the relative value of alternative treatments) for a specific patient. The patient is repeatedly given a treatment and placebo, or different treatments, in successive time periods.[13]

RANDOMIZATION

Randomization is a procedure whereby the assignment of treatments is left to chance. The allocation is decided by tossing a coin or some other strictly random method. Randomization does not guarantee that the groups will be identical, but it makes misleading results less likely, by ensuring that the only differences between the groups are those that occur by chance. This applies both to known risk and protective factors and to unsuspected ones. Unless the groups are very small, marked differences become unlikely.

The procedure of random assignment should be applied to *all* the subjects included in the study—to all the volunteers entering a prophylactic trial, or to all the patients whose diagnosis, clinical condition and other features make them eligible for inclusion in a therapeutic trial, and who have agreed to participate in it (Table 32.1). Exclusion criteria (too old, too ill, etc.) should be laid down in advance and, if possible, applied before the subjects are assigned to groups. If there is an objection to putting a subject in any one of the groups, he should be excluded from the trial before he is

---

Table 32.1 A typical randomized controlled trial

1. Eligible? ⟶ If not, exclude
2. Consent? ⟶ If not, exclude
3. Randomize to Groups A and B
4. Treat (subjects may be blinded to treatment)
5. Follow up all members of Groups A and B
6. Compare outcomes or changes in Groups A and B

allocated. Such exclusions do not bias the results of the comparison (internal validity), although they may limit the applicability of the results (external validity). The results of a well conducted RCT can validly be applied to the kind of person who entered the trial ('no bias is caused by exclusion, even if for silly reasons')[14], but not to anyone else.

Sometimes, as a convenient and theoretically adequate alternative to randomization, a systematic method of assignment is used, such as the allocation of alternate patients to treatment and control groups. Such methods have been criticized on the grounds that they are too easily manipulated by well-meaning clinicians. In a controlled trial of anticoagulant therapy for myocardial infarction, in which the patient's treatment was determined by whether he was admitted on an odd- or even-numbered day of the month, it was found that the physicians (convinced of the value of the treatment) saw to it that more patients were admitted on odd-numbered days.[15]

Another simple and valid alternative to ordinary randomization, appropriate only in small trials, is *minimalization*. Subjects are assigned in turn, using a modified randomization process that weights the scales in favour of a decision that will minimize the differences between the groups with regard to important prognostic factors.[16]

Whichever of these methods of allocation is used, it is wise before drawing conclusions to compare the groups to check whether they were similar before the trial started. In a large-scale trial of the effect of extra milk on the height and weight of schoolchildren, for example, the children allocated to the experimental group turned out to be shorter and lighter than the control children.[17]

Randomization may be achieved by tossing a coin or throwing a die, using tables[18] of random numbers or random permutations, or letting a computer[19] do the work. Use may be made of *balanced randomization*, which imposes a constraint on the randomization process so as to prevent the allocation ratio from diverging (by chance) from the intended ratio of, say, 1:1 or 2:1. Various methods are available for this purpose.[20]

Blocked (or stratified) randomization is sometimes used—the subjects are divided into 'blocks', and randomization (usually balanced) is carried out separately in each block. (This word comes from agricultural experiments in which a field was divided into blocks, in each of which a number of treatments was tried.)

The purpose of blocking (also called *prestratification*) is generally to control for the effects of important prognostic factors that may be confounded with the effects of the treatment—the blocks are pairs or sets of matched subjects. The candidates are stratified according to characteristics that may affect the outcome, such as age, severity of the disease, or month (if seasonal factors are deemed important), and randomization (usually balanced) or systemic assignment is then performed separately in each stratum. Blocking is often used in studies where the accrual of patients continues over a long period (with separate randomization of each pair or set of successively enrolled subjects) and in multicentre trials (with separate randomization at each centre). If the strata are large enough, the effects in different strata can be compared.

Matching and prestratification may be useful in small studies, but statisticians disagree about their value in large studies (the collective noun for statisticians is 'a variance of statisticians'). The grounds for opposition are that these procedures complicate the trial unnecessarily, and the effects of important prognostic factors can just as well be taken into account during the analysis, by *post-stratification* ('retrospective stratification')—i.e. stratifying the subjects according to characteristics that are found to be related to the outcome—or other methods.[21]

MAKING THE TRIAL EASIER

Randomized controlled trials are often unfeasible, and are always difficult. The constraints include ethical problems, insufficiency of resources or subjects, and the rapid evolution and obsolescence of treatments in some fields. 'It is hard to argue with the concept that every medical therapy should be evaluated in an RCT', says one expert, who also points out that the method 'is slow, ponderous, expensive, and often stifling of scientific imagination and creative changes in treatment protocols', and declares that it 'is a last resort for the evaluation of medical interventions'.[22]

There are a number of designs that try to lessen logistic or ethical difficulties, while still endeavouring to limit potential bias; special precautions are needed in their analysis or interpretation. For example:

1. Assign fewer patients to the less favourable therapy ('response adaptive randomization').[23] In a trial that compares treatments whose success can be adjudged rapidly, each patient's treatment

may be determined by the previous patient's result ('Play the winner') or by the cumulative results for all previous subjects (the 'two-armed bandit' method). Or two treatments may be tried in a half or third of the patients, and the more successful of the two can then be used in the remaining subjects.

2. Reduce the number of randomized concurrent controls, but compensate for this by also using historical controls who were treated at the same institution with the same eligibility criteria and methods of appraisal, and use both sets of controls in the analysis.[24]

3. Stop accepting new subjects as soon as there is a definitive answer. A *sequential design* of this sort is practicable if subjects enter the trial serially and results are available soon. It requires the prior establishment of 'stopping rules', and ongoing analysis.[25]

4. Assign all subjects who are at higher risk to the new treatment, and either assign subjects at lower risk randomly, or assign them to the standard treatment (or placebo). Statistical modelling is used to make sense of the results.[26]

5. In a trial comparing a new treatment with the best current standard therapy, randomize the subjects before obtaining their consent (this is Zelen's *prerandomized* or '*randomized consent*' design;[37] see Table 32.2) Give Group A the standard therapy, and ask the members of Group B for their consent to the new treatment. If they consent, give them the new treatment; if not, give them the standard treatment. (Alternatively, ask the members of Group B to choose between the two treatments.) Then compare the outcomes in Group A (all of whom received the standard treatment) and Group B (some of whom received the new treatment). This is a valid comparison of randomized groups, although the design 'dilutes' the difference between the treatments (but this may be offset by the higher participation rate that may be expected in such studies). The only ethical problem is that members of Group A are not offered the experimental treatment. This is overcome in the *double prerandomized design*, where (in addition) members of Group A are asked for their consent to the standard therapy (otherwise, they are given the new therapy); if they tend to consent, the comparison of Groups A and B remains useful. Disadvantages of prerandomized trials are that the subjects cannot be kept unaware of their treatment, and that it becomes difficult to examine the modifying effects of factors that are associated with the patient's decisions; the latter difficulty can be partly overcome by using

Table 32.2 Prerandomized controlled trial

1. Eligible? ⟶ If not, exclude
2. Randomize to Groups A and B
3. Consent? (requested in one or both groups)
   If refused, give treatment preferred by subject
4. Treat (subjects cannot be blinded to treatment)
5. Follow up all members of Groups A and B
6. Compare outcomes or changes in Groups A and B

'blocking' for selected factors when randomizing. These designs and their analysis are vigorously debated by statisticians.

6. Let the patient select his own form of treatment, and then control for the confounding effects of differences between the groups by using appropriate analytic methods. The potential biases of this kind of quasi-experiment are the same as those of nonexperimental studies, and the results cannot be expected to be as convincing—or necessarily the same—as those of randomized trials. This approach is advocated by opponents of randomization ('One is uncomfortable with a randomized protocol that lets chance dictate the medical care a human being receives'), who also plead for data banks for the accumulation of clinical experience, to provide material for evaluative studies ('One randomized trial with 100 patients can dramatically change physician behavior, whereas the experience of 100 000 patients might be neglected').[28]

PLANNING AND RUNNING A CLINICAL TRIAL

For a clinical trial to yield convincing conclusions it must be designed and conducted with meticulous attention to detail.[21] Unless the effects of the intervention are very marked and specific, they can be convincingly attributed to the intervention (and not to extraneous factors) only if special precautions are taken. These include the use of controls (discussed in Ch. 7) and 'blind' methods (see p. 165), and (where appropriate) matching and prestratification (see p. 360), as well as suitable methods of analysis.[21]

Study objectives should be formulated precisely, in the form of clear and specific hypotheses (see Chs 4 and 5). The study population should be defined explicitly (Ch. 6) and eligibility and exclusion rules formulated (as in case-control studies—see p. 106). Attention must be given to intervention allocation methods, the size of the groups (p. 97), the selection and precise definition of variables (Chs 10–12) (including the outcome variables), the use of reliable and valid methods of data collection (Chs 15–17), quality control (p. 281), surveillance of compliance, and data monitoring.

Running a trial is not easy, and is beset with day-to-day problems that can easily overshadow the study's *raison d'etre*; trials 'lack glamour; they strain our resources and patience, and they protract to excruciating limits the moment of truth; ... [but] if ... the alternative is to pay the cost of perpetual uncertainty, have we really any choice?'[29] Successful trial management requires careful attention to the rules of the game,[30] the first of which is 'Thou shalt know and follow thy rules'. A written study protocol[31] is generally desirable, and is essential in multicentre trials.[32] The protocol of a therapeutic trial should include a detailed description of the treatment and its permissible modifications.

The selection of a study population for a trial is determined by the reference population the investigator has in mind, i.e. to whom does he want to apply the results? This is the basis for decisions on the source of subjects and the method of enrolling them, and the formulation of eligibility and exclusion criteria. The results of a trial of the treatment of middle-aged adults with moderate hypertension may not be applicable to patients with mild hypertension, or to the elderly.

The generalizability of results depends on who is studied. The results of a trial conducted on volunteers, such as a trial of immunization performed by comparing outcomes in randomly allocated groups of volunteers, may not be directly applicable to the population at large. In all trials there are selective factors—the subject's wishes, the views of his treating physician, family, etc.—that the investigator cannot control. It is therefore important to try to appraise the importance and nature of selection bias by determining what proportion of eligible people enter the trial and how those who enter differ from those who do not. The rules and actual reasons for exclusions should of course be recorded, so that it is clear to what kinds of subject the results of the trial do not apply. If many people withhold consent, so that possible *non-consent bias* is an important consideration, it may be enlightening to follow up and compare the progress of nonrandomized as well as randomized subjects; this may be done by a *comprehensive cohort design* (a cohort study with a randomized subcohort)[33] or by parallel trials, one randomized and one nonrandomized (where patients who are eligible for randomization choose their own treatment).[34]

In a typical RCT the sequence of steps is: determine eligibility; request informed consent; assign randomly; treat; and follow up. In a prerandomized study, consent and randomization are reversed. In some studies, e.g. where compliance with the taking of medications is regarded as an essential condition for participation, it may be necessary to have a 'run-in' period before eligibility can be finally determined; this period may precede or follow randomization. In the Physicians' Health Study, which tested the prophylactic effect of aspirin and beta-carotene, all participants eligible for randomization were sent packs of aspirin and a beta-carotene placebo, and after an 18-week run-in period those who reported side-effects to aspirin or had taken less than two-thirds of their pills were excluded from the trial.[35] In studies where treatment cannot be delayed until all diagnostic test results are available, eligibility may not be certain before treatment is started. In principle, randomization should be done as late as possible—i.e. when eligibility is certain and, in a trial where the initial treatment is the same for all patients, only after the initial treatment phase.[21]

In randomized trials, clinicians may be asked to consult a list showing how successive subjects should be treated, or to open a sealed envelope specifying the next patient's treatment, or to contact a coordinator and be told what treatment to give. It may not be easy to avoid divergence from the random allocation, even if sealed envelopes are used.[36] Drugs should look the same and their containers should not have distinctive labels, if the clinician is to be kept unaware of the treatment.

Rules for withdrawals from the randomized treatment should be laid down in advance. 'Escape hatches' must always be provided, to enable patients to be withdrawn whenever this is in their best interests—if, for example, they develop worrisome side-effects, illnesses or complications, or whenever (in a double-blind study) it becomes necessary for the clinician to know what treatment is being administered. Subjects may also be withdrawn because they turn out to be ineligible.

Follow-up should be as complete as possible. Subjects who are withdrawn from the study and those who drop out may be highly selected groups, and if they are numerous their exclusion from the analysis may cause serious bias. Wherever possible, the reasons for drop-outs should be ascertained. In a trial with defined endpoints, such as death, the occurrence of a disease or complication, recovery, etc., the aim should be to follow up every member of every study group until the occurrence of an endpoint, the lapse of a predetermined study period, or the conclusion of the study. Patients who turn out to be misdiagnosed or ineligible for other reasons are exceptions to this rule; they can usually be withdrawn without causing bias.

Every trial needs a 'policeman'[37]—an investigator, co-ordinator or co-ordinating committee who will keep an eye on the study, ensure smooth running and the avoidance of bias, and protect subjects' interests. It may be important to check adherence to randomization plans and 'blind' techniques, and monitor patients' compliance and the completeness and quality of data. In some trials, ongoing monitoring of data is undertaken in order to see whether the study can or should be stopped early, e.g. because of harmful effects or unexpectedly large beneficial effects; this function is best performed by an independent individual or committee, not the investigators; 'stopping rules' should be laid down in advance.

In the analysis,[21] use should be made of methods that take account of the duration of the subject's participation and the times of endpoint events or repeated appraisals. Confounding can be reduced by appropriate analytic techniques, e.g. by subdividing the groups so that similar subjects can be compared (stratification).

Even in the best-run of randomized therapeutic trials, it is unusual for all subjects to have their allocated treatment throughout the study—inevitably, there are withdrawals (generally in the patient's interests), non-compliers and drop-outs. In trials of interventions aimed at changing lifestyles there are always subjects who fail to change their habits, or who change them despite being in a control group. Bias due to withdrawals and drop-outs can be avoided by comparing the outcomes in all the subjects originally allocated to each group (*intention-to-treat analysis*). This stringent approach may underestimate the efficacy of the treatment, and an *on-randomized-treatment analysis* may be performed as well, comparing the experience of subjects while they were still on their allocated treatment.

Clinical trials often yield inconclusive or inconsistent results because of their small size. Results of different trials can, however, be integrated so as to yield firmer conclusions about the effects of the intervention, their consistency, and the factors that influence them (including characteristics of the subjects, variations in the intervention, and the circumstances and methods of the trial). A *meta-analysis*[38] or overview of this sort requires the use of suitable statistical methods. Meta-analysis may be applied to observational

as well as experimental studies. It typically includes an appraisal of
the quality of the studies ('qualitative meta-analysis'), an analysis
of the factors modifying their findings, and (if there are no important modifying effects) a summary statement of the findings in the
various studies. Applied to trials, a meta-analysis might review
studies that test a specific effect of a specific intervention, or it
might compare the effects of different interventions or the various
effects of an intervention.

NOTES AND REFERENCES

1. Schwartz D, Flamart R, Lellouch J 1980 (Clinical trials. Academic Press,
   London) describe in detail how the purpose of a trial (explanatory or
   pragmatic?) can influence planning, conduct and analysis. In a pragmatic trial
   the treatment is administered in the manner in which it would be used in
   practice, to subjects similar to those to whom it would be applied in practice,
   and appraised in terms of outcomes that are important to patients, rather
   than biological effects. Also, see Roland M, Torgerson D J (1998a)
   Understanding controlled trials: what are pragmatic trials? British Medical
   Journal 316: 285; and (1998b) Understanding controlled trials: what
   outcome should be measured? British Medical Journal 317: 1075–1080).
2. The patients for this study were recruited from 198 centres in 23 European
   countries. After an average follow-up period of two years the incidence of
   stroke was 42% lower (95% confidence interval, 14 to 63% lower) in the
   treatment group, 72% of whom continued their treatment throughout. The
   trial was then stopped on the grounds that it would be unethical to continue
   it. Total cardiovascular mortality was 27% lower (95% confidence interval,
   48% lower to 2% higher) in the treatment group (Staessen J A, Fagard R,
   Thijs L et al 1997 Randomised double-blind comparison of placebo and
   active treatment for older patients with isolated systolic hypertension. Lancet
   350: 757).
3. Symptoms generally attributed to adenoidal hypertrophy (nasal obstruction,
   snoring, rhinorrhoea, etc.) were very prevalent in both groups before
   operation, and were seldom found after operation. They were equally
   common in both groups, both before and after operation. The study was
   'blind', i.e. the examiner did not know what operation the child would have
   or had had (Hibbert J, Stell P M 1978 Critical evaluation of adenoidectomy.
   Lancet 1: 657).
4. The proportions who were cured or improved were very similar among
   patients taking antihistaminic and placebo tablets. This applied to people
   who started treatment within a day of the onset of symptoms, 1 day after
   onset, 2 days after, and 3 or more days after onset (Hill A B 1962 Statistical
   methods in clinical and preventive medicine. Churchill Livingstone,
   Edinburgh, pp 105–119).
5. Internal mammary ligation was performed on 304 'unselected' patients with
   angina pectoris and/or a history of myocardial infarction, and symptomatic
   improvement was reported in 95% (Battezzatti, M, Tagliaferro A, Cattaneo
   A D 1959 Clinical evaluation of bilateral internal mammary artery ligation as
   treatment of coronary heart disease. American Journal of Cardiology 4: 180).
   In a randomized trial in 17 patients with angina pectoris, the results
   (significant improvement in just over half the cases) were very similar in the
   patients who had this operation and in those who had a sham operation. One
   patient, previously unable to work because of his heart disease, was almost

immediately rehabilitated and returned to his former occupation, and reported 100% improvement after 6 months; his arteries had not been ligated. The patients were told only that they were participating in a trial of the procedure, and the clinicians who appraised progress did not know which operation had been done (Cobb L A, Thomas G T, Dillard D H, Merendino K A, Bruce R A 1959 An evaluation of internal-mammary-artery ligation by a double-blind technic. New England Journal of Medicine 260: 1115).

6. This experiment was forced on Ambroise Paré one day in 1537, when he ran out of boiling oil. The next morning the soldiers he had treated with boiling oil 'were feverish with much pain and swelling about their wounds', whereas the others had 'but little pain, their wounds neither swollen nor inflamed'; cited by Bull J P 1950 (The historical development of clinical therapeutic trials. Journal of Chronic Diseases 10: 218). The trial was not blind, the treatments were not allocated at random, and statistical significance was not tested; but the difference was so convincing that Paré determined 'never again to burn thus so cruelly the poor wounded'; and boiling oil is eschewed to this very day in the treatment of arquebus wounds.

7. 'At the end of ten days their countenances appeared fairer and fatter in flesh than all the children which did eat the portion of the king's meat' (The Book of Daniel 1: 15). Mosteller F, Gilbert J P, McPeek B 1983 (Controversies in design and analysis of clinical trials. In: Shapiro S H, Louis T A, eds. Clinical trials: issues and approaches. Marcel Dekker, New York, pp 13–64) point out methodological flaws in this biblical clinical trial: sample too small, duration too short, no randomization, no control of extraneous factors such as physical activity, ill defined endpoint, no information about countenances at start of trials.

8. *Study designs for clinical trials*, and their pros and cons, are described by many authors. See, for example, Altman D G 1991 (Practical statistics for medical research. Chapman & Hall, London, pp 441–455); Mosteller F, Gilbert J P, McPeek B (1983; see note 7). For *parallel designs*, see Lavori P W, Louis T A, Bailar J C III, Polansky M 1983. (Designs for experiments—parallel comparisons of treatment. New England Journal of Medicine 309: 1291). For *crossover and self-controlled designs*, see Louis T A, Lavori P W, Bailar J C III, Polansky M 1984 (Crossover and self-controlled designs in clinical research. New England Journal of Medicine 310: 24). The use of *historical controls* is discussed by Bailar J C III, Louis T A, Lavori P W, Polansky M 1984 (Studies without internal controls. New England Journal of Medicine 311: 156) and Dupont W D 1985 (Randomized vs historical clinical trials: are the benefits worth the cost? American Journal of Epidemiology 122: 940.

On the Internet, types of experimental and quasi-experimental design are described by Trochim W M K 1996 (Trochim.human.cornell.edu/kb/design.htm).

9. The statistics of *factorial experiments* that examine more than two factors and their interaction and Latin squares are discussed by Fleiss J L 1986 (The design and analysis of clinical experiments. John Wiley, New York).

10. Stampfer M J, Buring J E, Willett W, Rosner B, Eberlein K, Hennekens C H 1985 The 2×2 factorial design: its application to a randomized trial of aspirin and carotene in US physicians. Statistics in Medicine 4: 111; Steering Committee of the Physicians' Health Study Research Group 1989 Final report on the aspirin component of the ongoing Physicians' Health Study. New England Journal of Medicine 321: 129; Hennekens C H, Buring J E, Manson J E et al 1996 Lack of effect of long-term supplementation with beta carotene on the incidence of malignant neoplasms and cardiovascular disease. New England Journal of Medicine 334: 1145.

11. Pocock S J 1977 (Randomised clinical trials. British Medical Journal 1: 1661) found variations of up to 46% in the death rates of control groups (who had

the same treatment) used by the same investigators in different cancer chemotherapy trials.

12. Taylor W R 1983 An evaluation of supplementary feeding in Somali refugee camps. International Journal of Epidemiology 12: 433.

13. *Single-patient trials*, like RCTs, are applications of Pickering's counsel to clinicians: 'If we take a patient afflicted with a malady, and we alter his conditions of life, either by dieting him, or by putting him to bed, or by administering to him a drug, or by performing on him an operation, we are performing an experiment. And if we are scientifically minded we should record the results' (Pickering G 1949 Physician and scientist. Proceedings of the Royal Society of Medicine 42: 229).

A typical 'N of 1' trial is based on successive pairs of treatment periods, a treatment being given in one period and another treatment (or a placebo) in the other; the sequence within each pair is decided randomly; where possible, 'blind' methods are used. The greater the number of time periods, the more convincing the results. The method is appropriate for chronic, stable conditions and treatments that act fast and stop acting soon after they are discontinued.

Methods are described by (among others): Cook D J 1996 (Randomized trials in single subjects: the N of 1 study. Psychopharmacology Bulletin 32: 363); Guyatt G, Sackett D, Adachi J, Roberts R, Chong J, Rosenbloom D, Keller J 1988 (A clinician's guide for conducting randomized trials in individual patients. Canadian Medical Association Journal 139: 497); and Johannessen T, Petersen H, Kristensen P, Fosstvedt D 1991 (The controlled single subject trial. Scandinavian Journal of Primary Health Care 9: 17).

Reports of the clinical usefulness of these trials include: Larson E B, Ellsworth A J K, Oas J 1993 (Randomized clinical trials in single patients during a 2-year period. Journal of the American Medical Association 270: 2708); and Mahon J, Laupacis A, Donner A, Wood T 1996 (Randomised study of n of 1 trials versus standard practice. British Medical Journal 312: 1069).

14. Peto R, Pike M C, Armitage P et al 1976 Design and analysis of randomized clinical trials requiring prolonged observation of each patient. I. Introduction and design. British Journal of Cancer 34: 585; II. Analysis and examples. British Journal of Cancer 1977 35: 1.

15. Wright I S, Marple C D, Beck D F 1954 Myocardial infarction: its clinical manifestations and treatment with anticoagulants. Grune & Stratton, New York, pp 9–11.

16. Because *minimalization* ensures the similarity of the groups compared in a trial, its protagonists say that 'if randomization is the gold standard, minimalization may be the platinum standard' (Treasure T, MacRae K D 1998 British Medical Journal 317: 362). Simple instructions are provided by Altman D G 1991 ([see note 8], pp 443–445). RANDOM, in the PEPI package, provides a dice-loading procedure to assist in the process; see note 7, p. 292.

17. 'Student' 1931 Biometrika 23: 398.

18. *Using random numbers*. If all the subjects are known in advance, random sampling methods (see p. 91) can be used to assign them randomly. If candidates are continuously enrolled during the trial, or if balanced randomization is desired, blocks of subjects can be randomized separately. If the subjects are paired, single-digit random numbers can be used as substitutes for tossing a coin; an even number might mean 'Treat the first member of the pair', and an odd number 'Treat the second'. A similar method can be used for allocating successive cases in a list or series; successive random numbers are used, odd and even numbers being interpreted as 'Group A' and 'Group B' respectively. If the required

allocation is 2:1, numbers 1 to 6 might be used for one group, and 7 to 9 for the other (zeros being ignored). If subjects are to be allocated equally to three groups, 1–3 might be taken to mean Group A, 4–6 Group B, and 7–9 Group C (zeros ignored).

Random permutations are easier to use than random numbers, because each number appears once only. Fleiss J L (1986; see note 9) supplies a table (Table A.7) and instructions (pp 47–51).

19. RANDOM, in the PEPI package, does simple, balanced and stratified randomization; see note 7, page 292.

20. Simple instructions for *balanced randomization*, using allocation ratios of 1:1, 1:2 or 1:1:1, are given by Peto et al (1976; see note 14). To obtain a balanced 1:1 allocation to two groups (A and B), for example, list all 30 of the possible arrangements of three As and three Bs (AAABBB, AABABB, etc.) and then (using random numbers) choose which of these sequences will be applied to each successive set of six subjects.

When allocating patients to three treatments, the groups can be kept equal by ensuring that three of each successive nine patients go into each group. This might be done by denoting treatment A as 1, 2 or 3, treatment B as 4, 5 or 6, and treatment C as 7, 8 or 9. One-digit random numbers are then chosen. Going from left to right in the top line of the table on p. 99, the first number is 9. This means that the first case should go into group C. The second number is 6, and the third 2; i.e. the second case should be put in group B, and the third in group A. The fourth number, 2, is ignored, as we have already had a 2. The next number is 7, so the fourth case goes into group C. And so on for the whole series of nine cases; the final sequence is C,B,A,C,B,C,A,A,B (Hill A B 1977 A short textbook of medical statistics. Hodder & Stoughton, London, pp 303–304).

21. See Altmann D G 1991 ([see note 8], pp 440–476) for a discussion of the design and analysis of controlled trials; a simple guide is provided by Peto et al 1976 and 1977 (see note 14).

Practical issues are discussed by (among others) Margitic S E, Miles N L 1998 (Ten commandments of successful trial management. Preventive Medicine 27: 84); Lavin P T 1983 (In: Shapiro S H, Louis T A, eds [see note 7], pp 129–154); and Friedman L W, Furberg C D, DeMets D L 1983 (Fundamentals of clinical trials. John Wright, Boston).

Statistical analysis is considered by (among many others) Fleiss J L 1986 (see note 9); Altman D G 1991 ([see note 8], pp 461–471); Bailey A, Crook A, Machin D 1994 (Statistical methods for clinical trials. Blood Reviews 8: 105); and Meier P 1983 (In: Shapiro S H, Louis T A [see note 7], pp 155–190).

22. Bailar J C III 1983 Introduction In: Shapiro S H, Louis T A 1983 ([see note 7], pp 1–12).

23. *Response adaptive randomization* has been little used in practice. See Berry D A, Eick S G 1995 (Adaptive assignment versus balanced randomization in clinical trials: a decision analysis. Statistics in Medicine 14: 231); Rosenberger W F, Lachin J M 1993 (The use of responsive-adaptive designs in clinical trials. Controlled Clinical Trials 14: 471); and Friedman L W, Furberg C D, DeMets D L 1983 ([see note 21], pp 51–56).

24. Pocock S J 1976 (The combination of randomized and historical controls in clinical trials. Journal of Chronic Diseases 29: 175) suggests combining the data for the randomized and historical controls in different ways, based on varying degrees of mistrust of the historical data. In a review paper, Louis T A, Shapiro S H 1983 (Critical issues in the conduct and interpretation of clinical trials. Annual Reviews of Public Health 4: 25) warn that the inclusion of historical controls 'can compromise a trial's validity, even if the investigators are convinced that it is valid'. See note 11.

25. Armitage P 1975 Sequential medical trials, 2nd edn. Blackwell, Oxford.
26. Finkelstein M O, Levin B, Robbins H 1996 Clinical and prophylactic trials with assured new treatment for those at greater risk: I. A design proposal. American Journal of Public Health 86: 691; Finkelstein M O, Levin B, Robbins H 1996 Clinical and prophylactic trials with assured new treatment for those at greater risk: II. Examples. American Journal of Public Health 86: 696; Mosteller F 1996 Editorial: The promise of risk-based allocation trials in assessing new treatments. American Journal of Public Health 86: 622.
27. Zelen M 1990 Randomized consent designs for clinical trials: an update. Statistics in Medicine 9: 645; Zelen M 1979 A new design for randomized clinical trials. New England Journal of Medicine 300: 1242. See debate in 'Variance and dissent' section, New England Journal of Medicine 1983 36: 609.
28. Weinstein M C 1974 Allocation of subjects in medical experiments. New England Journal of Medicine 291: 1278.
29. Fredrickson D S 1968 The field trial: some thoughts on the indispensable ordeal. Bulletin of the New York Academy of Medicine 44: 985.
30. Margitic S E, Miles N L 1998 (see note 21).
31. For a specimen protocol outline, see Friedman L W et al 1983 ([see note 21], p. 6).
32. The organization of *multicentre trials* is described by Friedman L W et al 1983 ([see note 21], p. 211) and Stanley K, Stjernsward J, Isley M 1981 (The conduct of a cooperative clinical trial. Recent Results in Cancer Research no 77, Berlin. Springer-Verlag, Berlin). For statistical aspects, see Fleiss J L 1986 ([see note 9], p. 176).
33. Olschewski M, Schumacher M, Davis K B 1992 Analysis of randomized and nonrandomized patients in clinical trials using the comprehensive cohort follow-up study design. Controlled Clinical Trials 13: 226.
34. Marcus S M 1997 Assessing non-consent bias with parallel randomized and nonrandomized clinical trials. Journal of Clinical Epidemiology 50: 823.
35. Lang J M, Buring J E, Rosner B, Cook N, Hennekens C H 1991 Estimating the effect of the run-in on the power of the Physicians' Health Study. Statistics in Medicine 10: 1585.
36. One investigator, scarred by his experiences in collaborative (i.e. multiclinic) clinical trials, cautions that 'consecutive numbering of envelopes alone is inadequate protection against tampering with randomization. The envelopes, if used, should be serially numbered, opaque, and sealed with water-insoluble glue to prevent steaming them open, and all nonopened envelopes should be returned to the coordinating center which should check the integrity of the seal. Still better, the coordinating center should issue an assignment only after the clinic has identified the eligible patient by name' (Ederer F 1975 Practical problems in collaborative clinical trials. American Journal of Epidemiology 102: 111).
37. Mainland D 1960 The clinical trial—some difficulties and suggestions. Journal of Chronic Diseases 11: 484.
38. *Meta-analysis.* See Smith G D, Egger M, Phillips A N 1997 (Meta-analysis and data synthesis in medical research. In: Detels R, Holland W W, McEwen J, Omenn G S, eds. 1997 Oxford Textbook of public health, 3rd edn, vol 2. The methods of public health. Oxford University Press, New York, pp 631–649); a series of articles in the British Medical Journal (Egger M, Smith G D 1997 Meta-analysis: Potentials and promise. 315: 1371; Egger M, Smith G D, Philips A N 1997 Meta-analysis: Principles and procedures. 315: 1533; Smith G D, Egger M, Phillips A N 1977 Meta-analysis: Beyond the grand mean? 315: 1610; Egger M, Smith G D 1998 Meta-analysis: Bias in location and selection of studies. 316: 61; Egger M, Scheider M, Smith G D 1998 Meta-analysis: Spurious precision? Meta-analysis of observational studies. 316: 140; Smith G D, Egger M 1998 Meta-analysis: Unresolved issues and

future developments. 316: 221); and Abramson J H 1990 (Meta-analysis: A review of pros and cons. Public Health Reviews 18: 1).

Meta-analysis software is reviewed by Egger M, Smith G D 1998 (Meta-analysis: Meta-analysis software. Available on the Internet: http://www.bmj.com/archive/7126/7126ed9.htm).

Programs in the PEPI package (see note 7, p. 292) can perform most of the basic meta-analytic computations.

33 Programme trials

Programme trials are experiments or quasi-experiments that test hypotheses concerning the effects of health programmes. The programme may be one directed at a specific problem or population category (e.g. mass screening, anti-smoking, clean air, prevention of AIDS, care of stroke patients or the elderly), or it may be an organizational form—a programme trial may appraise day-care hospitals, health centres, the work of a category of health personnel (nurse practitioners, chiropodists, village health workers), etc.

A programme trial endeavours not only to appraise outcomes, but to determine whether these can be attributed to the intervention rather than to extraneous factors. The aim is to obtain generalizable knowledge, applicable to settings like the one in which the trial was performed, about the value of a *type* of programme. In these respects a programme trial differs from a simple programme review (see p. 27), which is an observational study (generally descriptive, sometimes with an analytic component) that aims to appraise the implementation and/or outcome of a specific programme provided for a specific group or community, without necessarily seeking conclusive evidence that the outcome can be ascribed to the programme; such evidence may require the rigorous techniques used in trials.

Most studies of public health interventions are nonexperimental or quasi-experimental.[1] The importance of these studies should not, however, be minimized—they are more practicable than true experiments, and may provide useful and sometimes generalizable lessons.[2]

Programmes are sometimes evaluated by using a case-control design, as explained on pages 350–351. In the Netherlands, for example, the value of a cancer screening programme was confirmed by a study of women who died of breast cancer and matched living controls, comparing their history of participation in the programme.[3]

OBJECTIVES OR PROGRAMME TRIALS

A programme trial usually focuses on the outcome of care, and its variation in different population groups or different circumstances. There may also be interest in economic efficiency. Appraisals of performance, compliance, satisfaction, facilities and settings (see Ch. 5) usually have the specific purpose of explaining effectiveness or its lack, except in studies that focus on feasibility or acceptability.

Effectiveness can be convincingly demonstrated only if the outcomes used as criteria are clearly desirable ones—i.e. worthwhile 'end-results' in their own right, or stepping-stones to such end-results. In instances where the benefits to be expected from an activity are certain (e.g. immunization), a measure of its performance may be used as a criterion of effectiveness.

The outcomes selected for appraisal are generally those that the programme tries (explicitly or implicitly) to achieve. The goal attainment model[4] is illustrated in Figure 33.1. Every programme goal (G_2) may imply one or more subgoals or intermediate goals (G_1) that must be achieved if the programme goal is to be attained. Activities (A_1 and A_2) are performed in order to achieve the goals. As an example, attaining a reduced prevalence of hypertension (G_2) as a result of antihypertensive treatment (A_2) requires the achievement of an intermediate goal, the identification of hypertensives in the population (G_1), as an outcome of screening activities (A_1).

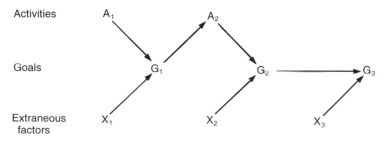

Fig. 33.1 Goal attainment model

These activities (A_1 and A_2), which aim at achieving goals G_1 and G_2, constitute the programme. (This is of course an oversimplification; most programmes comprise a number of longer, branched, and interconnecting chains.) It may also be possible to define 'ultimate goals' or end-results (G_3) that may result from the operation of the programme, but without further programme activities, e.g. a reduction in mortality from stroke.

Any outcome that is inherently desirable—in this instance, G_2 or G_3—is a satisfactory criterion of effectiveness in a programme trial. But extraneous factors (X_1, X_2 and X_3) may contribute to each outcome, and their confounding effects must be controlled.

A trial may, of course, aim to appraise undesired as well as desirable outcomes.

A trial that appraises an outcome may become more meaningful if it also opens the programme's 'black box' by examining the performance of activities and the attainment of intermediate goals leading up to the outcome. Success in attaining the desired outcome can be convincingly attributed to the programme only if the programme activities were performed satisfactorily, and failure to achieve this outcome may be explained by failure to perform these activities. A randomized controlled trial indicating that a programme providing extensive health examinations produced no change in mortality over the next 20 years,[5] for example, would be more meaningful if information was provided on the extent to which the examinations led to the provision of therapeutic and preventive care.

Here are three examples of programme trials. The study objectives were:

1. To compare the changes in (a) attitudes to smoking and (b) the prevalence of smoking among boys in the 10th to 12th grades in two schools, one with an anti-smoking programme and one without; controlling for grade, membership of sports teams, parents' smoking habits, and other variables.[6]
2. To compare the incidence of diarrhoea in children's day-care centres in which a handwashing programme was introduced (handwashing after toilet activities and before handling food or eating) with the incidence in control day-care centres.[7]
3. To compare the incidence of trachoma (an eye disease spread by eye discharges) in Tanzanian villages in which mass treatment with an antibiotic ointment was followed by an intensive educational programme to encourage facewashing, and in villages that received mass treatment only.[8]

STUDY DESIGNS

Programme trials may be individual-based or group-based.

In the former, individuals are allocated (preferably randomly) to groups that are exposed (or not exposed) to the programme under study. These trials do not differ in their design from other clinical trials.

In group-based trials the experimental units are groups or communities that are exposed (or not exposed) to the programme. These may be called *community trials*. The basic experimental or quasi-experimental designs are the same as for clinical trials (see p. 357): i.e. parallel, externally controlled, and 'self-controlled' (including crossover) studies. Since investigators seldom have the power to decide where or when programmes will be established, most programme trials are quasi-experiments.

Individual-based (clinical) and parallel, externally controlled and 'self-controlled' community trials will be discussed in more detail below.

Community trials may be undertaken to test aetiological hypotheses, not only to evaluate programmes. A classic example is Goldberger's demonstration of the nutritional origin of pellagra, based on experimental dietary changes in orphanages and a mental hospital.[9]

CLINICAL TRIALS TO EVALUATE PROGRAMMES

It is sometimes feasible to conduct a randomized clinical trial in which some individuals are allocated to a programme and others are used as controls, or individuals are allocated to different programmes.

For example, in a trial of breast cancer screening, members of the Health Insurance Plan of New York were randomly allocated to two groups; some women were offered four annual screening examinations (clinical and mammographic), and others continued to receive their usual medical care. Rates of mortality and other endpoints in the two groups were compared. This demonstrated a considerably lower rate of breast cancer mortality in the group assigned to the screening programme, among women aged 50 or more.[10]

As another example, rates of compliance with antihypertensive drug treatment were compared in workers randomly allocated to treatment by industrial physicians during working hours, or by their family doctors. This trial also compared the rates of compliance among men exposed and not exposed to an educational programme (slide-audiotape and booklet) about hypertension. No differences in compliance were found; an unexpected finding was that there was a dramatic increase in absenteeism among workers who were told they had hypertension, especially in the group exposed to the educational programme.[11]

Trials of this kind cannot be 'blind'. Bias caused by the Hawthorne effect (see p. 84) may be reduced if an alternative programme is offered to the control subjects. In a trial that showed the effectiveness of physical fitness classes as a way of preventing recurrences of low back pain in hospital workers, for example, a 'back school' (providing instruction on the prevention of back strain) was arranged for the control subjects.[12]

As in other clinical trials, more than one outcome may be studied. In a trial in Seattle, for example, individuals were randomly assigned to a prepaid health maintenance organization or to insurance plans requiring the payment of a fee-for-service, and the outcomes that were compared included changes in blood pressure, functional visual capacity, cholesterol, smoking habits, weight, physical functioning, role functioning, bed-days, serious symptoms, mental health, and other indices of general health.[13]

In trials where there are nonparticipants, outcomes must of course be measured in the total groups, including their nonparticipant members. Nonparticipants are likely to differ from participants, and their exclusion may introduce bias. As an example, if women who did not accept the offer of breast screening made in the Health Insurance Plan study were excluded from the analysis, the results indicated that screening produced a sizeable (but spurious) reduction in mortality from causes other than breast cancer.[10] The crucial comparison in such a study is not between those who participate in the programme and those who do not, but between the randomized groups ('intention-to-treat' analysis; see p. 366).

In trials of programmes that require active participation by the subjects, the extent of participation in the trial (as well as in the programme) may have an important bearing on the conclusions. This applies to community as well as clinical trials. In a trial of worksite smoking cessation programmes, where workers at a large installation who consented to participate were randomly allocated to different programmes, the proportions of the randomized groups who quit smoking (measured 12 months later) ranged from

16 to 26% (as compared with a spontaneous quit rate of 5%). But about 64% of the smokers at the plant had not expressed interest in the smoking cessation project, and another 25% had expressed interest but did not agree to participate.[14] Although the results led to a decision to offer the best of the programmes on a regular basis, the overall impact on smoking habits was likely to be small.

When a programme trial is conducted in a single health service, randomization of individuals is generally difficult or impossible. Making a programme available to some patients and not others may be ethically unacceptable, or resented by the patients; this difficulty can sometimes be overcome if the programme is introduced in stages (a shortage of resources may justify this) and will eventually be available to everyone. In a small practice, where patients know and talk to one another, there is likely to be 'contamination' that may interfere with the evaluation of programmes that have an educational component (i.e. that call for changes in behaviour).

PARALLEL COMMUNITY TRIALS

In *parallel community trials* two or more independent groups or communities are studied prospectively and compared (see the three illustrative studies on p. 375). More groups are preferable to fewer, even if they are smaller.[15,16] The groups should be selected (randomly if possible, but this is seldom feasible) in such a way that they represent the reference population.[17]

As in clinical trials, randomization (see p. 359) is the best way of reducing bias in these trials. Published examples include the random allocation of towns (for fluoridation of water supplies), factories (for programmes for the control of cardiovascular risk factors), villages (for fly control measures), families (for the provision of primary care by nurse practitioners or physicians), and orthodontic clinics.[18] If such studies have few experimental units, randomization may not prevent marked differences. Randomization is of little importance if only two communities are compared—the communities have the same differences, whatever the assignment, and these must be taken into account in the analysis. The analysis of randomized group trials may require special precautions.[16]

Unfortunately, randomization is seldom feasible, since investigators seldom have the power to decide where or when programmes will be established. Most community trials of programmes are quasi-experiments, in which the control groups are purposively selected to be as similar as possible to the intervention groups. The greater this similarity, and the more convincingly it can be demonstrated, the more persuasive are the conclusions. Similarity to the intervention group and the feasibility of obtaining satisfactory data are the main considerations when choosing control groups. There is often a very restricted choice concerning controls.

As in clinical trials, follow-up should be complete; people who do not actively participate in the programme should not be excluded.

'Postmeasure only' studies, where the findings in an intervention group (after exposure to a programme) are compared with those in a control population, are useful only if it can be assumed that the groups were similar before the institution of the programme.[19] A mobile coronary-care service, for example, was evaluated by comparing case fatality rates in two demographically similar communities in Northern Ireland, one of which had such a service. Fatality was higher in the community without a mobile service, although hospital facilities and hospital treatment were similar. The difference could not be attributed to differences in severity or other characteristics of the cases. The results would be more convincing, however, if there was direct evidence that the risk of dying was the same in both communities before the service was instituted or, as the authors point out, if this risk is found to decrease in the control community when such a service is started there.[20]

The minimal requirement is generally a 'premeasure—postmeasure' design, with 'before' and 'after' measurements for both populations. The longer the time series the better, as this permits a fuller comparison of *trends* in both populations. A long follow-up may also permit the cumulation of enough outcome events (diseases and deaths) to permit comparisons of incidence and mortality. On the other hand, long-term comparisons are beset with problems, as the differences in intervention may be attenuated by changes in health care and other influences affecting outcomes, or blurred by changes in the composition of the groups and by difficulties with follow-up. Several controlled community cardiovascular risk reduction reduction trials have failed to show substantial effects on health, and this has been attributed to the spread of interventions and educational messages to the comparison populations,[21] either from the intervention populations ('contamination') or because of wider societal, institutional or cultural changes. As an illustration, in 1975–76 an appreciably steeper decrease in the prevalence of cardiovascular risk factors was demonstrated in a Jerusalem population exposed since 1970 to such a programme (the CHAD programme) than in a neighbouring community receiving ordinary medical care from another agency. Risk factor status continued to improve in the exposed population, but it did so in the comparison population also, and in 1985–87 the differences were smaller than in 1975–76. Risk factor control had improved very considerably in the comparison population, partly as a result of a policy decision stimulated by the success of the CHAD programme, partly as a result of greater nationwide awareness by the media, public, and medical profession of the importance of these risk factors. By then 21% of adults 50 years or older in the control population were being treated for hypertension, 48% reported a blood cholesterol test within the last year, and 70% of hypertensives were under control. No one was very surprised that a 23-year follow-up of mortality revealed no significant differences between the populations.[22]

A feasible manoeuvre if a service is expanding to a progressively larger population is to compare the 'before' data for each newly admitted chunk with the contemporaneous 'after' data for the population admitted previously (on the assumption that the populations were initially similar), and later with its own 'after' data. In a study in Africa, this technique showed that a reduction in infant mortality could be attributed to a health centre's efforts.[23] In a city in the United States, it demonstrated that a programme for increasing the availability of medical care (by providing services free) apparently led to increased sickness, as measured by self-appraisals of health, the number of symptoms, and limitation of activities because of poor health.[24] A more ambitious multiple-group time-series design (i.e. the use of serial observations in different communities as a basis for both inter-community and within-community comparisons) has been used in community trials of cardiovascular disease prevention programmes.[25]

EXTERNALLY CONTROLLED COMMUNITY TRIALS

In an externally controlled community trial the investigator limits his investigation to groups or communities that are exposed to the programme, and compares the findings with data obtained from other sources. National data may be used, or published reports of surveys or trials in other populations.

The validity of such studies is often in serious doubt. Definitions and study methods may be different, the study population may differ in its characteristics or circumstances from the population from which the control data are derived, and the data may refer to different times.

'SELF-CONTROLLED' ('BEFORE—AFTER') COMMUNITY TRIALS

In 'self-controlled' community trials, observations before and after the institution of the programme are compared. The group or community is its own control. As in clinical trials of this sort, the main biases (see p. 358) are those connected with extraneous events or changes that occur between the observations, nonspecific effects caused by the trial itself, and changes in methods of measurement. 'Before—after' experiments of this sort, without external controls, are common in public health. 'Infant mortality dropped after the introduction of the programme' is adduced as evidence of effectiveness, although the same change might have occurred without the programme. Salutary testimony to the weakness of this reasoning is provided by McKeown's demonstration that although the introduction of specific immunization procedures and antibiotic treatment was followed by reductions in rates of mortality from tuberculosis, pneumonia, whooping cough, measles and other infective diseases, these changes were continuations of trends that had been observed for many years prior to the introduction of these procedures.[26]

To be reasonably convincing, the 'before—after' trial should be replicated in different populations or at different times—does infant mortality invariably or almost invariably drop when the programme is instituted? It is also helpful to examine data for a number of years *before* the institution of the programme—is there evidence of a *change* in the time trend?

It is also helpful if a 'before—after' study can be extended to an examination of what happens when the programme is withdrawn. It must be very rare, however, for an investigator to have the power or ethical justification for a decision to discontinue a programme that has shown an apparent effect. Such studies are therefore generally opportunistic quasi-experiments. In a rare example of a quasi-experimental crossover community trial, the effects of a programme to encourage the performance of Pap smears were observed in two Indian communities in the United States—one in which such a programme was instituted in 1978, and one in which it was discontinued in the same year.[27]

A WORD OF WARNING

Programme trials are important. Their topics are seldom trivial, and their practical implications may be prodigious. The importance of careful planning and rigorous methods of study and analysis can hence not be underestimated. The fact that most programme trials are quasi-experimental community trials, where the investigator does not have the power to make decisions on the allocation of study groups or (in some instances) on the collection of data, does not mean that the rules can be relaxed. On the contrary, the appraisal of bias and its analytic control become especially important.

Two major principles have been specified for the use of quasi-experimental designs.[28] The first requires that 'all plausible alternative explanations of the relationship between cause and effect or treatment and outcome be specified, and evidence to counter these rival explanations considered or demonstrated'. The second is that of 'assessing the consistency of findings from studies across times and across research settings, methods, and populations'.

The provision of sound scientific evidence about the value of health care programmes cannot ensure that policy for health care will be based on sound scientific evidence, or indeed that there will be *any* policy for health care.[29] But the provision of unsound scientific evidence can hardly improve matters.

NOTES AND REFERENCES

1. An analysis of studies dealing with preventive interventions, published in six community health journals in 1992, revealed that 30% were RCTs; a further 29% could and should have been RCTs (Smith P J, Moffatt M E K, Gelskey S C, Hudson S, Kaita K 1997 Are community health interventions evaluated appropriately? A review of six journals. Journal of Clinical Epidemiology 50: 137). This distribution is influenced by publication bias: programme reviews are generally of interest only to those concerned with the particular programme reviewed, and are much less likely to be published than programme trials. If a paper's 'subject is of local interest only or is not generalizable' the American Journal of Public Health rejects it on sight (Northridge M E, Susser M 1994 Annotation: Seven fatal flaws in submitted manuscripts. American Journal of Public Health 84: 718).
2. Susser M 1995 Editorial: The tribulations of trials—intervention in communities. American Journal of Public Health 85: 156.
3. Collette H J A, Day N E, Rombach J J, De Waard F 1984 Evaluation of

screening for breast cancer in a non-randomised study (the DOM project) by means of a case-control study. Lancet 1: 1224.

4. The classic paper on the evaluation of programme effectiveness, which presents the *goal attainment model*, is by Deniston O L, Rosenstock L M, Getting V A 1968 (Evaluation of program effectiveness. Public Health Reports 83: 323).

5. The investigators concluded that general health examinations 'are of little value in preventing diseases leading to death'. In this programme (in Stockholm in the early 1970s) people with a need for intervention were referred for care, but there was no follow-up. The unanswered question is whether mortality remained unaffected despite appropriate care, or because of inadequate care (Theobald H, Bygren L O, Carstensen J, Hauffman M, Engfeld P 1998 Effects of an assessment of needs for medical and social services on long-term mortality: a randomized controlled study. International Journal of Epidemiology 27: 194).

6. Using an increased awareness that 'smoking is dangerous to health' as a criterion, the programme was effective. Using changes in smoking habits as a criterion, it was ineffective (Monk M, Tayback M, Gordon J 1965 Evaluation of an antismoking program among high school students. American Journal of Public Health 55: 994; reprinted in Schulberg H C, Sheldon A, Baker F, eds. 1969 Program evaluation in the health fields. Behavioural Publications, New York, pp 345–359).

7. This study was done in suburban Atlanta, Georgia. During the 35 weeks of the trial the incidence of diarrhoea in the centres where hands were washed was half that in the control centres. Before the handwashing programme was started the incidence was higher in the experimental than in the control centres (Black R E, Dykes A C, Anderson K E 1981 American Journal of Epidemiology 113: 445).

8. Three pairs of villages (matched for maternal education, cleanliness of children's faces, and baseline prevalence of trachoma) participated in this study. The face-washing programme was administered to randomly chosen households in one randomly chosen village in each pair. The programme increased the prevalence of clean faces and reduced the incidence of severe trachoma in two villages but not in the third, in which there was 'a very strong ethos of disapproval for families who tried to be better than other families or "put on airs"' (West S, Munoz B, Lunch M, Kayongoya A, Chilangwa Z, Mmbaga B B O, Taylor H R 1995 Impact of face-washing on trachoma in Kongwa, Tanzania. Lancet 345: 155).

9. Goldberger J, Waring C H, Tanner W F 1923 Public Health Reports 38: 2361.

10. Shapiro S, Venet W, Strax P, Venet L, Roeser R 1982 Ten- to fourteen-year effect of screening on breast cancer mortality. Journal of the National Cancer Institute 69: 349.

11. Sackett D L, Haynes R B, Gibson E S et al 1975 Randomised clinical trial of strategies for improving medication compliance in primary hypertension. Lancet 1: 1205; Haynes R B, Sackett D L, Taylor D W, Gibson E S, Johnson A L 1978 Increased absenteeism from work after detection and labeling of hypertensive patients. New England Journal of Medicine 299: 741.

12. Donchin M, Woolf O, Kaplan L, Floman Y 1989 Secondary prevention of low back pain. Abstracts: Kyoto, Japan, May 15–19, 1989. International Society for the Study of the Lumber [sic] Spine, Toronto, p. 18.

13. This study (part of the Rand Health Insurance Study) found that the outcome of care by an HMO (where costs are lower, mainly because of reduced hospital admissions and hospital days) differed for poor and well-off individuals who had health problems at the outset. Among the well-off,

cholesterol levels and general health improved significantly more than in the
fee-for-service system; among the poor, those assigned to the HMO had more
bed-days and more serious symptoms (Ware J E Jr, Brook R H, Rogers W H
et al 1986 Comparison of health outcomes at a health maintenance
organisation with those of fee-for-service care. Lancet i: 1017).

14. Omenn G S, Thompson B, Sexton M et al 1988 A randomized comparison
of worksite-sponsored smoking cessation programs. American Journal of
Preventive Medicine 4: 261.

15. See Blackburn H 1991 (Community programmes in coronary heart disease
prevention and health promotion: changing community behaviour. In:
Marmot M, Elliott P, eds. 1991 Coronary heart disease epidemiology: from
aetiology to public health. Oxford University Press, Oxford, pp 495–514).

16. Murray D M 1997 Design and analysis of group-randomized trials: a review
of recent developments. Annals of Epidemiology 7: S70.

17. The design of programme trials is discussed by Hoffmeister H, Mensink
G B M 1997 Community-based intervention trials. In: Detels R, Holland
W W, McEwen J, Omenn G S, eds. 1997 Oxford Textbook of public health,
3rd edn, vol 2. The methods of public health. Oxford University Press, New
York, pp 571–584).

18. A trial of an anti-smoking programme, delivered by orthodontists, was
conducted by randomizing 154 orthodontic offices to experimental and
control groups (Slymen D J, Hovell M F 1997 Cluster versus individual
randomization in adolescent tobacco and alcohol studies: illustrations for
design decisions. International Journal of Epidemiology 26: 765).

19. The lack of baseline information about mortality, morbidity, growth and
nutritional status is a serious problem in trials of new patterns of grass-roots
primary health care in developing countries. Even discounting ethical
considerations, it is difficult to collect such data before community health
workers, on whom these care programmes are based, start to function. In the
Narangwal project in India, for example (an important controlled study of the
comparative effectiveness of nutritional care, medical care, and their
combination), no 'before' measurements were available in the villages
studied. Information on births and deaths was not collected in a uniform way
until the second year of the project. The validity of the conclusions rests on
the assurance that the villages were similar in such features as size, education,
the distribution of occupational groups, and access to previously available
health services (Kielmann A A, Taylor C E, Parker R L 1978 The Narangwal
Nutrition Study: a summary review. American Journal of Clinical Nutrition
31: 2040).

20. Mathewson Z M, McClockey B G, Evans A E, Russell C J, Wilson C 1985
Mobile coronary care and community mortality from myocardial infarction.
Lancet 1: 441.

21. Fineleib M 1996 Editorial: New directions for community intervention
studies. American Journal of Public Health 86: 1696.
    The capacity of cardiovascular risk reduction programmes, in many
instances, to reduce the prevalence of risk factors is not in question. See
reviews by Schooler C, Farquhar J W, Fortmann S P, Flora J A 1997
(Synthesis of findings and issues from community prevention trials. Annals of
Epidemiology 7: 554) and Stone E J, Pearson T A, Fortmann S P, McKinlay
J B 1997 (Community-based prevention trials: challenges and directions for
public health practice, policy, and research).

22. Abramson J H, Gofin J, Hopp C, Schein M H, Naveh P 1994 The CHAD
program for the control of cardiovascular risk factors in a Jerusalem
community: a 24-year retrospect. Israel Journal of Medical Sciences 30: 108.

23. Kark S L, Cassel J 1952 The Pholela Health Centre: a progress report. South
African Medical Journal 26: 101, 132; Kark S L 1981 The practice of

community oriented primary health care. Appleton-Century-Crofts, New York, pp 243–245.

24. Diehr P K, Richardson W C, Shortell S M, LoGerfo J P 1979 Increased access to medical care: the impact on health. Medical Care 17: 989.
25. Salonen J T, Kottke T E, Jacobs D R Jr, Hannan P J 1986 Analysis of community-based cardiovascular disease prevention studies—evaluation issues in the North Karelia project and the Minnesota Heart Health program. International Journal of Epidemiology 15: 176.
26. McKeown T 1979 The role of medicine: dream, mirage or nemesis? Blackwell, Oxford.
27. Freeman W L 1987 In: Nutting P A (ed) Community-oriented primary care: from principle to practice. Health Resources and Services. Administration, Public Health, Washington, D C, pp 410–416. In both communities the Pap screening rate was considerably higher when the programme was operative.
28. Patrick D L 1985 Sociological investigations. In: Holland W W, Detels R, Knox G (eds) Oxford Textbook of public health, vol 3. Oxford University Press, Oxford, Ch 11.
29. 'Do situations exist in which there is health policy without scientific evidence? In fact there are only a few situations in which there is any kind of policy.' (Ibrahim M A 1985 Epidemiology and health policy. Maryland, Aspen, Rockville, p. 183).

34 Community-oriented primary care

This chapter is written for practitioners of primary health care (doctors, nurses, health educators, managers and others) who try to 'treat the community as a patient' by appraising the health needs of a population and establishing programmes to deal with these in a systematic way, as well as caring for the needs of its individual members or their families.

This kind of integrated practice, which has been termed *community-oriented primary care (COPC)*,[1] requires the systematic collection and use of information as a basis for the planning, implementation, monitoring and evaluation of these community health programmes. The community orientation is expressed in a cyclic process (see Fig. 34.1), analogous to the examination—diagnosis—treatment—follow-up—reassessment cycle in the care of a patient. In this cycle, activities are continuously influenced by epidemiological and other information—what may be called an 'evidence-based'[2] approach. Without this use of information, a community orientation is likely to remain a well-meaning aspiration rather than a means of effecting demonstrable improvements in health. Studies of population health, it has been said, 'can be both the alpha and omega of health care by being the vehicle for both the discovery of need and the evaluation of the outcome of care and treatment.'[3]

A distinction is made in Figure 34.1 between a preliminary examination aimed at 'getting to know' the community and deciding which of its health problems merit detailed study and possible action, and a more detailed investigation ('community diagnosis') of selected problems. If a convincing case for action is revealed, these explorations lead to the development of an appropriate

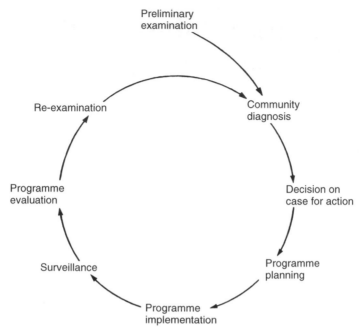

Fig. 34.1 The COPC cycle

programme or programmes. Subsequent monitoring of programme implementation, surveillance of changes in the community's status, and systematic evaluation of the programme permit re-examination of the situation, leading to decisions about the continuation or modification of the programme and about new issues for study or action.

COPC programmes (which have been called *'emphasis programmes')*[4] can deal with selected health problems of the whole population served or of defined subgroups, and may involve health promotion, primary or secondary prevention, curative, alleviative or rehabilitative care, or any combination of these activities. They may focus on specific disorders or specific risk or preventive factors, may involve individual counselling or clinical care, group or community health education, and other activities, and may require community action or inter-agency co-operation.

The prime purpose for which information is collected to COPC is to promote the health of the individuals and community served by the practice, by developing intervention based on the answers to what Kark has called the cardinal questions of community medicine:[5]

- What is the state of health of the community?
- What are the factors responsible for this state of health?
- What is being done about it by the health care system and by the community itself?
- What more can be done, what is proposed, and what is the expected outcome?
- What measures are needed to continue health surveillance of the community and to evaluate the effects of what is being done?

The information-collection process can also serve to promote community development and the community's involvement in its own care, which may be defined as aims of COPC. Meetings with community leaders, designed to learn their opinions about health problems and their solutions (see Ch. 20), can stimulate interest and promote community action, as can surveys and feedbacks of survey findings (using meetings, newsletters, local broadcasts, etc.). Community self-surveys can be especially fruitful in this regard.

Studies in a COPC framework can also provide generalizable new knowledge. There are opportunities for research on, for example, the aetiology, natural history and care of disorders handled in the primary care context, growth and development, and the effects of family processes and psychosocial factors on health and health care. Also—and this is possibly the most important research challenge facing COPC practitioners today—COPC itself can be evaluated; how feasible are specific kinds of COPC programmes in different populations and different health care systems? how effective are they in comparison with non-community-oriented care? what is their extra cost? and what hospital or other costs do they save?

This chapter will discuss the application in COPC of the principles and techniques described in previous chapters, with which the reader is now assumed to be familiar. (If not, return to Square 1.) Consideration will be given to the definition of the community, the preliminary examination ('getting to know the community'), community diagnosis, evaluation, and some aspects of data collection in COPC.

DEFINING THE COMMUNITY

The community may be easy or hard to define. Its definition is easiest if the COPC practice cares for the residents of a specific neighbourhood (whether or not they constitute a true community in the sociological sense), workers in specific places of employment, children in specific schools, or other specific groups. People registered as potential users of the services of a given general practitioner, group practice, neighbourhood health centre or health maintenance organization may also be regarded as a 'community' for whose welfare the practice is responsible. Definition is most difficult where there is no defined responsibility for a specific population; in such instances the aggregate of people who seek care, or those who have sought care recently, or those who seek care repeatedly, or some defined group of them, may be regarded as the 'community' for COPC purposes. A family physician who does not have a list of registered patients might define his 'community' as all the members of families of which any single member is an active patient.[6]

However defined, this community—the *target population* for health care—is the study population for survey purposes. The criteria for inclusion require clear formulation. If the community is defined geographically, decisions are required about the inclusion of transient residents, such as migrant seasonal labourers and their families, and expectant mothers or ill people who come to live with relatives.

Information may be required about the target population as a whole or (for specific purposes) about defined subgroups for whom programmes are contemplated or provided, such as infants and their parents, people with a specific disease, or specific high-risk groups. Samples are sometimes used (see Ch. 8 and p. 344), but sampling is obviously an unsatisfactory technique in surveys that aim (as do many surveys in COPC) not only to obtain information at a group level, but also to identify individuals who need care, with a view to offering them this care. If the community is too large to be studied accurately, one approach is to start data collection in an 'initial defined area' and then gradually expand this defined segment.[7]

In addition to this prime definition of the community as the target population for whose health care the practice is responsible, it may sometimes be decided to designate the community of which the members of the target population (or a large number of them), form a part, as a study population. If a COPC practice serves part of the population of a town, for example, it may be decided also to seek information about the town as a whole, in order to learn about available facilities and services, environmental hazards, patterns of leadership and communication, and other relevant 'ecological' factors, and to find census and other easily accessible data that can be applied (even if with reservations) to the target population. This extension may also permit the collection of information required for the planning and evaluation of programmes, e.g. health education projects, that are not restricted to members of the practice's target population, but in which the practice participates.

GETTING TO KNOW THE COMMUNITY

A general descriptive picture of the community can serve several purposes, the main ones being to identify health problems that merit detailed study and possible action (a 'needs assessment')[8] and to learn about their possible causes and the resources and circumstances that may be relevant to their solution. Getting to know the community and its problems is unquestionably a first step; but it is a continuing process, often slow and gradual, and not a one-time transitory activity. Subsequent stages of the COPC process are generally started as soon as they have a sufficient basis, without waiting for a full community picture.

The preliminary examination of the community generally makes use of 'rapid' methods (see Ch. 31), using easily available sources and qualitative research procedures (see p. 166). A search may be made for published reports and ready-made statistics concerning the target population or its area of residence, based on data collected locally or on small area analysis[9] of information collected at a broader regional or national level. Discussions may be held with community members and professionals (see Ch. 20) concerning their interests and concerns and their perception of the community's problems and ways of solving them. In addition, easily available clinical and administrative records—especially the practice's own records—may be gathered and analyzed in order to obtain information about the use of services, reasons for attendance, infant growth patterns, causes of hospitalization, mortality and its causes, etc. In drawing conclusions from these analyses it is usually necessary to consider the effects of selection bias, the lack of standardized criteria and methods, incomplete recording, and other shortcomings of the data. A household health survey is sometimes practicable, especially if the COPC practice is a new one, when the survey can also serve to introduce the public to the services offered to them. Home visits provide an excellent opportunity for

becoming acquainted with the community, as does direct observation in the field ('using the five senses and touring the community's streets, houses, workplaces, parks, schools, restaurants,
stores and service institutions').[10] Use of a combination of these
methods is recommended.[11]

It is important to obtain information about the size and demographic characteristics of the population. Not only is this an essential basis for the calculation of disease rates and other community
health indices, but it carries its own implications for health and
health care. Even the simplest of data, concerning only the population's age and sex distribution, may be of help in planning the
allocation of resources. It may be important to appraise mobility;
if there is much flux in the population, this will have obvious
implications for the planning of services.

Demographic information may be available from the registration
system used by the practice for administrative or fiscal purposes,
from other records (e.g. an age-sex register) maintained as a routine
in the practice, or from official sources (national census, population register, school registers, etc.). If not, a basic demographic
survey may be required; this is often combined with a health survey.
Sometimes the best that can be done is to use estimates derived
from census data for a broad area that includes the practice population, or (by extrapolation) from information about the patients
who use the service in a given period.[12]

Consideration should be given to the establishment of a register
of the target population, which may be useful not only as a basis
for analyses but as a sampling frame and as a tool for use in the
provision of care—for example, as a checklist for identifying elderly
people or infants who are not receiving care. Maps may also be
helpful.

'Getting to know the community' is a preliminary stage, in the
sense that it must start before the 'community diagnosis' stage can
commence. But the latter more intensive (and selective) investigation can start as soon as there is sufficient information to permit
this, while the 'getting to know' process continues in parallel with
other stages of the COPC cycle, and merges into the surveillance
stage in which the community picture is updated both by continued use of the methods of the preliminary description phase and
by special procedures such as the reporting of births and deaths
and other demographic changes.

No rules can be laid down concerning the scope of the community appraisal. This must obviously depend on the COPC practice's

focus of interest and its resources. A case can be made for the routine collection of a standard set of basic data, but the major part of the data should be selected to meet the practice's specific requirements.

The checklist in Appendix A (p. 403) may be helpful. It is not presented as a blueprint for a study, but as a reminder of topics that may be thought relevant.

COMMUNITY DIAGNOSIS

In the context of COPC, the community health diagnosis provides detailed information about selected health problems and their determinants, and can be narrow in its scope, often dealing with only a single subgroup of the population or with a single topic. The topic or topics are generally chosen on the basis of the preliminary examination of the community, but may also be expressions of a national or institutional health policy, not based on findings in the specific community. The community diagnosis may be descriptive, analytic, or both.

The community diagnosis has three main purposes. It permits a decision on the case for action directed at specific problems (is a community programme justified?), it helps in the planning and implementation of programmes, and it provides baseline data for the measurement of changes produced by programmes. The required study procedures may also serve the needs of patient care more directly; a prevalence survey, for example, can identify individuals who need care, providing a register of cases for use as a framework for the organization and monitoring of a programme.

The community diagnosis may include qualitative elements, especially to provide a basis for the *case for action*, which depends on the importance of the problem, the feasibility of intervention, and the likelihood that intervention will be effective. An appraisal of the importance of the problem sometimes requires detailed epidemiological data on its extent (incidence, prevalence) and impact (e.g. complications, disability, mortality) in the specific community, but it may be obvious without such data. If the problem is regarded as important, the decision on whether a programme is justified will depend largely on information about the community's felt needs and demands and its readiness and capacity to participate in the programme, prevalent attitudes and practices relevant to health care, and the nature and extent of the care presently given. Information on the use and availability of time, manpower and other resources, and the published results of evaluative studies of care procedures and programmes tested elsewhere also play an important part in decisions about the case for intervention.

One way of bringing these elements together so as to permit comparisons of alternative programmes for dealing with the problem, or of programmes to handle competing problems, is to compute a priority score.[13] This is the sum of ratings allotted to different elements, such as:

a. The *relative importance* of the problem: 1, low; 2, moderate, 3, high. This rating is based on the nature, extent and impact of the problem, and is founded both on the epidemiological picture in the community and on general knowledge about the effects of the disorder or risk factor under consideration.

b. The *feasibility and cost* of intervention: 1, low feasibility and/or high cost; 2, intermediate; 3, high feasibility and low cost. This rating is based on practical considerations, such as cost, the availability of trained and interested personnel, facilities and other resources, and the possible participation of volunteers or community bodies or other agencies.

c. The *predicted effectiveness* of intervention (should it be implemented): 1, ineffective; 2, moderate; 3, very effective. This rating is based both on an appraisal of local factors that may influence effectiveness (the community's interest, probable compliance, etc.) and on the results of evaluative studies elsewhere.

Despite the arbitrary features of such a score (subjectivity of ratings, equal weight given to each component), it serves to emphasize that the presence of a problem is not in itself enough to warrant intervention at the community level.

The other purposes of the community diagnosis necessitate more detailed epidemiological investigation. This may include measurement of the occurrence or distribution of the disease (or other problem under consideration) and its known risk and protective factors and risk markers, the identification of groups requiring special care because of their high risk or prevalence of disease or complications, a high case fatality rate, poor access to care, poor compliance, poor use of services, etc. Consideration may be given to causal relationships—specifically, what is the importance in this community of the various known causes of the disorders under consideration? (but a creative mind may also find opportunities for research into new causes). The community diagnosis may include measures of impact on bed disability, time lost from work, etc., as well as attributable, prevented or preventable fractions. The diagnosis may include the identification of *community syndromes*,[14] i.e. sets of associated diseases or other health characteristics that are causally interrelated or have shared or related causes. It may be more effective or efficient to design a programme to handle such a syndrome as a whole, rather than dealing separately with each component.

If the problem under consideration is hypertension, for example, the community diagnosis might include answers to the following questions: What are the frequency distributions of systolic and diastolic pressures in the community? What is the prevalence rate of hypertension? How does it vary in different population subgroups? How common are complications? What contribution do hypertension and hypertension-related diseases make to mortality? How strong is the association with overweight in this community? How prevalent is overweight? What are the community's attitudes to hypertension and overweight? How many of the hypertensives smoke cigarettes, or have other risk factors for coronary heart disease? What proportion of the community has been screened for hypertension? How many of the known hypertensives are under treatment? Do they take their medication? How many are under adequate control? Do people with borderline hypertension have regular blood pressure checks?

The value of the community diagnosis is generally enhanced if it includes appraisal of the care currently given, asking such questions as: What services are available? How adequately are they used? What are the current care procedures? What is the quality of care? How effectively is the problem prevented or treated?

To provide a useful baseline for the subsequent measurement of change, and hence for appraising the effectiveness of intervention, the minimal requirement is information on the incidence or prevalence of the diseases or other problems at which the programme is directed. Adequate outcome evaluation may be difficult or impossible if appropriate initial data are not available. In order to permit a process evaluation (is the programme running well?—see p. 59) it is also advisable to include measures that will provide baselines for appraising the attainment of the programme's activities and intermediate goals (see p. 374).

In COPC, community diagnosis is often a slow and gradual process, based as it generally is on information continuously collected in the clinical situation, supplemented from time to time by surveys performed outside this situation. If the population is small it may be necessary to cumulate several years' experience before satisfactory data, especially on mortality and disease incidence, are available. Moreover, some studies—e.g. of predictors of mortality in the COPC population—are intrinsically long-term. At some point, however, usually sooner rather than later, it is decided that enough information is available to permit the planning and introduction of an intervention programme. This does not halt the process of community diagnosis, which merges imperceptibly into the phase of health surveillance. During this phase, continued appraisal of specific problems and monitoring of the operation of specific community programmes are combined with ongoing general surveillance (broad or narrow in its scope) of the community's health and health care, designed to detect and measure changes in the community's health status and its exposure to risk and protective factors.

EVALUATION

In COPC, evaluation is always motivated by concern with the welfare of the specific community served. This kind of evaluation, aimed mainly at determining whether the programme is running well and whether outcomes are satisfactory, is what we have called a *programme review* (see p. 27). Evidence may also be sought that the outcomes can be attributed to the intervention (rather than to other factors), using an experimental or quasi-experimental design (see Ch. 33). This may require study of a control population as well. If a programme trial is contemplated, it is usually wise to attempt to reduce bias—or accusations of bias—by obtaining the assistance of impartial independent co-investigators and (for data obtained outside the ordinary clinical context) of independent observers.

The evaluation may embrace the COPC practice as a whole, or it may be limited to a specific programme or programmes, or to specific aspects of programmes. All the basic evaluative questions listed on page 56 may be asked. Questions about the process and outcome of care usually focus on the performance of the activities and the achievement of the goals specified in the plan of the intervention programme. The scope of the inquiry may vary from simple monitoring procedures (Are people with borderline hypertension having regular blood pressure checks? Are hypertensive patients taking their medication?) through a fuller evaluation including the measurement of immediate outcomes and the detection of obvious undesirable effects (What proportion of the known hypertensives have been brought under control? How many of the patients treated with hypotensive drugs complain of impaired sexual functioning?) to a comprehensive appraisal that may include the measurement of long-term outcomes (Have the frequency distributions of systolic and diastolic pressures or the prevalence of hypertension in the community changed? Has the incidence of stroke or other defined complications fallen?).

Real-time information about activities and intermediate outcomes may be useful as a trigger for immediate corrections to the intervention plan and the way it is implemented, and as a basis for prompt reports to the community. An evaluation of community health promotion programmes has shown that feedbacks on the immediate impact of a programme (without waiting to measure long-term changes) can stimulate the development of partnership with the community.[15]

Programmes that aim to change community behaviour can be expected to extend over a long period (marathons rather than sprints),[16] and the evaluation of such programmes, or any evaluation that measures long-term outcomes, will be a long-term affair, fusing with the continuing surveillance of changes in the community picture.

For practitioners with a crusading interest in the extension of COPC, the importance of evaluative studies cannot be over-emphasized. Pleading for a 'vibrant and compelling data base with which to make a case for COPC', Rogers[17] has pointed out that it may not be enough to demonstrate effects on mortality or morbidity rates. 'Such statistics ... lack immediacy and emotional impact ... A community or a nation will willingly and instantly spend millions to rescue a trapped coal miner ... but it is much harder to get that same community or nation to spend similar sums to reduce infant mortality rates ... As with olives or oysters, a taste for vital statistics is an acquired one.' He suggests that new yardsticks, such as measures of the restoration of crippled people to full functioning, may be needed to excite compassion and interest.

DATA COLLECTION IN COPC

The collection of information that is accurate enough to be useful for epidemiological purposes is far from easy, and a COPC practice ordinarily has limited resources to devote to this task. Attention should therefore be concentrated on data that are of obvious relevance to the practice's needs. There is no point in creating a database that is a cemetery for the interment of useless information, even if some of it will occasionally be exhumed for annual reports or other ritual observances. While the collection of some routine 'basic data' may be considered, the data set should in the main be custom-made to meet the practice's specific needs, particularly those related to its community health programmes.

Data collection in COPC has special features because of the clinical context. First, information is collected to fulfill a double function, meeting the practice's dual responsibilities for individual and community care. When a baby is weighed or a disease is diagnosed —whether in the course of ordinary clinical care or in a special survey—the result may be used both in caring for the individual and at a group level. An audit of records of the performance and results of investigations and the provision of specific advice and other care procedures may provide a basis for decisions both about individual patients and about the overall programme. Secondly, a good deal of the information needed for community diagnosis and surveillance and programme evaluation can be collected in the course of clinical care, either as part of the ordinary diagnostic investigation and surveillance of patients, or by adding tests and questions to clinic procedures for epidemiological purposes. In a practice where periodic health examinations are conducted, these provide an especially useful opportunity for the collection of such information.

The use of clinical data for epidemiological purposes demands methods that are no less rigorous than those in any epidemiological study, and this may not be easy to achieve. The information to be analyzed should be as valid and complete as possible. Careful preparations are needed. Operational definitions of diseases and disabilities should be standardized (especially if diagnoses are made by more than one clinician), at least for the conditions selected for epidemiological study; for these it may be wise to record the presence or absence of each diagnostic criterion, to permit ongoing or spot checks of conformity with the definition. Standardized procedures should be laid down for the collection of data, expecially if questions are asked or examinations done by more than one person. Written instructions are desirable, documenting the procedures and operational definitions, especially if there are frequent changes of personnel. Record forms should be convenient to use, and permit easy retrieval of data for the purposes of analysis; the use of personal computers in the clinic may facilitate the epidemiological use of clinical data. Quality control procedures and tests of validity and reliability should be instituted where necessary; even simple checks on the completeness of recording may yield startling findings.[18]

The integration of epidemiological data collection into a clinical context has both advantages and disadvantages. It provides opportunities for doing elaborate tests, for asking questions about delicate matters, and for long-term follow-up. But it may also produce bias. Not only may patients seeking care not be representative, but their illness or apprehension may affect their responses or measurements, and they may tend to give answers they think their health advisers expect. Moreover, observations may be biased by the clinician's prior knowledge of the patient (see 'halo effect', p. 166); this bias may be reduced by the use of standardized objective measures and by making measurements (say of blood pressure) without first referring to the patient's previous values.

Bias caused by the nonrepresentativeness of patients is likely to diminish in time, as more and more of the target population attend. In some subgroups coverage may become so high that the bias can be ignored; this may occur with infants and their mothers, pregnant women, the elderly, and hypertensives or other groups for whom periodic health examinations or special care programmes are organized. Often, however, there is a need for supplementary survey procedures; nonattenders may be identified and invited to attend, or visited at home, or asked to respond by mail or telephone.

The information required in COPC may be collected not only in the clinical situation, but by any appropriate and practicable method. It may be obtained by special surveys, conducted in the clinic context or outside it. These may range in scope from a small follow-up study of a group of patients to a comprehensive community health survey. A community survey can provide information that clinical records cannot or do not; it can appraise the health status and needs of people who have not sought care, can measure the use of other health services by the practice population, and may provide the COPC practice with a considerable amount of new information about its patients.[19] Response rates are generally high in surveys performed by or under the auspices of a COPC practice that has a good relationship with the community.

Feedback of the results to the community can be regarded as an important element of a community health survey—which takes us

full circle, back to the opening sentence of this book: 'The purpose
of most investigations in community medicine ... is the collection
of information that will provide a basis for action ...' And how can
this be done better than by stimulating the community itself to take
the action required to improve its health?—in accordance with the
principle of the WHO 'Health for All' policy[20] that

> Health for all will be achieved by people themselves. A well informed,
> well motivated and actively participating community is an element for
> the attainment of the common goal.

NOTES AND REFERENCES

1. The concept and practice of *community-oriented primary care* are described by
Kark S L 1981 (The practice of community-oriented primary care. Appleton-
Century-Crofts, New York); Kark S L, Abramson J H (eds) 1981
(Community-focused health care. Israel Journal of Medical Sciences 17: 65);
Abramson J H, Kark S L 1983 (Community oriented primary care: meaning
and scope. In: Connor E, Mullan F, eds. 1983 Community oriented primary
care: new directions for health services delivery. National Academy Press,
Washington, D C, pp 21–59); Connor E, Mullan F 1983 (see above);
Nutting P A (ed) 1987 (Community oriented primary care: from principle to
practice. Health Resources and Services Administration, Public Health
Services, Washington, D C); Abramson J H 1988 (Community-oriented
primary care—strategy, approaches and practice: a review. Public Health
Reviews 16: 35); Kark S L, Kark E, Abramson J H, Gofin J (eds) 1994
(Atencion primaria orientada a la comunidad [APOC], Ediciones Doyma
S A, Barcelona); Tollman S, Friedman I 1994 (Community-orientated
primary health care—South African legacy. South African Medical Journal
84: 646); Gillam S, Plamping D, McClenaham J, Harries J, Epstein L 1994
(Community-oriented primary care. King's Fund, London); Nevin J E, Gogel
M M 1996 (Community-oriented primary care. Primary Care 23: 1), and
Gillam S, Miller R 1997 (COPC—a public health experiment in primary
care. King's Fund, London).
   COPaCetic, a semiannual newsletter about COPC trends, is available free
from the Department of Family Medicine, Case Western Reserve University
School of Medicine, 10900 Euclid Avenue, Cleveland, Ohio.
2. The 'evidence' used in COPC includes not only information about the
community, but also the results of epidemiological studies and programme
trials conducted elsewhere, as cited by, for example, Blackburn H 1997
(Epidemiological basis of a community strategy for the prevention of
cardiovascular diseases. Annals of Epidemiology 7: S7).
3. Acheson R M, Hall D J 1976 Epilogue. In: Acheson R M, Hall D J, Aird L
(eds) Seminars in community medicine, vol 2: Health information, planning,
and monitoring. Oxford University Press, London, pp 145–164.
4. Nutting P A (ed) 1987 (see note 1), pp 248–249.
5. Kark S L 1981 (see note 1), p. 11.
6. Nutting P A, Wood M, Connor E M 1985 Community-oriented primary care
in the United States: a status report. Journal of the American Medical
Association 253: 1763.
7. Kark S L 1966 An approach to public health. In: King M (ed) Medical care
in developing countries. Oxford University Press, Nairobi, Ch 5; Kark S L
1981 (see note 1), pp 199–200; Nutting 1987 (see note 1), p. xxi.

8. See Trompeter T 1992 (Community responsive primary care: a basic guide to planning and needs assessment for community and migrant health. National Association of Community Health Centers, Washington, D C) and other references on *needs appraisal* (see note 9, p. 32).

9. *Small area analysis* derives community-specific information from broad databases, such as census, hospital discharge and cancer incidence data sets, with the idea of providing 'good data for good care' (Millman M L 1991 Consensus conference on small area analysis: summary. In: Consensus conference on small area analysis: proceedings. DHHS publication HRS-A-PE 91-1(A), US Public Health Service, pp 3–7).

In two of the other useful papers in the above publication, Nutting P A 1991 (Community-oriented primary care and small areas analysis, pp 85–87) points out that the information needed by a COPC practice can be helpful even if obtained by methods that are 'perhaps not rigorous enough for publication in the *New England Journal*', and Lashof J C, Hughes D C 1991 (Small area analysis and program evaluation, pp 143–151) stress the value of having data both about users of services (the 'clinic population') and about the total target population.

Computer-produced maps may be helpful for displaying the distribution of health indicators (Williams R L, Flocke S A, Zyzanski S J, Mettee T M, Martin K B 1995 A practical tool for community-oriented primary care community diagnosis using a personal computer. Family Medicine 27: 39) and comparing morbidity data for the COPC practice and the total area (Mettee T M, Martin K B, Williams R L 1998 Tools for community-oriented primary care: a process for linking practice and community data. Journal of the American Board of Family Practice 11: 28).

Data derived from small area analysis have obvious limitations if only part of the people living in the area are in the practice population. This has been shown for estimates of the socio-economic characteristics of general practices (Buckingham K 1996 Using census information to estimate GP practice morbidity. Public Health 110: 191).

Hospital admission rates do not necessarily reflect the prevalence of specific diseases. A study of 22 small areas in an English district showed moderate positive correlations only for respiratory disease and depression, and none for digestive disease, musculoskeletal disorders, or obesity (Payne J N, Coy J, Patterson S, Milner P C 1994 Is use of hospital services a proxy for morbidity? A small area comparison of the prevalence of arthritis, depression, dyspepsia, obesity and respiratory disease with inpatient admission rates for these disorders in England. Journal of Epidemiology and Community Health 48: 74).

10. Mettee T M 1987 Community diagnosis: a tool for COPC. In: Nutting P A (ed) 1987 (see note 1), pp 52–59.

11. Four methods of collecting data on health needs were compared in a study of a neighbourhood in Edinburgh: rapid participatory appraisal, a postal survey, analysis of routinely available small area statistics, and collation of information held in the practice. The methods were found to be complementary, serving different purposes—'a composite method may be most informative' (Murray S A, Graham L J 1995 Practice based health needs assessment: use of four methods in a small neighbourhood. British Medical Journal 310: 1443).

12. The number of people who use a service during (say) a year can be estimated from information about those who attend during a short survey period, and whether and when they attended previously (Laska E, Lin S, Meisner M 1997 Estimating the size of a population from a single sample: methodology and practical issues. Journal of Clinical Epidemiology 50: 1143). Extrapolations from users to the total target population, e.g. by 'using a fudge

factor of about 30 percent to account for non-attenders', are unlikely to be accurate (Hearst N 1987 The denominator problem in community-oriented primary care. In: Nutting P A, ed. 1987 [see note 1], pp 71–75).

13. This is the scoring scheme recommended by Vaughan J P, Morrow R H 1989 Manual of epidemiology for district health management. World Health Organization, Geneva.

     An alternative 'priority score' is the sum of the scores (1–3) allocated to six criteria: Prevalence/incidence, severity of problem, effective intervention, acceptability/feasibility, community involvement, and costs and resources (Gillam S et al. 1994 [see note 1]).

14. The *community syndrome* concept was introduced by Kark S L 1974 (Epidemiology and community medicine. Appleton-Century-Crofts, New York, section 4), who emphasized its potential importance for the development of community health programmes. For an example of a study designed to detect community syndromes, see Abramson J H, Gofin J, Peritz E, Hopp C, Epstein L M 1982 (Clustering of chronic disorders—a community study of coprevalence in Jerusalem. Journal of Chronic Diseases 35: 221).

15. Cheadle A, Beery W, Wagner E et al 1997 Conference report: community-based health promotion—state of the art and recommendations for the future. American Journal of Preventive Medicine 13: 240.

16. The 'marathon' metaphor is used in a paper that points out the importance of measuring change at various milestones in the race between the effects of a health promotion programme and the effects of social, cultural, organizational and policy changes extrinsic to the programme (Green L W 1997 Community health promotion: applying the science of evaluation to the initial sprint of a marathon. American Journal of Preventive Medicine 13: 225).

17. Rogers D E 1982 Community-oriented primary care. Journal of the American Medical Association 248B: 1622.

18. Checks have found primary care practices where less than half the contacts with patients were recorded (Weitzman S, Bar-Ziv G, Pilpel D, Sachs E, Naggan L 1981 Validation study on medical recording practices in primary care clinics. Israel Journal of Medical Sciences 17: 213), diagnoses were recorded for as few as 9% of episodes (Dawes K S 1972 Survey of general practice records. British Medical Journal 3: 219), and over half the patients did not live at their registered addresses (Hannay D R 1972 Accuracy of health-centre records. Lancet 2: 371).

19. As an example, a survey of the target population of a primary care practice revealed numerous cases of coronary heart disease, diabetes and hypertension who were not known to the practice, and provided the first systematic picture of the prevalence of obesity and smoking (Abramson J H, Epstein L M, Kark S L, Kark E, Fischler B 1973 The contribution of a health survey to a family practice. Scandinavian Journal of Social Medicine 1: 33).

     A household health survey in a neighbourhood in the Bronx, New York, revealed that about half the residents had no personal health provider; the results were used to develop a number of COPC outreach efforts (Taylor B R 1996 The use of household surveys in community-oriented primary care health needs assessments. Family Medicine 28: 415).

20. World Health Organization 1985 Targets for health for all. World Health Organization, Copenhagen.

Appendix A: Community appraisal: a checklist

APPENDIX A: COMMUNITY APPRAISAL: A CHECKLIST

Information on the following topics may be helpful in the appraisal of a community's health needs and ways of meeting them. Some of the items in this list are relevant only to a true community; this may be the community served by a COPC practice (see Ch. 34) or the community from which the practice's patients, or many of them, are drawn. Other items are relevant to any target population of a community-oriented practice, however this is defined.

The items in the list are not exhaustive or mutually exclusive, and they are not arranged in order of importance. Some of the information is qualitative.

1. Definition of the community/population:
   - eligibility criteria, exclusions
2. Demographic characteristics:
   - population size
   - distribution by age, sex, social class, economic status, educational level, occupation, religion, ethnic group, race, marital status, parity
   - population mobility
   - trends of change in size and demographic composition
   - vital statistics:
     — mortality, birth and fertility rates
     — life expectancy
3. General information:
   - history of the community

- physical and climatic characteristics of the neighbourhood
- economic activities, economic development, occupations
- affluence/poverty: prevalence of unemployment, household crowding, and other indices of deprivation
- social attributes: social structure, cohesiveness, social networks, family values and living patterns, formal and informal leadership, political structure
- crime and security

4. Facilities and services:
   - housing, water supply, sanitation, roads, transportation, shops, schools
   - available health services (including traditional healers)
   - information about health services: location, personnel, facilities, fiscal arrangements, accessibility, coverage, quality and effectiveness of care
   - health insurance: types and coverage
   - other welfare services
   - current health and welfare programmes: mother and child health, immunization, family planning, elderly, screening, control of specific diseases, meals-on-wheels, etc.
   - discontinued health programmes and the reasons for their failure
   - inter-agency and inter-sectoral co-operation in health-related services

5. Utilization of services:
   - consultation rates and reasons for attendance
   - use of antenatal, child care, dental and other specific services
   - hospitalization rates and reasons for hospitalization
   - differential use of services by various groups
   - barriers to use of services: language, cultural, geographic, financial

6. The community's involvement in its own health care:
   - the community's interests and concerns: felt needs, expectations of services, demand for services, satisfaction with services
   - organized action groups and their activities
   - actual and potential participation by community bodies and volunteers in activities run by health agencies
   - self-care

7. Health-relevant knowledge, attitudes and practices:
   - lifestyle: e.g. diet, infant feeding, family planning, smoking, drinking, drugs

- knowledge about disease causation, prevention of common diseases, and health maintenance and promotion
- health and illness behaviour
- compliance with medical advice
- trends of change in health-relevant behaviours

8. Health and disease status:
    - causes of death
    - common or important diseases (including behavioural and emotional disorders) and disabilities: incidence and prevalence rates, sickness absenteeism
    - nutritional status
    - growth and development of children
    - distribution of health-relevant characteristics, such as weight and blood pressure
    - trends of change in health status

9. Risk and protective factors:
    - prevalence of personal risk factors for important disorders (smoking, obesity, teenage pregnancy, etc.)
    - environmental health hazards
    - immunization status
    - measures of impact of risk and protective factors (attributable, prevented or preventable fractions)

Appendix B: Random numbers

```
53 74 23 99 67   61 32 28 69 84   94 62 67 86 24   98 33 41 19 95   47 53 53 38 09
63 38 06 86 54   99 00 65 26 94   02 82 90 23 07   79 62 67 80 60   75 91 12 81 19
35 30 58 21 46   06 72 17 10 94   25 21 31 75 96   49 28 24 00 49   55 65 79 78 07
63 43 36 82 69   65 51 18 37 88   61 38 44 12 45   32 92 85 88 65   54 34 81 85 35
98 25 37 55 26   01 91 82 81 46   74 71 12 94 97   24 02 71 37 07   03 92 18 66 75

02 63 21 17 69   71 50 80 89 56   38 15 70 11 48   43 40 45 86 98   00 83 26 91 03
64 55 22 21 82   48 22 28 06 00   61 54 13 43 91   82 78 12 23 29   06 66 24 12 27
85 07 26 13 89   01 10 07 82 04   59 63 69 36 03   69 11 15 83 80   13 29 54 19 28
58 54 16 24 15   51 54 44 82 00   62 61 65 04 69   38 18 65 18 97   85 72 13 49 21
34 85 27 84 87   61 48 64 56 26   90 18 48 13 26   37 70 15 42 57   65 65 80 39 07

03 92 18 27 46   57 99 16 96 56   30 33 72 85 22   84 64 38 56 98   99 01 30 98 64
62 95 30 27 59   37 75 41 66 48   86 97 80 61 45   23 53 04 01 63   45 76 08 64 27
08 45 93 15 22   60 21 75 46 91   98 77 27 85 42   28 88 61 08 84   69 62 03 42 73
07 08 55 18 40   45 44 75 13 90   24 94 96 61 02   57 55 66 83 15   73 42 37 11 61
01 85 89 95 66   51 10 19 34 88   15 84 97 19 75   12 76 39 43 78   64 63 91 08 25

72 84 71 14 35   19 11 58 49 26   50 11 17 17 76   86 31 57 20 18   95 60 78 46 75
88 78 28 16 84   13 52 53 94 53   75 45 69 30 96   73 89 65 70 31   99 17 43 48 76
45 17 75 65 57   28 40 19 72 12   25 12 74 75 67   60 40 60 81 19   24 62 01 61 16
96 76 28 12 54   22 01 11 94 25   71 96 16 16 88   68 64 36 74 45   19 59 50 88 92
43 31 67 72 30   24 02 94 08 63   38 32 36 66 02   69 36 38 25 39   48 03 45 15 22

50 44 66 44 21   66 06 58 05 62   68 15 54 35 02   42 35 48 96 32   14 52 41 52 48
22 66 22 15 86   26 63 75 41 99   58 42 36 72 24   58 37 52 18 51   03 37 18 39 11
96 24 40 14 51   23 22 30 88 57   95 67 47 29 83   94 69 40 06 07   18 16 36 78 86
31 73 91 61 19   60 20 72 93 48   98 57 07 23 69   65 95 39 69 58   56 80 30 19 44
78 60 73 99 84   43 89 94 36 45   56 69 47 07 41   90 22 91 07 12   78 35 34 08 72

84 37 90 61 56   70 10 23 98 05   85 11 34 76 60   76 48 45 34 60   01 64 18 39 96
36 67 10 08 23   98 93 35 08 86   99 29 76 29 81   33 34 91 58 93   63 14 52 32 52
07 28 59 07 48   89 64 58 89 75   83 85 62 27 89   30 14 78 56 27   86 63 59 80 02
10 15 83 87 60   79 24 31 66 56   21 48 24 06 93   91 98 94 05 49   01 47 59 38 00
55 19 68 97 65   03 73 52 16 56   00 53 55 90 27   33 42 29 38 87   22 13 88 83 34
```

```
53 81 29 13 39    35 01 20 71 34    62 33 74 82 14    53 73 19 09 03    56 54 29 56 93
51 86 32 68 92    33 98 74 66 99    40 14 71 94 58    45 94 19 38 81    14 44 99 81 07
35 91 70 29 13    80 03 54 07 27    96 94 78 32 66    50 95 52 74 33    13 80 55 62 54
37 71 67 95 13    20 02 44 95 94    64 85 04 05 72    01 32 90 76 14    53 89 74 60 41
93 66 13 83 27    92 79 64 64 72    28 54 96 53 84    48 14 52 98 94    56 07 93 89 30

02 96 08 45 65    13 05 00 41 84    93 07 54 72 59    21 45 57 09 77    19 48 56 27 44
49 83 43 48 35    82 88 33 69 96    72 36 04 19 76    47 45 15 18 60    82 11 08 95 97
84 60 71 62 46    40 80 81 30 37    34 39 23 05 38    25 15 35 71 30    88 12 57 21 77
18 17 30 88 71    44 91 14 88 47    89 23 30 63 15    56 34 20 47 89    99 82 93 24 98
76 69 10 61 78    71 32 76 95 62    87 00 22 58 40    92 54 01 75 25    43 11 71 99 31
```

Reproduced with permission from Fisher R A, Yates F 1974 Statistical tables for biological, agricultural and medical research. Longman, London.

Index